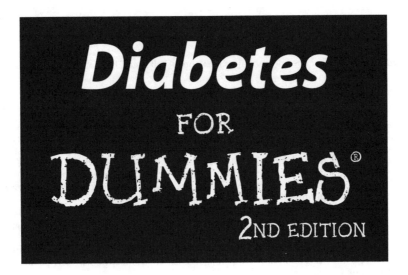

Diabetes
FOR
DUMMIES®
2ND EDITION

by Dr Sarah Jarvis, GP, and Alan L Rubin, MD

BICENTENNIAL
BICENTENNIAL
1807
WILEY
2007
BICENTENNIAL
BICENTENNIAL

John Wiley & Sons, Ltd

Diabetes For Dummies®, 2nd Edition

Published by
John Wiley & Sons, Ltd
The Atrium
Southern Gate
Chichester
West Sussex
PO19 8SQ
England

E-mail (for orders and customer service enquires): cs-books@wiley.co.uk

Visit our Home Page on www.wiley.com

Copyright © 2007 John Wiley & Sons, Ltd, Chichester, West Sussex, England

Published by John Wiley & Sons, Ltd, Chichester, West Sussex

For general information on our other products and services, please contact our Customer Care Department within the U.S. at 800-762-2974, outside the U.S. at 317-572-3993, or fax 317-572-4002.

For technical support, please visit www.wiley.com/techsupport.

Wiley also publishes its books in a variety of electronic formats. Some content that appears in print may not be available in electronic books.

British Library Cataloguing in Publication Data: A catalogue record for this book is available from the British Library

ISBN: 978-0-470-05810-7

Printed and bound in Great Britain by Bell & Bain Ltd, Glasgow

10 9 8 7 6 5 4 3 2

WILEY

About the Authors

Dr Sarah Jarvis is a GP, GP trainer, and Fellow of the Royal College of General Practitioners. Since qualifying at Cambridge and Oxford, she has combined her clinical life with a writing and medical broadcasting career. Her particular interest has been in educating and empowering patients. She has been lunchtime news doctor for ITN and doctor for *Today* newspaper, and has regular columns in several magazines. She is a regular guest on Radio 5 Live, and has published over 500 patient information leaflets. Her practice has a high proportion of patients with diabetes, and she has a special interest in their care.

Alan L Rubin, MD, is one of the foremost experts on diabetes in the US. He is a professional member of the American Diabetes Association and the Endocrine Society and has been in private practice specialising in diabetes and thyroid disease for 30 years. Dr Rubin has been on numerous radio and television programmes, and has spoken to medical audiences and non-medical audiences around the world. He was Assistant Clinical Professor of Medicine at University of California Medical Center in San Francisco for 20 years.

Dedication

This book is dedicated to my mother, who passed away while it was being written. She was my role model, and her kindness, boundless energy, and enthusiasm were an inspiration to all who knew her.

– Sarah Jarvis

Authors' Acknowledgements

My biggest debt of gratitude must be to my best friend, my closest confidant, my personal shopper, and my number one fan, who come all rolled into one in the shape of my beloved husband, Simon. Thank you, Simon, for your unfailing support and loyalty – and your mouthwatering cooking! A great big thank you to my children, Seth and Matilda, who make my life a constant joy. They have put up with the closed study door between them and their mother with (almost) unfailing good humour and patience. And thank you to Joan, who has been the best of friends for far more years than either of us care to remember, and who introduced me to the wonderful team at Wiley. Finally, thank you to Marc Evans, consultant diabetologist extraordinaire – even if I do have to translate your pearls from Medical into English occasionally!

A second edition also gives me the opportunity to thank the thousands of people who have themselves thanked me for *Diabetes For Dummies*. You know who you are. You have given me a sense of enormous gratification for writing this book, having shared your stories with me and permitting me to laugh and cry with you. One of the best stories is the following from Andrea in Canada:

'My three-year-old daughter was recently diagnosed with diabetes type one. It has been a rough time. To help us out, my brother and his wife bought us your book, *Diabetes For Dummies*. One day my daughter saw this bright yellow book and asked what I was reading. I told her the book was called *Diabetes For Dummies*. As soon as the words came out of my mouth, I regretted them. I didn't want her to think that dummies got diabetes so I quickly added, "I am the dummy." Without missing a beat, she then asked, "Am I the diabetes?"

'The story doesn't just end there. The other day she was relaxing on the couch. She looked at me and said, "I don't want to have diabetes any more." Feeling terrible I responded, "I know sweetie; I don't want you to have it any more either." I then explained that she would have diabetes for the rest of her life. With a very concerned look she then asked, "Will you be the dummy for the rest of your life?"'

As sad as it is, I guess you're right. We must look for humour in everything, otherwise we break down.

– Sarah Jarvis

Publisher's Acknowledgements

We're proud of this book; please send us your comments through our Dummies online registration form located at www.dummies.com/register/.

Some of the people who helped bring this book to market include the following:

Acquisitions, Editorial, and Media Development

Project Editor: Steve Edwards

(Previous Edition: Daniel Mersey)

Executive Editor: Jason Dunne

Copy Editor: Sally Lansdell

Proofreader: Helen Heyes

Executive Project Editor: Martin Tribe

Special Help: Daniel Mersey

Cover Photos: GettyImages/davies & starr

Cartoons: Ed McLachlan

Composition Services

Project Coordinator: Jennifer Theriot

Layout and Graphics: Denny Hager, Stephanie D. Jumper, Laura Pence

Proofreaders: Susan Moritz, Dwight Ramsey

Indexer: Techbooks

Publishing and Editorial for Consumer Dummies

> **Diane Graves Steele,** Vice President and Publisher, Consumer Dummies

> **Joyce Pepple,** Acquisitions Director, Consumer Dummies

> **Kristin A. Cocks,** Product Development Director, Consumer Dummies

> **Michael Spring,** Vice President and Publisher, Travel

> **Kelly Regan,** Editorial Director, Travel

Publishing for Technology Dummies

> **Andy Cummings,** Vice President and Publisher, Dummies Technology/General User

Composition Services

> **Gerry Fahey,** Vice President of Production Services

> **Debbie Stailey,** Director of Composition Services

Contents at a Glance

Table of Contents

Introduction

● ●

*W*hat's funny about diabetes? It's a disease, isn't it? Yes, it's a disease, but the people who have it at the start of the 21st century are the most fortunate group of diabetes sufferers in history.

You may know the story of the doctor who called his patient to give him the results of his blood tests. 'I have bad news and worse news,' said the doctor.

'Gosh,' said the patient. 'What's the bad news?'

'Your blood tests indicate that you have only 24 hours to live,' said the doctor.

'What could be worse than that?' said the patient.

'I've been trying to reach you since yesterday,' said the doctor.

Those of you with diabetes have a decade or more in which to avoid the long-term complications of the disease. In a sense, a diagnosis of diabetes is both good news and bad news. It is bad news because you have a disease you would happily do without. It is good news if you use it to make some changes in your lifestyle that can not only prevent or minimise complications, but also help you to live a longer and higher-quality life.

As for laughing about it, at times you probably feel like doing anything but laughing. Nevertheless, scientific studies are clear about the benefits of a positive attitude. In a very few words: He who laughs, lasts. Another point is that people learn more and retain more when humour is part of the process.

If you have experienced something funny during the course of your diabetes care, we hope you share it with others. Our goal is not to trivialise human suffering by being comic about it, but to lighten the burden of a chronic disease by showing that it is not all gloom and doom.

About This Book

The book is not meant to be read from cover to cover, although if you know nothing about diabetes, that may be a good approach. This book is intended to serve as a source of information about the problems that arise over the years. You can find the latest facts about diabetes and the best sources for discovering any information that comes out after the publication of this edition.

So much has changed in the five years since the first edition was written that a second edition was clearly necessary. We have new medicines (see Chapter 10), new glucose meters (see Chapter 7), new ideas about diet and exercise (Chapters 8 and 9), new information about diabetes in certain ethnic groups (Chapter 2), and plenty of new material concerning diabetes in children (Chapter 13), and the occupational and insurance problems of people with diabetes (Chapter 15). In fact, you can find something new in just about every chapter, especially, obviously, Chapter 16, 'What's New in Diabetes Care.'

Conventions Used in This Book

Diabetes, as you may already know, is all about sugar. But sugars come in many types. So doctors avoid using the words *sugar* and *glucose* interchangeably. In this book (unless we slip up), we use the word glucose rather than sugar. (You may as well get used to it, sweetie.)

What You Don't Have to Read

Throughout the book, you find shaded areas, which we call sidebars. These sidebars contain material that is interesting but not essential. We hereby give you permission to skip them if the material inside them is of no particular interest to you. You can still understand everything else.

Foolish Assumptions

This book assumes that you don't know anything about diabetes. You don't suddenly have to face a term that is not explained and that you have never heard of before. Those who already know a lot can find more in-depth explanations. And while you can pick and choose how much you want to know about a subject, the key points are clearly marked.

How This Book Is Organised

This book divides into six parts to help you find out all you can about the topic of diabetes.

Part 1: Dealing with the Onset of Diabetes

To slay the dragon, you have to be able to identify it. This part clears up the different types of diabetes, how you get them, and if you can give them to others.

In this part, you find out how to deal with the emotional and psychological consequences of the diagnosis and an explanation of what all those big words mean. You also discover how to prevent the complications of diabetes.

Part II: How Diabetes Affects Your Body

In this part, you find out what you need to know about both the short- and long-term complications of diabetes. You also find out about some sexual issues related to diabetes and the problems of a diabetic pregnancy.

Part III: Managing Diabetes: The 'Thriving with Diabetes' Lifestyle Plan

In this part, you discover all the tools available to treat diabetes. You find out about the kinds of tests that you should be doing, as well as what tests your doctor should be ordering to determine how severe your diabetes is, what to do about it, and how to follow the success of your therapy.

You also discover the dietary changes that you need to make to control your blood glucose and how to get the most out of your exercise routine and medications. Finally, you find out about the huge amount of help that's available for you and your family.

Part IV: Special Considerations for Living with Diabetes

The way that diabetes develops is different for each age group. In this part, you discover those differences and how to manage them. You also find out about some of the special problems of people with diabetes, which relate to discrimination, driving, and jobs.

Lastly, this part covers all the new developments in diagnosing, monitoring, and treating diabetes and helps correct a lot of misinformation about diabetes treatment.

Part V: The Part of Tens

This part presents some key suggestions, the stuff you most need to know as well as the stuff you least want to know.

You discover the ten commandments of diabetes care and the myths that confuse many diabetic patients. You also find out how to get others to help you in your efforts to control your diabetes.

Part VI: Appendixes

This part of the book contains even more information about diabetes. Two special appendixes help you improve your diet by giving you recipes and diabetic exchanges. The other appendix points out hot spots to visit on the Internet, in case you want to continue finding out about diabetes when you've finished this book.

Icons Used in This Book

The icons tell you what you must know, what you should know, and what you may find interesting but can live without:

This icon marks a story about a diabetes patient.

This icon marks paragraphs where we define terms.

 When you see this icon, it means that the information is essential and you should be aware of it.

 This icon points out when you should see your doctor (for example, if your blood glucose level is too high or you need a particular test done).

 This icon marks important information that can save you time and energy.

 This icon warns against potential problems (for example, if you don't treat something).

Part I
Dealing with the Onset of Diabetes

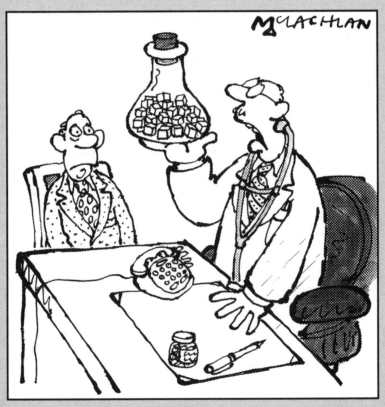

'It's only a guess, but judging by your sample,
I would say you are a diabetic.'

In this part . . .

You have found out that you or a loved one has diabetes. What do you do now? This part helps you deal with all the emotions that arise when you discover that you will not live forever – from wondering whether the diagnosis is correct to avoiding the complications associated with diabetes.

Chapter 1

Dealing with Diabetes

*O*ne of our patients told me that, when she was working at her first job out of university, the employees' tradition was to have a birthday cake and celebration for every birthday. She came to the first celebration and a colleague urged her to eat the cake. She refused and refused, until finally she had to say, 'I can't eat the cake because I have diabetes.' The woman trying to persuade her said, 'Thank God. I thought you just had incredible willpower.' Twenty years later, our patient clearly remembers being told that having diabetes is better than having willpower. Another patient told us, 'The hardest thing about having diabetes is having to deal with doctors who don't respect me.' Several times over the years, she had followed her doctor's recommendations exactly, but her glucose control still hadn't been ideal. The doctor blamed her for this 'failure'.

Although some people may try to define you by your diabetes, you know that you are more than the sum of your blood glucose levels. You have feelings, and you have a history. The way you respond to the challenges of diabetes determines whether the disease is a moderate annoyance or the source of major sickness for you.

Unless you live alone on a desert island, your diabetes doesn't affect only you. How you deal with your diabetes affects your family, friends, and colleagues, as does their desire to help you. This chapter shows you some coping skills to help you handle diabetes and your important relationships.

Diabetes in a Nutshell

What is diabetes? It's a disease in which the body does not produce or properly respond to insulin. And what is insulin? It's a hormone that you need in your body to convert sugar and other food into the energy needed for daily life. You can read more about how doctors define diabetes in Chapter 2, and about what type of diabetes you have in Chapter 3 (yes, more than one type of diabetes exists).

Because getting a diagnosis of diabetes depends on your having raised blood sugar, and because having very high blood sugar is so dangerous, doctors used to concentrate on the sugar side of diabetes. In recent years, the fact has become increasingly clear that diabetes doesn't just affect your blood sugar. If you have diabetes (and especially if you have type 2 diabetes), looking after your heart (by keeping your blood pressure and cholesterol under control) is every bit as important as looking after your blood sugar. But don't worry – this book gives you all the help you need to look after every bit of you.

You're Not Alone

Just because you have diabetes, you don't have to sit quietly in the corner and hope that no one notices. Many other people with diabetes are out there – most are ordinary people, but no shortage exists of famous ones either.

Steve Redgrave is the greatest British rower ever to have competed. He has so many Olympic and Commonwealth gold medals, he probably needs a whole room, rather than just a mantelpiece, to display them. He also has diabetes.

At the same time as Steve was rowing his way to fame, Will and Mike Cross, a father-and-son team, were walking to the South Pole. Their arrival on 17 January 2003 made Mike the oldest man ever to accomplish the feat. Even as these two reached their goal, another man on the other side of the world was working towards his. Douglas Cairns was in the middle of a five-month flight round the world, in a light twin aircraft. Will, Mike, and Douglas all have diabetes, too.

Diabetes is a common disease, so it's bound to occur in some very uncommon people. The list of people with diabetes is long, and you may be amazed at some of the names on it. The point is that every one of them lives or lived with this chronic illness, and every one of them was able to do something special with their life. Consider these other examples:

✔ **Politicians:** Politicians seem to be a group with a lot of diabetes. A well-recognised close link exists between type 2 diabetes and the size of your waist (Chapter 4 tells you more about diet and the onset of diabetes) – enough said for politicians! One of us was recently interviewing John Prescott about his diabetes, and he suggested that he had the sort of lifestyle that went with the illness. It was too good an opportunity to miss: we reminded him that, more to the point, he had the sort of waist-line that went with diabetes. Among the Russian premiers who have had diabetes are Yuri Andropov, Nikita Krushchev, and Mikhail Gorbachev. Former Israeli Prime Minister Menachem Begin had diabetes, as does Winnie Mandela, former head of the ANC Women's League in South Africa.

✔ **Entertainers:** Diabetes has also affected some of the most glamorous actors and actresses in the world. Halle Berry may have been calculating her blood glucose as she climbed the podium last year to accept her Oscar; Elizabeth Taylor, as famous for her marriages as for her luminous eyes and breathtaking acting ability, has diabetes, too. So did Mae West, who told men to 'Come up and see me some time.' Singers who lived with diabetes included Harry Secombe, Ella Fitzgerald, and Elvis Presley. John Peel, one of the best-loved broadcasters in Britain, was diagnosed with diabetes. And diabetes hasn't stopped Jimmy Tarbuck from being funny.

✔ **Writers:** Diabetes certainly isn't a bar to creativity in the world of writing, either. Ernest Hemingway and HG Wells were both diabetic. So are Colin Dexter, the author of the Inspector Morse books, and Sue Townsend, who penned the Adrian Mole series.

✔ **At least one famous marquess:** And for those of you worried that having diabetes will make you less attractive to the opposite sex, there's good news. Who hasn't marvelled at the exploits of the eccentric Marquess of Bath, with his wife and seventy-three 'wifelets'? Yes, you've guessed it, he has diabetes, too.

The names in the preceding paragraphs are just a partial list of those with diabetes who have achieved greatness. The point of these many examples is this: *Diabetes shouldn't stop you from doing what you want to do with your life.*

Perhaps the many people with diabetes who achieved greatness used the same personal strengths to overcome the difficulties associated with diabetes and to excel at their particular callings. Or maybe their diabetes forced them to be stronger, more perseverant, and therefore more successful. What *you* need to remember is that following the rules of good diabetic care is important (you can read more about why in Chapters 7 through 12). If you follow the rules of good diabetes care, you can, for the most part, be just as healthy as a person without diabetes. In fact, if you follow the rules, you may actually be healthier than people without diabetes who smoke, over-eat, under-exercise, or combine these and other unhealthy habits.

Even if you follow every bit of advice in this book about healthy living to the letter, you're unrealistic if you expect your diabetes not to have any effect on your health. Even with a healthy lifestyle, diabetes is likely to have some long-term effects on your eyes, kidneys, and nerves. It's also a major risk factor for heart disease. However, smoking, unhealthy eating, and lack of exercise can seriously damage your health even if you don't have diabetes. At least you have an added incentive to do something about your lifestyle at an early stage.

Chapter 15 shows you a few areas (such as piloting a commercial flight) in which certain people with diabetes can't participate – largely due to the ignorance of some legislators. As you show that you can safely and competently do anything that a person without diabetes can do, these last few obstacles to complete freedom of choice for those with diabetes will come down.

Dealing with Your Diagnosis

Do you remember what you were doing when you found out that you or a loved one had diabetes? Unless you were too young to understand, the news was quite a shock, yes? Suddenly you had a condition from which people die. Many of the feelings that you went through were exactly those of a person learning that she is dying. The following sections describe the normal stages of reacting to a diagnosis of a major medical condition such as diabetes.

You may experience the various stages of reacting to your diabetes in a different order than we describe in the following sections. Some stages may be more prominent, and others may be hardly noticeable.

The stage of denial

When your doctor first tells you that you've got diabetes, you probably begin by denying that you do, despite all the evidence. Your doctor may help your denial by saying that you have just 'a touch of diabetes', which is an impossibility equivalent to 'a touch of pregnancy'. You're probably looking for any evidence that the whole thing is a mistake. Ultimately, you have to accept the diagnosis and begin to gather the information needed to start to help yourself. But perhaps you've neglected to take your medication, follow your diet, or perform the exercise that is so important to maintaining your body.

Hopefully, you've not only accepted the diabetes diagnosis yourself, but have also shared the news with your family, friends, and people close to you. Having diabetes isn't something to be ashamed of, and it isn't something that you should hide from anyone. You need the help of everyone in your environment, from your colleagues, who need to know not to tempt you with treats that you can't eat, to your friends, who need to know how to give you *glucagon* (a treatment for low blood glucose) if you become unconscious from a severe insulin reaction.

Your diabetes isn't your fault – nor is it a form of leprosy or other diseases that historically or currently carry a social stigma. Diabetes isn't contagious, and no one can catch it from you.

If you accept that you have diabetes and are open about it, you're going to find that you're far from alone in your situation. If you don't believe us, read the section 'You're Not Alone', earlier in this chapter.

One of our patients told me about an uplifting experience she had. She arrived at work one morning and was very worried when she realised that she had forgotten her insulin. But she quickly found a source of comfort when she remembered that she could go to a colleague with diabetes and ask to borrow some insulin. Another time, she left the crowd at a party and stepped into a friend's bedroom to take an insulin injection, and she found a man there doing the same thing.

The stage of anger

When you pass the stage of denying that you or a loved one has diabetes, you may become angry that you're burdened with this 'terrible' diagnosis. But you quickly find that diabetes isn't so terrible and that you can't do anything to rid yourself of the disease. Your anger only worsens your situation, and it's detrimental in the following ways:

- ✔ If your anger becomes targeted at a person, who may get hurt.
- ✔ If you often feel guilty that your anger is harming you and those close to you.
- ✔ If your anger often keeps you from successfully managing your diabetes.

As long as you're angry, you are not in a problem-solving mode. Diabetes requires your focus and attention. Turn your anger into creative ways to manage your diabetes. For ways to manage your diabetes, see Part III.

The stage of bargaining

The reactions of anger that you may experience often lead to a stage when you or your loved ones become increasingly aware of the loss of immortality and bargain for more time. At this point, most people with diabetes realise that they have plenty of life ahead of them, but the talk of complications, blood tests, and pills or insulin starts to overwhelm them. You may experience depression, which makes good diabetic care all the more difficult.

Studies have shown that people with diabetes suffer from depression at a rate that is two to four times higher than the rate for the general population. Those with diabetes also experience anxiety at a three to five times higher rate than people without diabetes.

If you suffer from depression, you may feel that your diabetic situation creates problems for you that justify being depressed. You may rationalise your depression in the following ways:

- ✔ You're hindered by diabetes as you try to make friends.
- ✔ You don't have the freedom to choose your leisure activities because of your diabetes.
- ✔ You may feel that you're too tired to overcome difficulties.
- ✔ You may dread the future and possible diabetic complications.
- ✔ You don't have the freedom to eat what you want.
- ✔ You may feel a constant level of annoyance because of all the minor inconveniences of dealing with diabetes.

All the preceding concerns are legitimate, but they also are all surmountable. How do you handle your many concerns and fend off depression? The following are a few important methods:

- ✔ Try to achieve excellent blood glucose control.
- ✔ Begin a regular exercise programme.
- ✔ Recognise that every abnormal blip in your blood glucose is not your fault.

If you can't overcome the depression brought on by your diabetic concerns, you may need to consider therapy or antidepressant drugs. But you probably won't reach that point. Most people with diabetes don't.

Moving on

As you move through the stages of reacting to your diagnosis, don't feel that any emotion you experience – anger, denial, or depression – is wrong. These are natural coping mechanisms that serve a psychological purpose for a brief time. The key is to allow yourself to have these feelings – and then drop them. Move on and learn to live normally with your diabetes.

Maintaining the Good Life

You may assume that a chronic disease like diabetes leads to a diminished quality of life. But must this be the case? Several studies have been done to evaluate this question, and some of the more detailed findings can be seen in the sidebar 'The survey said . . .'. The evidence seems to suggest that quality of life is related directly to how well controlled the diabetes is. Those who have better control over their blood glucose levels and who maintain healthy lifestyles experience a better quality of life. A couple of other things seem to have a big impact as well: family support and whether you're dependent on insulin injections.

How to maintain quality of life

One factor that contributes to a lower quality of life is a lack of physical activity. This is one negative factor that you can alter immediately. Physical activity is a habit that you must maintain on a lifelong basis. (See Chapter 9 for advice on exercise.) The problem is that making a long-term change to a more physically active lifestyle is difficult; most people maintain their activity for a while but eventually fall back into inactive routines.

Perhaps you're afraid that intensified insulin treatment, which involves three or four daily injections of insulin and frequent testing of blood glucose, may keep you from doing the things that you want to do and diminish your daily quality of life (see Chapter 10 for more information about intensified insulin treatment). A study in *Diabetes Care* in November 1998 explored whether the extra effort and time consumed by such diabetes treatments had an adverse effect on people's quality of life. The study compared people with diabetes to people with other chronic diseases, such as gastrointestinal disease and hepatitis (inflammation of the liver), and then compared all of those groups to a group of people who had no disease. The diabetic group reported a higher quality of life than the other chronic illness groups. The people in the diabetic group were not so much concerned with the physical problems of diabetes, such as intense and time-consuming tests and treatments, as they were worried about the social and psychological difficulties.

The survey said . . .

Two studies published in 2002 and 2003 looked at the impact of people with diabetes monitoring their own glucose, with a view to tailoring and improving their own control. In other words, they looked at the impact of the person with diabetes being in day-to-day charge of their diabetes control. Both studies showed that improving their glucose control was linked to significant improvements in quality of life measurements, including depression and well-being.

Most of the other surveys of quality of life for people with diabetes have been long-term studies. In one study of more than 2,000 people with diabetes, receiving many different levels of intensity of treatment, the overall response was that quality of life was lower for the person with diabetes than for the general population. But several factors separated those with the lower quality of life from those who expressed more contentment with life.

Many other studies have examined the different aspects of diabetes that affect a person's quality of life. The studies had some useful findings:

- **Insulin injections for adults:** Do adults with diabetes who require insulin injections experience a diminished quality of life? A report in *Diabetes Care* in June 1998 found that insulin injections don't reduce the quality of life: The person's sense of physical and emotional well-being remains the same after beginning insulin injections as it was before injections were necessary.

- **Insulin injections for teenagers:** Teenagers who require insulin injections don't always accept the treatment as well as adults do, so teenagers more often experience a diminished quality of life. However, a study of more than 2,000 such teenagers in *Diabetes Care* in November 2001 showed that as their diabetic control improved, they showed greater satisfaction with their lives and felt in better health, while they felt themselves to be less of a burden to their family.

- **Stress management:** When patients were divided into two groups, one of which received diabetes education alone and the other diabetes education plus five sessions of stress management, the latter group experienced significant improvement in diabetic control compared to those with only diabetes education. This study, in *Diabetes Care* in January 2002, showed that lowering stress lowers blood glucose. How can you lower your level of stress?

- **Family support:** People with diabetes greatly benefit from their family's help in dealing with their disease. But do people with diabetes in a close family have better diabetic control? One study in *Diabetes Care* in

February 1998 attempted to answer this question and found some unexpected results. Having a supportive family didn't necessarily mean that the person with diabetes in the study would maintain better glucose control. But a supportive family did make the person with diabetes feel more physically capable in general and much more comfortable with her place in society.

✔ **Quality of life over the long term:** How does a person's perception of quality of life change over time? As they age, do most people with diabetes feel that their quality of life increases, decreases, or persists at a steady level? The consensus of studies is that most people with diabetes experience an increasing quality of life as they get older. People feel better about themselves and their diabetes after dealing with the disease for a decade or more. This is the healing property of time.

Putting all this information together, what can you do to maintain a high quality of life with diabetes? Here are the steps that accomplish the most for you:

✔ Keep your blood glucose as normal as possible (see Part III).

✔ Look after your blood pressure and cholesterol (see Chapter 5).

✔ Make exercise a regular part of your lifestyle.

✔ Get plenty of support from family, friends, and medical resources.

✔ Stay aware of the latest developments in diabetes care.

✔ Maintain a healthy attitude. Remember that some day you will laugh about things that bug you now, so why wait?

When you're having trouble coping

You wouldn't hesitate to seek help for your physical ailments associated with diabetes, but you may be very reluctant to seek help when you can't adjust psychologically to diabetes. The problem is that sooner or later, your psychological maladjustment ruins any control that you have over your diabetes. And, of course, you can't lead a very pleasant life if you're in a depressed or anxious state all the time. The following symptoms are indicators that you're past the point of handling your diabetes on your own and may be suffering from depression:

✔ You can't sleep.

✔ You have no energy when you are awake.

✔ You can't think clearly.

✔ You can't find activities that interest or amuse you.

✔ You get tearful very easily.

✔ You feel worthless.

✔ You feel guilty.

✔ You have frequent thoughts of suicide.

✔ You have no appetite, or too great an appetite.

✔ You find no humour in anything.

If you recognise several of these symptoms as features of your daily life, you need to get some help. Your sense of hopelessness may include the feeling that no one else can help you – and that simply isn't true. Your GP or diabetes specialist is the first place to go for advice. She may help you to see the need for some short-term or long-term therapy. Well-trained therapists – especially therapists who are trained to take care of people with diabetes – can see solutions that you can't see in your current state. You need to find a therapist whom you can trust, so that when you're feeling low you can talk to this therapist and feel assured that she is very interested in your welfare.

Your GP or therapist may decide that your situation is appropriate for medication to treat the anxiety or depression. Currently, many drugs are available that are proven to be safe and low in side effects. Even if the medication causes side effects at first, these often wear off within a couple of weeks. Sometimes a brief period of medication is enough to help you adjust to your diabetes.

You can also find help in a support group. The huge and continually growing number of support groups shows that positive things are happening in these groups. In most support groups, participants share their stories and problems, which helps everyone involved to cope with their own feelings of isolation, futility, or depression.

You can get excellent support, whether you're suffering from depression or looking after someone who has it, from MIND. Look the organisation up on www.mind.org.uk for details of your local branch. Your GP may also be able to tell you about other self-help or support groups in your area.

Chapter 2

It's the Glucose

In This Chapter

▶ Defining diabetes by the blood glucose

▶ Finding treatments for diabetes

▶ Tracking diabetes around the world

▶ Meeting actual patients and their stories

*T*he Greeks and Romans knew about diabetes. Fortunately, the way they tested for the condition – by tasting the urine – has gone by the wayside. By this method, the Romans discovered that the urine of certain people was *mellitus,* the Latin word for *sweet*. The Greeks noticed that when people with sweet urine drank, the fluids came out in the urine almost as fast as they went in the mouth, like a siphon. They called this by the Greek word for *siphon – diabetes*. This is the origin of the modern name for the disease, *diabetes mellitus*.

In this chapter, we cover the not-so-fun stuff about diabetes – the big words, the definitions, and so on. But if you really want to understand what's happening to your body when you have diabetes, then you don't want to skip this chapter.

Recognising Diabetes

When you have diabetes, your body can't process sugar the way it needs to (Chapter 3 gives you details on why), and the unprocessed sugar passes through your system. The sweetness of the urine comes from *glucose,* also known as blood sugar. Many different kinds of sugars are in nature, but glucose is the sugar that has the starring role in the body, providing a source of instant energy so that muscles can move and important chemical reactions can take place. Sugar is a carbohydrate, one group of the three sources of energy in the body. The others are protein and fat, which we discuss in greater detail in Chapter 8.

One lump or two?

Table sugar (or *sucrose),* the sort you use in a recipe or put in your tea, is actually two different kinds of sugar – glucose and *fructose* – linked together. Fructose is the type of sugar found in fruits and vegetables. It's sweeter than glucose, which makes sucrose sweeter than glucose as well. Your taste buds require less sucrose or fructose to get the same sweetening power of glucose.

Diabetes mellitus is associated with thirst and frequent urination. But it's not the only disease with these symptoms. Another condition in which fluids go in and out of the body like a siphon is called *diabetes insipidus.* Here, the urine is not sweet. Diabetes insipidus is an entirely different disease that you should not mistake for diabetes mellitus. In diabetes mellitus, the hormone insulin plays a major part. In diabetes insipidus, the problem lies with a different hormone called vasopressin. If you have symptoms of thirst, frequent urination, and passing water at night, your doctor should first check you out for diabetes mellitus. If tests for diabetes mellitus are negative, your doctor checks for the much rarer diabetes insipidus. The diagnosis of diabetes insipidus is made on the basis of repeated blood tests and weight measurements while you avoid drinking any fluids for eight hours.

How do doctors define diabetes?

The standard definition of diabetes mellitus is excessive glucose in a blood sample – in other words, you have too much sugar in your blood. For years, doctors set this level fairly high. The World Health Organisation (WHO) lowered the standard for a normal glucose level in 1997, and now almost everyone in the UK uses this new standard for diagnosis. Why did the WHO decide to lower the standard level? Because too many people were experiencing complications of diabetes even though their glucose level wasn't high enough to be diagnosed with diabetes. The new definition of diabetes includes symptoms of diabetes, along with any one of the following three criteria:

- ✔ A random plasma sugar level greater than 11 mmol/l (millimoles per litre)

- ✔ A fasting plasma sugar level greater than or equal to 7 mmol/l (or 6.1 mmol/l in whole blood)

- ✔ A plasma sugar level greater than 11 mmol/l two hours after drinking 75 grams of glucose dissolved in water in an oral glucose tolerance test (OGTT)

WHO – who are they?

The World Health Organisation is the specialised agency for health of the United Nations. It was established in 1948 and aims to help people around the world to achieve the highest possible level of health. The WHO is governed by 192 member states through the World Health Assembly.

Health is defined by the WHO as a state of complete physical, mental, and social well-being – not merely the absence of disease or infirmity. You can contact its European headquarters at:

Regional Office for Europe (EURO)
8, Scherfigsvej
DK-2100 Copenhagen 0, Denmark
Telephone: +(45) 39 17 17 17
Facsimile: +(45) 39 17 18 18
www.who.int

Mmol/l stands for millimoles per litre. This way of measuring blood glucose concentrations is used almost all over the world, except in America. Over there, most glucose measurements are in mg/dl, or milligrams per decilitre. To translate mmol/l into mg/dl, multiply your figure in mmol/l by 18. So if you're travelling in the United States and need to speak to a doctor, make sure that one of you has a calculator to hand!

And how accurate are their tests?

The WHO also recommends that if your blood tests show a high concentration but you haven't got any symptoms of diabetes (see the later section 'Controlling Your Glucose'), you shouldn't be diagnosed with diabetes on the basis of a single glucose measurement. In these cases, it recommends that you get another plasma glucose concentration done on another day to confirm the first test. This second test can be either fasting (nothing but water to eat or drink for eight hours beforehand), or from a random sample, or two hours after taking an oral glucose tolerance test. Finally, the WHO suggests that if the fasting or random levels aren't enough to give a diagnosis, you should get an oral glucose tolerance test. With several tests in place, you can be fairly sure that your final diagnosis is accurate.

For those of you who like the hard data, here's a useful list:

- ✔ FPG (fasting plasma glucose) below 6.1 mmol/l is a normal fasting glucose.

- ✔ FPG at least 6.1 mmol/l but less than 7.0 mmol/l is impaired fasting glucose.

✔ FPG equal to or greater than 7.0 mmol/l gives a provisional diagnosis of diabetes.

✔ 2-h PG (plasma glucose two hours after an oral glucose tolerance test) less than 7.8 mmol/l is normal glucose tolerance.

✔ 2-h PG greater than or equal to 7.8 mmol/l but less than 11 mmol/l is impaired glucose tolerance.

✔ 2-h PG above 11 mmol/l gives a provisional diagnosis of diabetes.

All these changing definitions may seem confusing, but there's more change on the way! Type 2 diabetes (see Chapter 3), as we see later on, isn't a condition that comes on quickly. Insulin resistance usually increases over years rather than months, and your body becomes gradually less efficient at keeping your blood sugar steady. So between 'no diabetes' and 'type 2 diabetes' are stages called impaired fasting glucose and impaired glucose tolerance. In 2005, the International Diabetes Federation decided that for the condition called metabolic syndrome (see Chapter 3), the cut-off to define impaired FPG should be a fasting blood glucose above 5.6 mmol/l, rather than the 6.1 mmol/l that has traditionally been used.

Controlling Your Glucose

In order to understand the symptoms of diabetes, you need to know a little about the way the body normally handles glucose and what happens when things go wrong. The following sections explain the fine line that your body treads between control and lack of control of its glucose levels.

Hormones at the helm

A *hormone* is a chemical substance made in one part of the body that travels (usually through the bloodstream) to a distant part of the body where it performs its work. A hormone called *insulin* finely controls the level of glucose in your blood. Insulin acts like a key to open the inside of a cell, such as muscle or fat, so that your glucose can enter. If your glucose can't enter the cell, it can provide no energy to the body from that cell.

Because of the important role it plays, insulin is essential for growth. In addition to providing the key to entry of glucose into the cell, scientists consider insulin the 'builder hormone' because it does the following:

✔ It enables fat and muscle to form.

✔ It allows storage of glucose in a form called *glycogen* for use when fuel is not coming in.

✔ It blocks breakdown of protein.

Without insulin, you can't survive for long. With the fine-tuning that insulin gives, the body manages to keep the level of glucose in your body pretty steady at about 3.3 to 6.4 mmol/l all the time.

Symptoms and signposts

Your glucose starts to rise in your blood when your body doesn't produce enough insulin or when the body is not working effectively. Once your glucose rises above about 10.0 mmol/l (sometimes higher as you get older), glucose begins to seep into your urine and make it sweet. Up to that point, your kidney – the filter for your blood – is able to extract glucose before it enters your urine. Losing glucose into the urine leads to many of the short-term complications of diabetes (you can read about these short-term complications in Chapter 4).

The following list identifies the most common early symptoms of diabetes and how they occur. One or more of the following symptoms may be present when diabetes is diagnosed:

✔ **Frequent urination and thirst:** The glucose in your urine draws more water out of your blood, so more urine forms. More urine in your bladder makes you feel the need to urinate more frequently during the day and to get up at night to empty the bladder, which keeps filling up. As the amount of water in your blood declines, you feel thirsty and drink much more frequently.

✔ **Fatigue:** Because glucose can't enter cells that depend on insulin as a key for glucose (the most important exception is the brain, which does not need insulin), glucose can't be used as a fuel to move muscles or to facilitate the many other chemical reactions that have to take place to produce energy. Before you're diagnosed with diabetes, you often feel tired, and you're likely to feel much stronger once treatment allows glucose to enter cells again.

✔ **Weight loss:** Weight loss is common among some people with diabetes because they lack insulin, which is the builder hormone. When insulin is lacking for any reason, the body begins to break down. You lose muscle tissue. Some of the muscle converts into glucose even though it cannot get into cells. It passes out of your body in the urine. Fat tissue breaks down into small fat particles that can provide an alternate source of energy. As your body breaks down and you lose glucose in the urine, you often experience weight loss. However, most people with diabetes are heavy rather than skinny (we explain why in Chapter 3). Weight loss is much more likely to be a symptom of type 1 rather than type 2 diabetes (more about the differences between these types of diabetes in Chapter 3).

✔ **Persistent vaginal infection among women:** As your blood glucose rises, all the fluids in your body contain higher levels of glucose, including the sweat and body secretions such as semen in men and vaginal secretions in women. Many bugs, such as bacteria and fungi, thrive in the high glucose environment. Women may begin to complain of itching or burning, an abnormal discharge from the vagina, and sometimes an odour.

In the UK, all patients who register with a new general practitioner will be offered a new patient registration check, which may include a dipstick test of your urine for glucose and protein. The idea is to pick up diabetes early in people who don't have any symptoms. Unfortunately, the level of blood sugar at which your body lets glucose 'overflow' into your urine varies from person to person, and at different times of your life. As you get older, for instance, you can usually have much higher levels of blood glucose without getting sugar in your urine. That makes the urine-screening test for diabetes notoriously inaccurate. If you (or someone you know) think you might have diabetes but your urine is negative for sugar on testing, make sure you ask to have a fasting blood test (which is explained above in the section 'And how accurate are their tests?').

Discovering Ways to Treat Diabetes

A condition that must have been diabetes mellitus appears in the writings of China and India more than 2,000 years ago. The description is the same one that the Greeks and Romans reported – urine that tasted sweet. Scholars from India and China were the first to describe frequent urination. But not until 1776 did researchers discover the cause of the sweetness – glucose. And only in the nineteenth century did doctors develop a new chemical test. Later discoveries showed that the pancreas produced a crucial substance, called insulin, which controlled the glucose in the blood (for more on insulin, see the 'Hormones at the helm' section earlier in this chapter). Since that time, insulin has been extracted and purified – and it's still a real life saver today. Oral drugs have been available for the past 40 years and stand alongside injected insulin in the fight to reduce blood glucose.

Once insulin was discovered, diabetes specialists, led by Elliot Joslin and others, recommended three basic treatments for diabetes that are as valuable today as they were when first suggested in 1921:

- Diet (see Chapter 8)
- Exercise (see Chapter 9)
- Medication (see Chapter 10)

The discovery of insulin has not solved the problem of diabetes, although it saves the lives of thousands. Before the use of insulin became widespread, the only treatment had been starvation; as people treated in this way aged, they had unexpected complications in the eyes, the kidneys, and the nervous system (see Chapter 5 to find out why). And insulin did not address the problem of the much larger group of people with diabetes now known as type 2 (see Chapter 3 to find out more about the different types of diabetes). Their problem was not lack of insulin but resistance to its actions. Fortunately, doctors now have the tools to bring the disease under control.

The next major discovery was the group of drugs called *sulphonylureas* (Chapter 10 tells you more about these), the first drugs that could be taken by mouth to lower the blood glucose. But the only way to know the level of the blood glucose was still by testing the urine, which was entirely inadequate for good diabetic control (see Chapter 7).

Around 1980, the first portable meters for blood glucose testing became available. This offered the possibility, for the first time, of relating treatment to a measurable outcome. This has led, in turn, to the discovery of other great drugs for diabetes like rosiglitazone, pioglitazone, acarbose, repaglinide, nateglinide, and others.

Typical Patient Stories

Diabetes is a huge problem in the United Kingdom, where it already uses up more than 10 per cent of the National Health Service's total resources. The facts and figures that we use to diagnose diabetes don't begin to reflect the human dimensions of the disease. People end up with these tests after days or months (or even years) of minor discomforts that reach the point where they can no longer tolerate them. Some people are diagnosed completely by accident, when they have a urine or blood test for an unrelated reason.

Diabetes in the United Kingdom

In the United Kingdom, probably at least 3 million people are thought to have diabetes. Only 1.8 million of them, however, have been diagnosed with the disease. As we show in later chapters, much of the damage caused by diabetes has already taken place by the time a diagnosis of type 2 diabetes is made. Many doctors hoped that nationwide initiatives, such as the recently published National Service Framework (NSF) on diabetes, would provide guidance on screening to find the 'missing million'

undiagnosed diabetics in Britain. Unfortunately, the NSF has concentrated on developing services for people already diagnosed with diabetes. However, new projects concentrating on quality of care, such as the New General Practitioner Contracts of 2004 and 2006, may well redress the balance. In the meantime, we must rely on identifying people at high risk of diabetes (head to Chapter 3 to find out what your family's risks are) and persuading them to come forward for testing sooner rather than later.

The next few stories of real (though renamed) patients can help you understand that diabetes is a disease that happens to people – people who are working, relaxing, travelling, sleeping, and doing many other things that make life so complex.

The Steadmonsons – John, Mary, daughter Rachel, 9, and son Lyle, 5 – were on holiday in Spain in August. The heat made everyone extremely thirsty and forced them to drink lots of fluids. Lyle was also urinating a lot, but no one thought much about it. However, when they returned home, Lyle continued to complain of thirst and urinated excessively. He seemed to eat a lot of sweets but did not gain weight. Then Lyle wet his bed, which had not happened for years. Mary took him to the general practitioner, who did a random blood glucose, which was 26 mmol/l. The doctor told Mary and John that Lyle had type 1 diabetes. He was admitted to hospital the same day. This was the beginning of many changes in the Steadmonson household.

Eleanor Andrews, 34, had been diagnosed with schizophrenia in her 20s. For the last eight years, her condition had been well controlled with medication, but the medication had also caused her to put on three stone in weight. She blamed her constant tiredness on her weight. At a medication review, her GP checked her weight and told her that her weight put her into the category of obesity. He suggested doing a blood test for glucose and cholesterol. Her blood sugar was 13.2 mmol/l, and a repeat was 12.9 mmol/l. Her GP referred her to the diabetic clinic and to the dietician. The dietician was sympathetic to her difficulties with losing weight, both because of her medication and because of embarrassment over her size, which made exercise difficult. She worked with Elaine and the practice nurse to devise a diet and exercise regimen with fortnightly weight checks. Within two months, Elaine had lost 1 stone and her energy levels were improving.

Tracking diabetes around the world

Diabetes is a global health problem. A 1994 study estimated that approximately 100 million people around the world have diabetes and that by the year 2010, the number would rise to more than 215 million. These estimates were made before the current, more inclusive definition of diabetes was accepted in 1997. Under the new definition, the number of people in the world with diabetes was more like 130 million in 1994 and will be 300 million in 2025. In Europe alone, which had 21 million people with diabetes in 1995, it is estimated that the number of people with diabetes will reach 32 million by 2010 – and that 3 million of these will be in the United Kingdom.

In developing countries, however, diabetes is a potential catastrophe. It is projected that by 2015, developing countries in general will have three times more deaths from non-communicable diseases like diabetes than from communicable diseases like infections and parasitic disease. Even more worryingly, it seems likely that 75 per cent of people with diabetes in developing countries will be of working age, in the 45–64-year age group. That means that in less than 30 years from now, 170 million men and women in the developing regions of the world will be suffering from diabetes at the most productive time in their lives.

Diabetes is concentrated where food supplies allow people to eat more calories than they need, so that they develop obesity. Several different types of diabetes actually exist, but the type usually associated with obesity, called type 2 diabetes (see Chapter 3), accounts for about 95 per cent of all cases.

Diabetes is also increasing throughout the world because the age of the population is increasing (age is another major risk factor; see Chapter 3 for more risk factors). It is estimated that by 2020, more than 1,000 million people in the world will be over 60 – 70 per cent of them living in developing countries. As other diseases are controlled and the population gets older, more diabetes is being diagnosed. In addition, the longer people have diabetes, the more complications they suffer from.

One very interesting study traced people of Japanese ancestry as they went from living in Japan to living in Hawaii and finally the United States mainland. Those in Japan, where people customarily maintain a normal weight, tended to have a very low incidence of diabetes. As they moved to Hawaii, the incidence of diabetes began to rise along with their average weight. On the mainland, where food is most available, these Japanese had the highest rate of diabetes of all.

Not only the number of calories but the composition of the diet changes as people migrate. Before they migrate, they tend to consume a low-fat, high-fibre diet. Once they reach their new destination, they adopt the local diet, which tends to be higher in fat and lower in fibre. The carbohydrates in the new diet are from high-energy foods, which do not tend to be filling, promoting more calorie intake.

The Japanese provide another interesting lesson about the place of obesity as a factor in the onset of diabetes. Japanese Sumo wrestlers have to gain enormous quantities of weight in order to fight in a certain weight class. Even while they are still fighting, they demonstrate a high frequency of diabetes. Once they become more sedentary, the frequency goes up to 40 per cent, a huge prevalence.

(continued)

(continued)

In China, as the country becomes more affluent, doctors are seeing a significant increase in the incidence of diabetes. Migrant Chinese populations show even higher rates, especially where the environment allows them to gain more weight and be more sedentary.

The United States has the highest incidence of obesity in the world. In 2005, it was estimated that 36.5 per cent of men and 41 per cent of women in America were obese. The rise in the incidence of diabetes and its complications has mirrored these figures, and diabetes is now so common that in parts of Harlem, one in two hospital beds is taken up with someone affected by the complications of diabetes.

Leroy Groves was a 46-year-old black-belt judo instructor. Despite his very active lifestyle, he was not careful about his diet and had gained a stone in the last few years. He was more fatigued than he had been in the past but blamed this on his increasing age. His mother had diabetes, but he assumed that his physical fitness would protect him from this condition. He was finding that he could barely get through a one-hour class without excusing himself to visit the loo. His wife finally made him an appointment with the practice nurse at his doctor's surgery for a well-person check. She found glucose in his urine on dipstick testing and referred him to his general practitioner. Blood tests revealed a random blood glucose of 14.7 mmol/l. The following week, another random blood glucose was 16.0 mmol/l. The doctor told Leroy he had diabetes, but Leroy refused to believe it. He left the doctor's surgery in an angry mood but vowed to lose weight and did so successfully. On a repeat visit to the doctor, a random glucose was 9.3 mmol/l. Leroy told the doctor that he knew he did not have diabetes, but the resolve to eat carefully did not last, and he was back six weeks later with a glucose of 16.8 mmol/l. Finally, he accepted the diagnosis and started treatment. He rapidly returned to his usual state of health, and the fatigue disappeared.

Debbie O'Leary's active sex life with her husband was continually being interrupted by vaginal thrush infections, which resulted in an unpleasant smell, redness, and itching. Debbie (41) would go to the pharmacy and buy an over-the-counter preparation, which promptly cured the condition but did not stop it from returning. Finally, after three of these infections in two months, she decided to see her general practitioner. The doctor did a urinalysis and found glucose in her urine. A random blood test showed a glucose of 13.5 mmol/l. The doctor then ordered a variety of tests, including a fasting blood glucose, which was 8.3 mmol/l. He told Debbie she had diabetes and recommended exercise and diet to start with. He referred her to the in-house diabetic clinic at the surgery, where she got advice from the dietician and practice nurse. Following this advice, she lowered her blood glucose to the point that she no longer developed yeast infections. As an added bonus, the resulting weight loss and return of energy that she did not know was missing made her sex life with her husband even more satisfying.

Chapter 3

What Type of Diabetes Do You Have?

· ·

· ·

*Y*ou can prevent diabetes, but not quite as easily as you may like. Your best method for preventing diabetes would be to pick your parents carefully, but that's a little impractical, even with modern technology. In general, you can prevent a disease if it meets two requirements. First, you have to be able to identify individuals who are at high risk for getting the disease. Second, the disease must have at least some treatments or actions that you can take to definitely reduce your chance of getting it. You can meet both of these requirements in an effort to prevent diabetes. This chapter shows you how to identify whether you're at risk of type 1 or type 2 diabetes, and it covers definite actions that you can take to prevent both of these types of diabetes.

This chapter also helps you get a clear understanding of your type of diabetes, how it relates to the other types of diabetes, and how the failure of your friendly pancreas to do its assigned job can lead to a host of unfortunate consequences. (We cover these consequences in greater detail in Part II.)

Getting to Know Your Pancreas

You may not think that having a personal relationship with one of your body organs is possible or even desirable, but don't disregard your pancreas. Your pancreas is a shy little organ that can rear its lovely head at entirely unexpected moments. You probably don't know that your pancreas has a head – and a tail – but it does. So now's the time to break the ice and get to know what it does for you! Most of the time, your pancreas hides behind your stomach, quietly doing its work, helping with digestion first, and then helping to make use of the digested food. And, in one way or another, the pancreas plays a role in all of the various types of diabetes.

You don't see your pancreas very often, but you hear from it all the time. It has two major functions:

✔ To produce *digestive enzymes,* which are the chemicals that your small intestine uses to help break down food. The digestive enzymes don't have much relation to diabetes, so we don't spend much time talking about them in this book.

✔ To produce the important hormone *insulin* and secrete it directly into the blood. This function is important to diabetes. Figure 3-1 shows the microscopic appearance of the pancreas. The insulin-producing pancreas cells are found in groups called *Islets of Langerhans.*

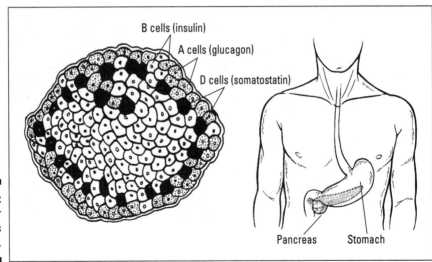

Figure 3-1: What your pancreas looks like.

B cells (insulin)

A cells (glucagon)

D cells (somatostatin)

Pancreas   Stomach

Conditions and hormones that can lead to diabetes

The following is a partial list of hormones caused by tumours and their associated conditions:

✔ Excessive adrenal gland hormone (your body's naturally occurring steroid) is present in Cushing's Syndrome. This steroid stimulates the liver to put out more glucose while it blocks the uptake of glucose by muscle tissue.

✔ Excessive prolactin is present in a prolactin-secreting tumour, or *prolactinoma*, of the pituitary gland. It blocks insulin action and glucose intolerance results.

✔ Excessive growth hormone is made by a tumour of the pituitary gland, resulting in a condition called *acromegaly*. Growth hormone reduces insulin sensitivity and forces the pancreas to make much more insulin.

✔ Excessive adrenaline is made by a *phaeochromocytoma* (a tumour of another part of the adrenal gland). It causes increased liver production of glucose, while it blocks insulin secretion.

✔ Excessive aldosterone is made by still another part of the adrenal gland in a condition called *primary hyperaldosteronism*. This condition causes glucose intolerance in a different way – by facilitating the loss of body potassium, which has a negative effect on insulin production.

✔ Excessive thyroid hormone found in hyperthyroidism causes the liver and other organs to produce excessive quantities of glucose. Hyperthyroidism is also a disease of autoimmunity, which may play a role in the loss of glucose tolerance.

✔ A glucagon-secreting tumour of the pancreas can create excessive glucagon. Glucagon has many properties that are opposite to insulin. This condition is rare, and only around 100 cases of it have been described in medical literature, so don't think you have it.

✔ A somatostatin-secreting tumour of the pancreas can create excessive somatostatin. *Somatostatin* is another hormone made in a cell present in the Islets of Langerhans. Somatostatin actually blocks insulin from leaving the beta cell, but it also blocks glucagon and other hormones, so the diabetes is very mild. This condition occurs even less often than the glucagon-secreting tumour.

If you understand only one hormone in your body, insulin should be that hormone, especially if you want to understand diabetes. Over the course of your life, the insulin that your body produces or the insulin that you inject into your body (as described in Chapter 10) affects whether or not you control your diabetes and avoid the complications of the disease.

Think of your insulin as an insurance agent, who lives in Brighton (which is your pancreas) but travels from there to do business in London (your muscles), Leeds (your fat tissue), Glasgow (your liver), and other places. This insulin insurance agent is insuring your good health.

Wherever insulin travels in your body, it opens up the cells so that glucose can enter them. After glucose enters, the cells can immediately use it for energy, store it in a storage form of glucose (called *glycogen*) for rapid use later on, or convert it to fat for use even later as energy.

After glucose leaves your blood and enters your cells, your blood glucose level falls. Your pancreas can tell when your glucose is falling, and it turns off the release of insulin to prevent unhealthy low levels of blood glucose, called *hypoglycaemia* (see Chapter 4). At the same time, your liver begins to release glucose from storage and makes new glucose from amino acids in your blood.

If your insurance agent (insulin, remember? – stick with me here!) doesn't show up when you need her (meaning that you have an absence of insulin, as in type 1 diabetes) or she does a poor job when she does show up (such as when you have a resistance to insulin, as in type 2 diabetes), your insurance coverage may be very poor (in which case, your blood glucose starts to climb). High blood glucose is the beginning of all your problems.

Doctors have proven that high blood glucose is bad for you and that keeping the blood glucose as normal as possible prevents the complications of diabetes (which we explain in Part II). Most treatments for diabetes are directed at restoring the blood glucose to normal.

Type 1 Diabetes and You

There is more than one form of diabetes. The main two forms are called *type 1* and *type 2 diabetes*. Each has its own symptoms, causes, and treatments. This section tells you all about type 1 diabetes (I bet you guessed that from the header!). If you need to know about type 2 instead, read the section 'Type 2 Diabetes and You'.

John Phillips, a 10-year-old boy, was always very active, and his parents became concerned when the teachers who had looked after him on his school field trip told them that he seemed not to have much energy. When he got home from the field trip, John's parents noticed that he was thirsty all the time and running to the toilet. He was very hungry but seemed to be losing weight, despite eating more than enough. John's parents took him to the GP, who did a blood glucose test and told them that their son had *type 1 diabetes mellitus,* which used to be called *juvenile diabetes* or *insulin-dependent diabetes.* This story has a happy ending because John's parents, though quite upset, were willing to do the necessary things to bring John's glucose under control. John is just as energetic as ever, but he has had to get used to a few inconveniences in his daily routine. You can read about these daily lifestyle changes in Part III.

Identifying the symptoms of type 1 diabetes

Type 1 diabetes used to be called *juvenile* diabetes because it occurs most frequently in children. However, so many cases are found in adults that doctors don't use the term *juvenile* any more. The disease isn't gender biased, either. Males and females get type 1 diabetes to an equal degree. The following sections list the general symptoms and give some important information on how and when these symptoms can manifest themselves in kids.

General symptoms

Before your doctor actually diagnoses you with type 1 diabetes, you may notice that you have some of the major signs and symptoms.

If you experience the following symptoms (or your child does), take time to ask your doctor about the possibility that you have diabetes:

- ✔ **Frequent urination:** You experience frequent urination because your kidneys can't return all the glucose to your bloodstream when your blood glucose level is greater than about 10 mmol/l (see Chapter 7 for all the details on blood glucose level testing). The large amount of glucose in your urine makes the urine so concentrated that water is drawn out of the blood and into the urine to reduce the concentration of glucose in the urine. This fills up the bladder repeatedly.

- ✔ **Increased thirst:** Your thirst increases because you lose so much water in your frequent urination that your body begins to dehydrate.

- ✔ **Weight loss:** You lose weight as your body loses glucose in the urine and your body breaks down muscle and fat looking for energy.

- ✔ **Increased hunger:** You notice that you're increasingly hungry. Your body has plenty of extra glucose in the blood, but your hunger is a result of your cells becoming malnourished because you lack the insulin required to allow the glucose to enter your cells. Your body is going through 'hunger in the midst of plenty'.

- ✔ **Weakness:** You feel weak because your muscle cells and other tissues don't get the energy that they require from glucose.

Special problems in children

Some children are diagnosed early in life, and other children have a more severe onset of the disease as they get a little older. With older children, parents or teachers may have missed the early signs and symptoms of diabetes. These kids have a great deal of fat breakdown in their bodies to provide energy, and this fat breakdown creates other problems.

✔ *Ketone bodies,* products of the breakdown of fats, begin to accumulate in the blood and spill into the urine. Ketone bodies are acidic and lead to nausea, tummy pain, and sometimes vomiting.

✔ At the same time, the child's blood glucose rises higher. Levels as high as 20 to 40 mmol/l are not uncommon, but levels as low as 16.6 mmol/l are possible. The child's blood is like thick maple syrup and doesn't circulate as freely as normal.

✔ The large amount of water leaving the body with the glucose depletes important substances such as sodium and potassium. The vomiting causes the child to lose more fluids and body substances.

All these abnormalities cause the child to become very drowsy and possibly lose consciousness. This situation is called *diabetic ketoacidosis,* and if it isn't identified and corrected soon, the child can die. See Chapter 4 for more details on the symptoms, causes, and treatments of ketoacidosis.

Other stuff to know

A few special circumstances affect the symptoms that you may see in people with type 1 diabetes. Remember the following factors:

✔ **The 'honeymoon' period** is a time after the diagnosis of diabetes, when the person's insulin needs decline for one to six months and the disease seems to get milder. The honeymoon period is longer when a child is older at the time of diagnosis, but the apparent diminishing of the disease is always temporary.

✔ **Warm weather** (well, warmer than the average British winter, anyway!) is associated with a decrease in the occurrence of diabetes compared to the winter months, particularly in older children. The probable reason for this is that a virus is involved in bringing on diabetes, and viruses spread much more when children are learning and playing together inside in the winter.

Investigating the causes of type 1 diabetes

When your doctor diagnoses you with diabetes, you almost immediately begin to wonder what may have caused you to acquire the disease. Did someone with diabetes sneeze on you (this isn't as silly as it sounds – take a look at the following section, 'Getting type 1 diabetes: Your chances')? Did you eat so much sugary food that your body reacted by giving you diabetes? Well, rest assured that the causes of diabetes aren't so simple or easily avoidable. Here is a list of the causes:

✔ **Problems with your immune system:** Type 1 diabetes is an *autoimmune disease,* meaning that your body is unkind enough to react against – and, in this case, destroy – a vital part of itself, namely the insulin-producing beta cells of the pancreas. Your immune system is what usually fights off infections, and you can't survive without it. It works by recognising 'intruders' in your body and attacking them. That attack is fine if the intruder is a germ causing a cold. Unfortunately, some people have an over-sensitive or faulty immune system. If it overreacts to dust or pollen, for instance, you can end up with asthma. If it overreacts to nickel touching your skin, you can end up with a form of eczema. If it mistakes your pancreas for an intruder and attacks it, you end up with diabetes.

One way that doctors discovered that type 1 diabetes is an autoimmune disease was by measuring proteins in the blood, called *antibodies,* which are literally substances directed against your body – and, in particular, against the islet cells in your pancreas. These specific antibodies are called *islet cell antibodies*, and they are found in relatives of those who have type 1 diabetes and in the people with diabetes themselves for a few years before the disease begins. Another clue that type 1 diabetes is an autoimmune disease is that treatments to reduce autoimmunity also delay the onset of type 1 diabetes. Also, type 1 diabetes tends to occur in people who have other known autoimmune diseases.

✔ **Abnormal characteristics on your chromosomes:** People who get type 1 diabetes more often have certain abnormal characteristics on their genetic material, their *chromosomes* (the DNA in each cell in your body that determines your physical characteristics), that are not present in people who don't get diabetes. Doctors can look for these abnormal characteristics on your DNA and wait to see whether you develop diabetes. But having these abnormal characteristics on your chromosomes isn't enough to guarantee that you get diabetes. Many people who have these specific abnormalities never get diabetes, so doctors need to consider other factors in addition to your DNA.

✔ **A virus:** Another essential factor in predicting whether you develop diabetes is your exposure to something in the environment, most likely a virus. If this virus infiltrates your body, it can attack your pancreas directly and reduce your ability to produce insulin. This can quickly create the diabetic condition in your body. The virus can also cause diabetes if it is made up of a substance that is also naturally present in your pancreas. If the virus and your pancreas possess the same substance, the antibodies that your body produces to fight off the virus also attack the shared substance in your pancreas. This, of course, leaves you in the same condition as if the virus itself attacked your pancreas.

Researchers haven't identified one particular virus that they can blame for type 1 diabetes. Research on patients who are at the beginning stages of type 1 diabetes has uncovered many different viruses that may be the culprit.

✔ **Other stuff:** Some doctors believe that certain chemicals in cow's milk bring on type 1 diabetes. Researchers are comparing breast-fed babies who are susceptible to type 1 diabetes to susceptible babies who are given cow's milk. They haven't yet determined whether cow's milk is a factor that causes type 1 diabetes.

Getting type 1 diabetes: Your chances

You may get type 1 diabetes if you have certain factors on your *chromosomes*. If you have several of these factors, your chance of getting type 1 diabetes is much greater than that of a person who has none of these factors. But just having these factors is not enough. You have to come into contact with something in your environment that triggers the destruction of your *beta cells,* the cells that make insulin. Doctors think that this environmental trigger is probably a virus, and they've identified several viruses that may be to blame. Doctors think they are the same viruses that cause the common cold. People with type 1 diabetes probably get the virus just like any cold virus – from someone else who has the virus who sneezes on them. But because they also have a susceptible genetic tendency, they get type 1 diabetes.

A small number (about 10 per cent) of patients with type 1 diabetes don't seem to need an environmental factor to trigger the diabetes. In these people, the disease is entirely an autoimmune destruction of the beta cells. If you fall into this category of people with diabetes, you may have other autoimmune diseases such as autoimmune thyroid disease. Your thyroid gland is on the front of your neck, and it produces another hormone called thyroxine, which tells your body how fast to 'tick over' and burn up energy. Diabetes itself doesn't affect your levels of thyroxine.

How likely are you to get type 1 diabetes if someone in your family has it? Studies of many families have provided fairly good answers to this question:

✔ If one of your parents has type 1 diabetes, the odds are only 3 to 4 per cent that you will get it. You get half of your total genetic material from each parent.

✔ If you and your sibling (brother or sister) have exactly the same genetic material, you are identical twins. The identical twin of a person with type 1 diabetes has about a 20 per cent chance of also getting type 1 diabetes.

✔ If you have only half of your genetic material in common with your sibling who has type 1 diabetes, your chance of getting type 1 diabetes drops to 5 per cent.

✔ If none of the genetic material associated with diabetes is the same as your sibling with type 1 diabetes, your chance of developing type 1 diabetes is less than 1 per cent.

Knowing your family's risks

We all want to protect our loved ones. If you have diabetes, one of the best ways you can do this is to remind them to get themselves checked out for diabetes regularly. Even if you are the only member of your family to have diabetes, that still increases the risk of all your first-degree relatives (parents, children, brothers and sisters) of developing diabetes too. As you can read in this chapter, much of the damage done by diabetes has already been done by the time type 2 diabetics are diagnosed. The sooner they're diagnosed, the sooner they can get treatment to prevent diabetic complications. Because there's no national screening programme for diabetes in the United Kingdom, it's largely up to you and them to take this step to look after their health.

Having diabetes in the family isn't the only risk factor for getting diabetes, but it's certainly a major one. If a member of your family has other risk factors, like the ones listed below, they're at even higher risk. Explaining the risks to them is well worth doing, so they can understand the importance of getting themselves checked out regularly.

The sort of risk factors to look out for include:

✔ If you have a first-degree relative with diabetes (especially type 2 diabetes).

✔ If you belong to a high-risk ethnic group. South Asians, for instance, are more than five times as likely as western Europeans to develop type 2 diabetes in middle age or beyond, and tend to get the condition at a younger age.

✔ If you have metabolic syndrome (see later in this chapter).

✔ If you are obese (especially abdominal obesity, described in this chapter).

✔ If you have impaired glucose tolerance or impaired fasting glucose.

✔ If you have a sedentary lifestyle.

✔ If you take drugs that predispose you to diabetes.

✔ If you have had gestational diabetes during pregnancy.

✔ If you had a low birth weight.

✔ If you are a smoker.

✔ If you have one of the hormone-related conditions that can lead to diabetes.

These relatively low chances of both siblings – even for identical twins – getting diabetes clearly show that more factors than your genetic inheritance from your parents are involved in acquiring type 1 diabetes. Otherwise, identical twins would both have type 1 diabetes almost 100 per cent of the time.

Preventing type 1 diabetes

In order to prevent diabetes, you have to undergo treatment before the disease starts, a method called *primary prevention*. Preventive treatment given to a person with diabetes after the disease is triggered but before it causes complications is called *secondary prevention*. In order to try secondary prevention, the doctor must be able to recognise that diabetes has begun, even though the patient is not yet unwell. And months to years must pass between diagnosis and onset of symptoms in order to have enough time for the treatment to prevent sickness.

In the realms of science fiction, diabetes would be a perfect candidate for both primary and secondary prevention. The way it develops makes it possible to pick up people at high risk, and in the future we may be able to provide them with primary prevention, as explained in the section 'Primary prevention measures'. In real life, secondary prevention, which you can read about in the section 'Secondary prevention measures', is well on the way.

Primary prevention measures

Doctors can analyse the genetic material (DNA) of someone who has a family history of diabetes to see whether that person has the genetic material most often found in people who have diabetes. Theoretically, a person diagnosed as having the potential for diabetes at that time can receive primary prevention to block the disease.

The Juvenile Diabetes Research Foundation is the world's largest funder in the voluntary sector for research into prevention of type 1 diabetes. In 2005, it set up a trial at the University of Bristol and King's College, London, looking into the possibility of a vaccine for the prevention of type 1 diabetes. It hopes to prove that the vaccine will work in humans by generating cells to protect the islet cells of the pancreas against the autoimmune response (where the body's immune system attacks itself) that causes type 1 diabetes. Of course, results are still some years off, but they could potentially lead to a vaccine for people at high risk of developing type 1 diabetes.

The Juvenile Diabetes Research Foundation also has regional groups that organise local meetings and fundraising events. You can find out more about its work by visiting its website at www.jdrf.org.uk, or you can contact the organisation at Juvenile Diabetes Research Foundation, 19 Angel Gate, City Road, London EC1V 2PT; Tel: 0207-713-2030.

Gene therapy?

You may think that all the recent scientific advances in gene research would allow doctors to change people's genetic material to prevent the onset of type 1 diabetes. Although scientists have made great strides in identifying the genes associated with diabetes, they haven't quite reached the point where they can change those genes. Such methods for primary prevention of type 1 diabetes are something for the future.

Secondary prevention measures

Lots of trials of secondary prevention are under way, though most show only partial success. Most of these trials make use of doctors' knowledge that patients whose bodies produce autoantibodies have type 1 diabetes and that the antibodies are gradually destroying their insulin-producing beta cells. In these patients, full-blown type 1 diabetes may take a couple of years to appear and create major problems, so the doctor has time to intervene. The most prevalent methods of secondary prevention for type 1 diabetes attempt to block the autoimmune disease from destroying all of your pancreas's beta cells. The following list shows some of the more promising secondary prevention trials and techniques:

- **Steroid drugs:** You can take steroid drugs such as prednisone to block autoimmune conditions. When doctors find islet cell antibodies in a person with type 1 diabetes, they give the person these steroids, which reduce the amount of islet cell antibodies and seem to prolong the period between the development of the antibodies and the onset of symptoms such as excessive thirst and urination. But this approach isn't 100 per cent successful, and steroids have many side effects – especially in small children, who are the usual victims of type 1 diabetes. Small children who use steroids suffer from growth problems, infections, and other unwanted side effects. If diabetes becomes active, the reason may be the failure of the steroid to prevent the autoimmune destruction of the pancreas as well as the glucose abnormalities caused by the steroid itself.

- **Cytotoxic drugs:** Another group of drugs used to increase the time between antibodies and disease consists of the so-called *cytotoxic drugs,* which act against the cells that may participate in the destruction of the pancreatic beta cells. Again, studies have shown only a slowing down of the time between antibodies and symptoms. Cytotoxic drugs destroy various types of cells – and not just the bad cells. Studies of cytotoxic drugs have all been complicated by side effects that were severe and damaging to some of the patients.

- **Nicotinamide:** In animal studies, nicotinamide (a B vitamin) protects the beta cells of mice that are diabetes prone. A similar trial in humans was somewhat successful, showing that 20 per cent of patients using nicotinamide didn't develop symptoms of diabetes and didn't lose as many beta cells. Doctors are surprised that a drug known to raise plasma glucose (see Chapter 2) may prevent diabetes.

- **Insulin:** In another study, small amounts of insulin were given to people who have islet cell antibodies, in an attempt to prolong the time between antibodies and symptoms. This has shown some promise, but the findings aren't yet definite.

The most important study of prevention ever done for type 1 diabetes was published in 1993 – the Diabetes Control and Complications Trial (DCCT). It shows that keeping very tight control over your blood glucose is possible but difficult. The difficult part of keeping your blood glucose close to normal is that you increase your risk of having low blood glucose, or hypoglycaemia (see Chapter 4). The study shows that you can significantly reduce the complications of diabetes – including eye disease, kidney disease, and nerve disease – by keeping your blood glucose as normal as possible. If you have already suffered from such complications, improving your blood glucose control very significantly slows the progression of the complications. Since this report, doctors generally treat type 1 diabetes by keeping the patient's blood glucose as close to normal as possible and practical.

Type 2 Diabetes and You

Type 2 diabetes has different symptoms and causes to type 1 diabetes. Despite sharing a common name, the different forms of diabetes have their own causes and effects. They do have several things in common, though. They both affect your body's blood sugar levels. They can both cause severe long-term complications if you don't treat them effectively. And you need to take both of them very seriously indeed.

Mary Darlington, a 46-year-old woman, has gained about a stone in the last two years, so that her 5-foot 5-inch body now weighs about 11 stone. Mary doesn't do much exercise. She has noticed that she feels more tired recently, but she blames her age and approaching menopause for this. One reason that Mary is more tired is that she gets up several times a night to urinate, which is unusual for her. She is especially disturbed because her vision is blurry, and she does a lot of work on a computer. Finally, Mary went to her general practitioner because she developed a rash and discharge in her vagina. When Mary described her symptoms, her doctor decided to do a blood glucose test. When her results came back, it turned out that her random blood glucose was 12.2 mmol/l.

Mary's general practitioner asked her whether other members of her family have had diabetes. She replied that her mother and a sister are both being treated for it. The doctor asked her to come back the next morning for a fasting blood glucose test. When this gave a result of 11.5 mmol/l the GP explained to Mary that she had type 2 diabetes.

The signs and symptoms that Mary has in this scenario, along with the results of the two blood glucose tests, provide a textbook picture of type 2 diabetes. But you should also remember that people with type 2 diabetes may have few or none of these symptoms. That explains the importance of getting your glucose checked regularly if you are at high risk of diabetes (see 'Knowing your family's risks' earlier in this chapter) or if you get any of the symptoms of diabetes listed in the following sections.

 These days, most doctors' surgeries also run 'well man' and 'well woman' checks, where you can get your general health checked out. When you register with a new general practitioner, you're invited to have a new patient registration check, where the same kind of checks are offered. You may find it worth taking a sample of your urine with you, so that the nurse can check it for sugar. Testing your urine isn't a foolproof way of excluding diabetes, but it often picks up type 2 diabetes long before you develop any symptoms.

Type 2 diabetes is a disease of gradual onset rather than the severe emergency that can herald type 1 diabetes. Because the symptoms are so mild at first, you may not notice them. You may ignore these symptoms for years before they become bothersome enough to consult your doctor. No autoimmunity is involved in type 2 diabetes, so no antibodies are found. Doctors believe that no virus is involved in the onset of type 2 diabetes – making it a very different kind of diabetes to type 1.

Recent statistics show ten to twenty times more people with type 2 diabetes than type 1 throughout the world. Type 2 diabetes used to be considered a 'mild' form of diabetes that didn't need to be treated as vigorously as type 1. Gradually, though, doctors have cottoned on to the fact that a disease complication is a disease complication, regardless of the cause. In fact, serious complications like heart and kidney disease are just as likely to occur in type 1 and type 2 diabetes patients.

The changing face of type 2 diabetes

Type 2 diabetes used to be known as adult onset diabetes, or non-insulin dependent diabetes, because it was rarely seen under the age of about 40. Sadly, as the incidence of obesity increases in the United Kingdom and more and more of the population are inactive, this type of diabetes is being seen earlier and earlier in life. A few years ago, most children and teenagers were out on their bikes or playing football in the school playground whenever they could escape the classroom. Now, you're more likely to find them crouched over a hot computer or video game. The combination of rising property prices and anxieties about child abduction has meant that parents no longer feel safe to let their children play in public places and are less likely to have big gardens for them to run free. Add this to the addictive properties of computer games and the rapid rise in digital television, with its all-day children's programmes, and you have a recipe for couch potato-dom.

Sadly, this has contributed not only to a rise in childhood obesity, but has also meant that type 2 diabetes is being seen in young adults and even in older children. As you get older, type 2 diabetes gets even more common.

In the United Kingdom, you're much more likely to have your type 2 diabetes looked after at your general practice than you are at the hospital. That doesn't mean your condition isn't taken as seriously as it would be if you had type 1 diabetes. Studies like the United Kingdom Prospective Diabetes Study have made it clear that keeping really tight control of your glucose, blood pressure, and cholesterol can reduce your risks of complications to a fraction of what they would be. You can find out more about different models of diabetic care in Chapter 7.

You may hear people talk about type 2 diabetes as a 'mild' form of diabetes. Don't listen to them. You're just as likely as a type 1 diabetic to develop kidney disease, and you may be even more likely to get heart disease. The good news, though, is that while the risks of type 2 diabetes are bigger than doctors thought, the benefits of tight control of glucose, blood pressure, and cholesterol are much greater than previously realised, too.

Identifying the symptoms of type 2 diabetes

We're pretty convinced that at least 3 million Britons have diabetes, but only 1.8 million of them know it yet. The rest make up the 'lost million' Britons who haven't yet been diagnosed.

The following signs and symptoms are good indicators that you have type 2 diabetes. If you experience many of these symptoms, check with your doctor:

- ✔ **Fatigue:** Type 2 diabetes makes you tired because your body's cells aren't getting the glucose fuel that they need. Even though there is plenty of insulin, your body is resistant to its actions. See the 'Getting to Know Your Pancreas' section for more explanation.

- ✔ **Frequent urination and thirst:** You find yourself urinating more frequently than usual, which dehydrates your body and leaves you thirsty.

- ✔ **Blurred vision:** The lenses of your eyes swell and shrink as your blood glucose levels rise and fall. Your vision blurs because your eye can't adjust quickly enough to these changes in the lens.

- ✔ **Slow healing of skin, gum, and urinary infections:** Your white blood cells, which help with healing and defend your body against infections, don't function correctly in the high-glucose environment present in your body when it has diabetes. Unfortunately, the bugs that cause infections thrive in the same high-glucose environment. So diabetes leaves your body especially susceptible to infections.

- ✔ **Genital itching:** Yeast infections, often called thrush, also love a high-glucose environment. So diabetes is often accompanied by the itching, creamy white vaginal discharge, and discomfort of yeast infections.

- ✔ **Numbness in the feet or legs:** You experience numbness because of a common long-term complication of diabetes, called neuropathy (the details of neuropathy are explained in Chapter 5). If you notice numbness and neuropathy along with the other symptoms of diabetes, you probably have had the disease for quite a while, because neuropathy takes more than five years to develop in a diabetic environment.

- ✔ **Heart disease:** Heart disease occurs much more often in people with type 2 diabetes than in people who don't have diabetes. But the heart disease may appear when you are merely glucose intolerant (which we explain in the next section), before you actually have diagnosable diabetes.

- ✔ **Obesity:** If you're obese, you are considerably more likely to acquire diabetes than you would be if you maintained your ideal weight. We tell you more about definitions of obesity later in this chapter.

The signs and symptoms of type 2 diabetes are similar in some cases (such as high blood glucose) to the symptoms of type 1 diabetes (which we cover in the 'Identifying the symptoms of type 1 diabetes' section, earlier in this chapter), but in many ways they are different. The following list shows some of the differences between symptoms in type 1 and type 2 diabetes:

- ✔ **Age of onset:** Those with type 1 diabetes are usually younger than those with type 2 diabetes.

- ✔ **Body weight:** Those with type 1 diabetes are likely to be thin or normal in weight, but obesity is a common characteristic of those with type 2 diabetes.

- ✔ **Level of glucose:** Those with type 1 diabetes have higher glucose levels at onset of the disease. Those with type 1 diabetes usually have blood glucose levels above 16.6 mmol/l, and those with type 2 diabetes usually have blood glucose levels of 11–14 mmol/l.

- ✔ **Severity of onset:** Type 1 diabetes usually has a much more sudden and dramatic onset, but type 2 diabetes gradually shows its symptoms.

Investigating the causes of type 2 diabetes

Although type 2 diabetes doesn't necessarily appear in your body until later in your life (as opposed to the early onset of type 1 diabetes), you're probably nonetheless shocked and curious about why you developed the disease.

Doctors have learned quite a bit about the causes of type 2 diabetes. For example, they know that type 2 diabetes runs in families. Usually, people with type 2 diabetes can find a relative who has had the disease. Therefore, doctors consider type 2 diabetes to be much more of a genetic disease than type 1 diabetes. In studies of identical twins, when one twin has type 2 diabetes, the likelihood that type 2 diabetes will develop in the other twin is nearly 100 per cent.

People with type 2 diabetes have some insulin in their bodies (unlike people with type 1 diabetes, who have none of their own insulin in their bodies), but their bodies respond to the insulin in abnormal ways. Those with type 2 diabetes are insulin resistant, meaning that their bodies resist the normal, healthy functioning of insulin. This insulin resistance, combined with not enough insulin to overcome the insulin resistance, causes type 2 diabetes, just like the absent insulin causes type 1 diabetes.

Before obesity or lack of exercise (or diabetes for that matter) is present, future type 2 patients already show signs of insulin resistance. First of all, the amount of insulin in the blood of these people is raised compared to normal people. Secondly, an injection of insulin doesn't reduce the blood glucose in these insulin-resistant people nearly as much as it does in people without insulin resistance. See Chapter 10 to find out more about insulin injections in diabetes.

Barking up the wrong diabetes tree

People often think that the following factors cause type 2 diabetes, but they actually have nothing to do with the onset of the disease:

- ✔ **Sugar:** Eating excessive amounts of sugar does not cause diabetes, but it may bring out the disease to the extent that it makes you fat. Eating too much protein or fat will do the same thing.

- ✔ **Emotions:** Changes in your emotions do not play a large role in the development of type 2 diabetes, but may be very important in dealing with your disease and your subsequent diabetic control.

- ✔ **Stress:** High stress levels don't cause diabetes.

- ✔ **Antibodies:** Antibodies against islet cells are not a major factor in type 2 diabetes. Type 2 diabetes isn't an autoimmune disease like type 1.

- ✔ **Gender:** Males and females are equally as likely to develop type 2 diabetes. Gender doesn't play a role in the onset of this disease.

When your body needs to make extra insulin just to keep your blood glucose normal, your insulin is, obviously, less effective than it should be – which means that you have *impaired glucose tolerance.* Your body goes through impaired glucose tolerance before you actually have diabetes, because your blood glucose is still lower than the levels needed (see Chapter 2) for a diagnosis of diabetes. When you have impaired glucose tolerance and you add other factors such as weight gain, a sedentary lifestyle, and ageing, your pancreas can't keep up with your insulin demands and you become diabetic.

Another factor that comes into play when doctors make a diagnosis of type 2 diabetes is the release of sugar from your liver, known as your *hepatic glucose output.* Why is your glucose high in the morning after you've fasted all night? You would think that your glucose would be low because you didn't eat any sugar to increase your body's glucose. In fact, your liver is a storage bank for a lot of glucose, and it can make even more from other substances in the body. As your insulin resistance increases, your liver begins to release glucose inappropriately and your fasting blood glucose rises.

Getting type 2 diabetes: Your chances

Genetic inheritance causes type 2 diabetes, but other factors, such as obesity and lack of exercise, trigger the disease. In contrast with type 1 diabetes, over 75 per cent of people with type 2 diabetes are overweight when they are diagnosed. People with type 2 diabetes are insulin resistant before they become obese or sedentary. Later, ageing, poor eating habits, obesity, and failure to exercise combine to bring out the disease.

Spouses of people with type 2 diabetes are at higher risk of developing diabetes and should be screened just like relatives of diabetics, because they share the environmental risk factors for diabetes such as diet and a sedentary lifestyle.

Inheritance seems to be a much stronger factor in type 2 diabetes than in type 1 diabetes:

- ✔ If your identical twin has type 2 diabetes, you have a 90 per cent chance of developing the same condition at some point in your life.

- ✔ If one of your parents has type 2 diabetes, you have a 40 per cent chance of developing type 2 diabetes at some time.

- ✔ If both of your parents have type 2 diabetes, your lifetime risk goes up above 50 per cent.

The metabolic syndrome – 1 in 4 and rising fast

Only a decade ago, even many doctors in the United Kingdom hadn't heard of the metabolic syndrome; now experts reckon that 1 in 4 adults in Britain suffers from it, and that the incidence of metabolic syndrome, like diabetes, is rising fast. Why is this such a concern? And what does it have to do with diabetes?

Metabolic syndrome is a combination of inter-related risk factors. Each of these risk factors on its own increases your likelihood of having a heart attack or stroke. But if you have several of these risk factors, your risk of heart attack or stroke rises dramatically. And metabolic syndrome also increases your risk of developing diabetes.

To have a diagnosis of metabolic syndrome, you have to have at least three of the risk factors shown here (according to the International Diabetes Federation, 2005):

✔ Abdominal obesity (waist >90 centimetres in males, >84 centimetres in females) if European, less if Asian

✔ Together with at least two of:

- Raised triglycerides ≥ 1.7 mmol/l

- Low HDL-cholesterol, < 1.04 mmol/l in males and < 1.29 mmol/l in females

- Blood pressure ≥ 130/85 mmHg

- Fasting hyperglycaemia (fasting glucose ≥ 5.6 mmol/l) or previous diagnosis of diabetes or impaired glucose tolerance

The only risk factor you have to have to receive a diagnosis is abdominal obesity, or a high waist circumference.

Some people are diagnosed with metabolic syndrome before they have diabetes. If you're one of them, now is the perfect time to take action and reduce your long-term risks. Reducing your weight, improving your diet, and getting more active can cut your risks of a heart attack and diabetes dramatically. You can find out more in the section 'Preventing type 2 diabetes'.

The thrifty gene theory

We've heard a lot about how your genetic make-up, or your genes, can affect your chances of getting type 2 diabetes. The thrifty gene theory sounds like a great treatment for shopaholics, but it isn't. This theory suggests that some people have a gene that lets them store up energy when food is plentiful, so increasing their chances of survival during times of famine. Obviously, people who had this gene would be more likely to survive long enough to have children if they lived in a time and a part of the world where food is often scarce. Over time, then, more and more of the surviving population would have inherited this thrifty gene.

The problem with having a thrifty gene is that once food supplies become more abundant, you're more likely to get fat. An ample supply of food often goes hand in hand with less physical exercise. The combination of reduced exercise and increasing obesity makes you more prone to diabetes. The side-bar about 'Tracking diabetes around the world' in Chapter 2 gives some examples of this.

The foetal origins theory

The foetal origins theory is a bit like the thrifty gene theory. A pair of scientists called Barker and Hales, from Southampton and Cambridge, came up with the theory, which suggests that, if you're malnourished in the womb, your body gets 'reprogrammed' for life to economise on energy. This idea is supported by the link between low birth weight and getting type 2 diabetes in middle age, especially if you put on a lot of weight later. Interestingly, other risk factors for your heart, like high blood pressure, have also been linked to low birth weight.

Preventing type 2 diabetes

Doctors can predict type 2 diabetes years in advance of its actual diagnosis by studying the close relatives of people who already have the condition. This early warning period offers plenty of time to try techniques of primary prevention (which we explain in the 'Preventing type 1 diabetes' section, earlier in this chapter). After doctors find high blood glucose in a person and diagnose type 2 diabetes, complications such as eye disease and kidney disease (see Chapter 5) can take ten or more years to develop in that person. During this time, doctors can apply secondary prevention techniques (you can read more about the various treatments in Part III).

Because so many people suffer from type 2 diabetes, doctors have had a wealth of people to study in order to work out the most important environmental (basically diet and lifestyle) factors that turn a genetic predisposition to type 2 diabetes into a clinical disease. The following are the major environmental factors. If you recognise any of these factors in your body or lifestyle, you can correct them. Type 2 diabetes allows the high-risk individual or the diagnosed person the time to work towards prevention or control of the disease. In Part III, you can find out specific ways to reduce your weight, increase your exercise, improve your diet, and prevent or reverse diabetes and diabetic complications.

High body mass index

The *body mass index (BMI)* is the way that doctors look at weight in relation to height. BMI is a better indicator of a healthy weight than just weight alone, because a person who weighs 11 stone and is 5 foot 2 inches tall is overweight, but a person who weighs 11 stone and is 5 foot 10 inches tall is thin. You can work out your BMI by using the table in Chapter 7.

Muscle is actually much heavier than fat, so if you're a weight trainer or an athlete, you can have a raised BMI without being fat. In fact, the reason doctors use BMI is because it is helpful for identifying people with abdominal obesity (see the section 'Abdominal obesity: The apple and pear debate' for more on this), which is a much more accurate predictor of risk than BMI.

The new definition of BMI states that a person with a BMI from 25 to 29.9 is overweight, and a person with a BMI of 30 or greater is obese. A BMI between 20 and 25 is considered normal weight.

To make matters more complicated still, your ideal weight depends not just on your height, but also on your age and ethnic background. That's because obesity-related complications are much more common, and start at a lower BMI, in some ethnic groups. The World Health Organisation defines obesity in Indo-Asians, for instance, at BMI over 27. If you're under 16, you are considered to be obese if your BMI is over 25.

In Chapter 7, you find a chart where we do the hard work for you. Just find out your weight in pounds and your height in feet and inches, plug the figures in to the chart, and voilà! Instant BMI.

Many studies have confirmed the great importance of the level of the BMI in determining who gets diabetes. A large study of thousands of nurses in the United States showed that the nurses with a BMI of greater than 35 had diabetes almost 100 times more often than nurses with a BMI of less than 22. Even among the women in this study considered to be lean, those with the higher BMI, though still in the category of lean, had three times the prevalence of diabetes compared to leaner nurses. Also, a large study of doctors in the United States found the same relationship of high BMI to high levels of type 2 diabetes. The same study also showed that the length of time that you're obese is important, because men who were obese ten years earlier more often had diabetes than men who weren't obese at that time.

Under the latest version of the General Medical Services Contract to which general practitioners work, all general practitioners have to keep an obesity register, which lists everyone in the practice with a BMI over 30. As we can see, this should be useful for identifying people at higher risk of diabetes and heart disease. However, the contract doesn't tell general practitioners what to do with people on this register. So if anyone you know is carrying a little too much weight, do tell them to get their BMI checked out when they next see their doctor or practice nurse. If their BMI is over 30 (or they have abdominal obesity, see the section 'Abdominal obesity: The apple and pear debate') they should talk to the nurse or general practitioner about getting a cholesterol and glucose test done.

Physical inactivity

Physical inactivity is closely linked with diabetes, as evidenced in many studies. Former athletes have diabetes less often than non-athletes. The same study of the health of nurses that we cite above showed that women who were physically active on a regular basis had diabetes only two-thirds as often as the couch potatoes. In a study in Hawaii, the occurrence of diabetes was greatest for the non-exercisers, and none of the people in the study was obese, so that was not a factor.

Prevention research: Possibilities for future prevention of diabetes

Researchers have performed many valuable studies on the prevention of type 2 diabetes. The results of these studies suggest that you can prevent diabetes, but probably only by making major lifestyle changes and sticking to them over a long period of time. Here are some important conclusions based on prevention research:

✔ If you take drugs that don't treat your insulin resistance, they don't help to prevent your diabetes or its complications.

✔ If you exercise regularly, you can delay the onset of diabetes.

✔ If you maintain a proper diet and exercise regularly, you can delay the onset of diabetes and slow the complications that may occur.

✔ Controlling your blood pressure and your blood glucose has substantial benefits for preventing the complications of diabetes.

A study reported in 1991 confirmed the above conclusions by looking at obese people who had close relatives with type 2 diabetes – which meant that these people were highly likely to develop diabetes. For six months, the researchers gave the participants extensive training in exercise routines and maintaining proper diet. Many of the participants lost significant amounts of weight, improved their overall health, and staved off the development of diabetes. But after six months, many of the people being studied were no longer participating as fully and sticking as closely to the diet and exercise regimens, and by 12 months, many had started to regain some of their lost weight. The people who were able to maintain the proper diet and exercise – which helped them not to gain weight – were least likely to develop diabetes. The main point that this study proves is the importance (and, for many people, the difficulty) of maintaining a programme of diet and exercise for a long period of time.

The results of the Diabetes Prevention Program were published in the *New England Journal of Medicine* in February 2002. They clearly showed that diet and exercise are effective in preventing type 2 diabetes. When this did not work alone, a drug called metformin was successful. More than 3,000 people took part in this study. People who were in the diet and exercise group reduced their chance of developing diabetes by 58 per cent, while the metformin group was successful 31 per cent of the time.

The Finnish Diabetes Prevention Study (*Diabetes Care*, December 2003) shows that lifestyle changes can be accomplished and sustained not only in a research setting like that of the Diabetes Prevention Program above, but in a community setting as well. They continue to be successful after three years, with the same 58 per cent reduction in onset of diabetes.

Another study looked at the question of restoration of insulin sensitivity in people at risk for prediabetes (see Chapter 2). It compared intensive lifestyle change, both diet and exercise, with moderate lifestyle change. The intensive group ate less fat and did more vigorous exercise. Only the intensive group increased their insulin sensitivity, thus holding off the development of diabetes. The study was published in *Diabetes Care* in March 2002. We all may have to cut our fat and increase our level of exercise to protect ourselves from diabetes.

Abdominal obesity: The apple and pear debate

When people with diabetes become overweight, they tend to distribute the extra weight inside the tummy, also known as *visceral fat*. Having a high level of visceral fat is known as abdominal obesity. You check for abdominal obesity when you measure your waistline, because this type of fat stays around your midsection. We're not talking about the fat just under your skin – so-called subcutaneous fat – the kind you measure when you 'pinch an inch'. The fat is actually inside your stomach wall. So a person with abdominal obesity is more apple shaped than pear shaped.

Visceral fat also happens to be the type of fat that probably comes and goes most easily on your body, and it is relatively easy to lose when you diet. Visceral fat seems to cause more insulin resistance than fat in other areas, and it is also correlated with the occurrence of coronary artery disease. If you have a lot of visceral fat, losing just 10 per cent of your weight can cut your visceral fat by as much as 30 per cent, and may very dramatically reduce your chance of diabetes or a heart attack.

Low intake of dietary fibre

Populations with a high prevalence of diabetes tend to eat a diet that is low in fibre. Dietary fibre seems to be protective against diabetes, because it slows down the rate at which glucose enters the bloodstream.

Gestational Diabetes and You

If you're pregnant (yes, that excludes you men) and you've never had diabetes before, during the course of your pregnancy you could acquire a form of diabetes called *gestational diabetes*. If you already have diabetes when you become pregnant, that is called *pre-gestational diabetes*. As Chapter 6 shows you, the difference between pre-gestational diabetes and gestational diabetes is very important in terms of the consequences for both mother and baby. Gestational diabetes occurs in about 2 per cent of all pregnancies.

During your pregnancy, you can acquire gestational diabetes because the growing foetus and the placenta create various hormones to help the foetus grow and develop properly. Some of these hormones have other characteristics, such as anti-insulin properties, that decrease your body's sensitivity to insulin, increase glucose production, and therefore cause diabetes.

At approximately your 20th week of pregnancy, your body produces enough of these hormones to block your insulin's normal actions and cause diabetes. After you give birth, the foetus and placenta are no longer in your body, so their anti-insulin hormones are gone and your diabetes disappears.

Be aware that, even though your diabetes subsides after you give birth, type 2 diabetes develops within 15 years after the pregnancy in more than half of the women who had gestational diabetes. This high likelihood of type 2 diabetes probably results from a genetic susceptibility to diabetes in these women that is magnified by the large amount of anti-insulin hormones in their bodies during pregnancy.

Every time you go for an antenatal check, your midwife or doctor probably wants to check your urine for, among other things, sugar. It may be really tough to wee into that tiny pot when your tummy is so big that you can't see where you're aiming, but the result is well worth the effort! The 'renal threshold' at which glucose passes from your bloodstream into your urine is often lower when you're pregnant. That means that you can have sugar in your urine even if you aren't diabetic. But if you do have sugar in your urine, your midwife or doctor will test your blood for sugar, too. You may also have a blood test done for gestational diabetes around the 24th to the 28th week of your pregnancy.

Could You Have Another Type of Diabetes?

Cases of diabetes other than type 1, type 2, or gestational are rare and usually don't cause severe diabetes in the people who have them. But occasionally one of these other types of diabetes is responsible for a more severe case of diabetes, so you should be aware that they exist. The following list gives you a brief rundown of the symptoms and causes of other types of diabetes:

- ✔ **Diabetes due to loss or disease of pancreatic tissue:** If you have a disease such as cancer that requires you to have some of your pancreas removed, you lose your pancreas's valuable insulin-producing beta cells, and your body becomes diabetic.

- ✔ **Diabetes due to other diseases:** Your body has a number of hormones that block insulin action or have actions that are opposed to insulin's actions. You produce these hormones in glands other than your pancreas. If you get a tumour on one of these hormone-producing glands, the gland sometimes produces excessive levels of the hormones that act in opposition to insulin. This can give you either simple glucose intolerance or diabetes.

- ✔ **Diabetes due to hormone treatments for other diseases:** If you're receiving hormones to treat a disease other than diabetes, those hormones can cause diabetes in your body. The hormone that is most likely to cause diabetes in this situation is *prednisolone* (similar drugs are hydrocortisone and dexamethasone), a steroid anti-inflammatory agent used in diseases of inflammation (such as arthritis, severe asthma, or inflammatory bowel disease). If you're taking prednisolone and you have the symptoms of diabetes listed in earlier sections of this chapter, talk to your doctor.

✔ **Diabetes due to other drugs:** If you're taking other commonly used drugs, be aware that some of them raise your blood glucose as a side effect. Some antihypertensive drugs, especially beta blockers and thiazide water tablets (the most commonly prescribed one in the United Kingdom is called bendrofluazide), raise your blood glucose level. Taking both a beta blocker and a thiazide increases your risk still further, and guidelines released in April 2006 recommend that you should avoid this combination. If you have a genetic tendency towards diabetes, taking these drugs may be enough to give you the disease. If you're taking a beta blocker and a thiazide together, talk to your doctor about the possibility of changing to a more suitable alternative.

Part II
How Diabetes Affects Your Body

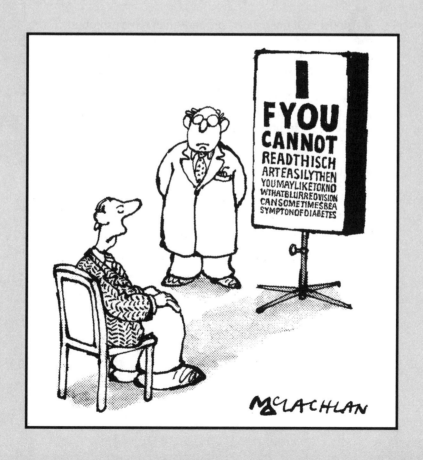

In this part . . .

Diabetes, if not treated properly, can have profound effects on your body. This part explains these effects, how they occur, the kind of symptoms they produce, and what you and your doctor need to do to treat them. You may be surprised at how many parts of your body can be affected by diabetes. Remember that everything we describe in this part is preventable, and even if you have not been able to prevent a particular problem, you can treat it.

With the pace of discovery in diabetes, most of the effects of the disease will be fit for exhibition in an ancient history museum in the not-too-distant future. Meanwhile, it is important that you know about the effects of diabetes and respond to them appropriately.

Chapter 4

Battling Short-Term Complications

• •

In This Chapter

▶ Understanding short-term complications

▶ Dealing with low blood glucose levels

▶ Handling very high blood glucose levels

▶ Coping with the highest blood glucose levels

• •

Chapters 2 and 3 tell you about how doctors make a diagnosis of diabetes and how they determine which type of diabetes you have. Those chapters cover some of the signs and symptoms of diabetes. You could consider these to be the shortest of the short-term complications of the disease, because they're generally mild and begin to subside when you start treatment. This chapter covers the more serious forms of short-term complications of diabetes, which occur when your blood glucose is out of control – reaching dangerously high or low levels.

Although the complications that we cover in this chapter are called short term, you may get them at any time during the course of your diabetes. Short term simply means that these complications arise rapidly in your body, as opposed to the long-term complications that take ten or more years to develop (see Chapter 5 for all the details about long-term complications).

With the exception of *hypoglycaemia* (low blood glucose), you should treat all the complications in this chapter as medical emergencies. Don't try to treat these complications at home. Keep in touch with your doctor and go to the hospital promptly if your blood glucose is uncontrollably high or you're unable to hold down food. You may need a few hours in the Accident and Emergency department or a day or two in the hospital to reverse your problems.

Solving Short-Term Complications

Generally, you experience the severe short-term complications associated with high blood glucose when you aren't monitoring your blood glucose levels. Small children and older people who live alone or have illnesses are susceptible to lapses in glucose monitoring and, therefore, to short-term complications. If you suffer an acute illness or trauma, you should monitor your glucose even more frequently than usual because you're more vulnerable to short-term complications.

The short-term complications of diabetes affect your ability to function normally. So you may have trouble driving your car properly. If you're a student, you may have difficulty studying or taking tests. Potential employers may question your ability to perform certain jobs. But most companies and government agencies are very enlightened about diabetes and do everything possible to accommodate you in these situations. (Chapter 15 shows you how to overcome some challenges that you may face with employment and with your driving licence.)

You don't have to feel limited in what you can do. You can have control over your diabetes, and all of the short-term complications are avoidable. If you take your medication at the appropriate time, eat the proper foods at the proper times, and monitor your blood glucose regularly, you're much less likely to suffer from any severe forms of the short-term complications. As you monitor and control your blood glucose closely, it may drop to lower than normal levels, but monitoring quickly alerts you to the drop, and you can treat yourself before the drop affects your mental and physical functioning. (See Chapter 7 for all the details on glucose monitoring and other testing.)

Short-term complications develop in days or even hours; fortunately, they respond to treatment just as rapidly.

Understanding Hypoglycaemia

The condition of low blood glucose is known as *hypoglycaemia*. If you have diabetes, you can get hypoglycaemia only as a consequence of your diabetes treatment. As a person with diabetes, you're in constant combat with *high* blood glucose, which is responsible for most of the long-term and short-term complications of the disease. Your doctor prescribes drugs and other treatments in an effort to fine-tune your blood glucose. (Part III explains many techniques that help you control your blood glucose levels.) But unfortunately, these drugs and treatments aren't always perfect. If you take too much of a drug, exercise too much, or eat too little, your blood glucose can drop to the low levels at which symptoms develop. The following sections explain more about hypoglycaemia's symptoms, causes, and treatment.

Symptoms of hypoglycaemia

Your body doesn't function well when you have too little glucose in your blood. Your brain needs glucose to run the rest of your body, as well as for intellectual purposes. Your muscles need the energy that glucose provides in much the same way that your car needs petrol. So when your body detects that it has low blood glucose, it sends out a group of hormones that rapidly raise your glucose. But those hormones have to fight the strength of the diabetes medication that has been pushing down your glucose levels.

At what level of blood glucose do you develop hypoglycaemia? Unfortunately, the level varies for different individuals, particularly depending on the length of time that the person has had diabetes. But most experts agree that a blood glucose of 3.3 mmol/l or less is associated with signs and symptoms of hypoglycaemia in most people.

Doctors traditionally put the symptoms of hypoglycaemia into two main categories:

✔ **Symptoms due to your brain not receiving enough fuel, so your intellectual function suffers.** This first category of symptoms is called *neuroglycopenic* symptoms, which is medical speak for 'not enough (*penic*) glucose (*glyco*) in the brain (*neuro*)'. Neuroglycopenic symptoms occur most often when your hypoglycaemia takes longer to develop. The symptoms become more severe as your blood glucose drops lower. The following neuroglycopenic symptoms are often signs that you're becoming (or already are) hypoglycaemic:

- Headache

- Loss of concentration

- Visual disorders, such as double vision

- Fatigue

- Confusion

- Convulsions

- Coma, or an inability to be awakened

✔ **Symptoms due to the side effects of the hormones (especially adrenaline) that your body sends out to counter the glucose-lowering effect of insulin.** The second category of symptoms is called *adrenergic* symptoms, because adrenaline comes from your adrenal gland. Adrenergic symptoms occur most often when your blood glucose falls rapidly. The following adrenergic symptoms may tip you off that you're hypoglycaemic:

- Whiteness, or pallor, of your skin

- Sweating

- Rapid heartbeat

- Palpitations, or the feeling that your heart is beating too fast

- Anxiety

- Sensation of hunger

People lose their ability to think clearly when they become hypoglycaemic. They make simple mistakes, and other people often assume that they're drunk.

One of our patients was driving when another driver noticed that she was weaving back and forth in her lane and reported her to the traffic police. A police officer stopped her, concluded that she was drunk, and took her to the police station. Fortunately, someone noticed that she was wearing a diabetic medical bracelet. After promptly receiving the nutrition that she needed, she rapidly recovered. She faced no charges, but clearly you want to avoid this kind of situation. If you're planning to drive a car, read Chapter 15 to find out how to avoid the situation. If you take insulin or a *sulphonylurea drug,* which squeezes more insulin out of your reluctant pancreas, for your own safety you need to wear or carry with you some form of identification, in case you unexpectedly develop hypoglycaemia. (See Chapter 10 for a full explanation of the insulin and sulphonylurea medications.) It's also a good idea to carry a supply of sugar cubes, glucose tablets, or a sugary drink with you at all times.

Causes of hypoglycaemia

Hypoglycaemia results from elevated amounts of insulin driving down your blood glucose to low levels, but an extra high dose of insulin or sulphonylurea isn't always the culprit that raises your insulin level. The amount of food you take in, the amount of fuel (glucose) that you burn for energy, the amount of insulin circulating in your body, and your body's ability to raise glucose by releasing it from the liver or making it from other body substances all affect your blood glucose level.

Hypoglycaemia occurs about 10 per cent of the time in type 1 diabetes, but is only symptomatic twice a week and is severe perhaps once a year. In type 2 diabetes, severe hypoglycaemia occurs only one tenth as often.

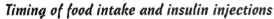
Timing of food intake and insulin injections

When you take insulin injections, you have to time your food intake correctly to raise your blood glucose as the insulin takes effect. Chapter 10 explains the different kinds of insulin and the proper methods for administering them. But remember that the different types of insulin are most potent at differing amounts of time (minutes or hours) after you inject them. If you skip a meal or take your insulin too early or too late, your glucose and insulin levels aren't in sync and you develop hypoglycaemia. If you go on a diet and don't adjust your medication, the same thing happens.

If you take sulphonylurea drugs, you need to follow similar restrictions. You and your doctor must adjust your dosage when your calorie intake falls. Other drugs don't cause hypoglycaemia by themselves, but when combined with sulphonylureas, they may lower your glucose enough to reach hypoglycaemic levels. Chapter 10 talks more about these other drugs.

Your diet plays a major role in helping you avoid hypoglycaemia if you take medication. You're better off having a snack in the middle of the morning and in the afternoon – in addition to your usual breakfast, lunch, and dinner – especially if you take insulin. A properly timed snack provides you with a steady source of glucose to balance the insulin that you're taking. Chapter 8 gives much greater detail about proper diet.

Exercise

Exercise generally lowers your blood glucose as well. Obviously, exercise burns more of your body's fuel, which is glucose. Some people with diabetes use exercise in place of extra insulin to get their high blood glucose down to a normal level. But if you don't adjust your insulin dose or food intake to match your exercise, exercise can result in hypoglycaemia. People who exercise regularly require much less medication and generally can manage their diabetes more easily than non-exercisers can. Chapter 9 covers much more about the benefits of exercise.

One of our patients is dedicated to exercise. He has taken insulin injections for years, but requires very little insulin to control his glucose because he burns so much glucose through exercise. He avoids hypoglycaemia by measuring his blood glucose level many times a day – especially before vigorous exercise. If his level is low at the beginning of exercise, he eats extra carbohydrates before he starts. Chapter 8 tells you which foods to eat (and when) in order to have the intended effect on your glucose levels.

As type 1 diabetes progresses, there is a decrease in the production of the hormones that counteract insulin when hypoglycaemia is present. This, plus the fact that the amount of injected insulin does not decrease in response to a lower blood glucose (as it would if no insulin injection had been given) leads to more severe hypoglycaemia later in type 1 diabetes. Those with type 2 diabetes who take insulin also develop this loss of protective hormones.

Lack of these hormones also leads to loss of the warning signs produced by these hormones, such as sweating, a rapid heartbeat, and anxiety, so you are not prompted to eat. This is called *hypoglycaemia unawareness*.

Alcohol

Several drugs that you may take that are unrelated to your diabetes can lower your blood glucose. One important and widely used drug, which you may not even think of as a drug, is alcohol (in the form of wine, beer, or spirits). Alcohol can block your liver's ability to release glucose. It also blocks hormones that raise blood glucose and increases the glucose-lowering effect of insulin. If you're malnourished for some reason or you simply haven't eaten in a while and you drink alcohol before going to bed, you may experience severe fasting hypoglycaemia the next morning.

If you take insulin or sulphonylurea drugs, don't drink alcohol without eating some food at the same time. Food counteracts some of the glucose-lowering effects of alcohol.

Aspirin

Be aware that aspirin (and all of the drugs related to aspirin, called *salicylates*) can lead you to hypoglycaemia. In adults who have diabetes, aspirin can increase the effects of other drugs that you're taking to lower your blood glucose. Children should never take aspirin anyway, because of rare but very serious complications. However, taking regular small doses of aspirin (usually about 75 milligrams a day) can significantly reduce your risk of having a heart attack or stroke, and carries only a very small risk for your blood sugar.

Prevention of hypoglycaemia

A number of techniques are used to prevent hypoglycaemia. Among them are:

 ✔ Frequent measurement of your blood glucose with your meter

 ✔ Maintaining a realistic goal for your blood glucose level

 ✔ Alteration in the timing of food and exercise

 ✔ Alteration of insulin and oral drug regimens

 ✔ Becoming totally aware of your own symptoms for low blood glucose

Treatment of hypoglycaemia

The vast majority of hypoglycaemia cases are mild. As soon as you (or a friend or relative) have noticed that you have the symptoms, you can treat the problem with a small quantity of glucose in the form of sugar cubes, two or three glucose tablets, a small amount of a sugary soft drink, or anything that has about 15 grams of glucose in it. (Glucose tablets are available in any pharmacy, and any person with diabetes who may develop hypoglycaemia should carry them.) Eight fluid ounces of milk or six fluid ounces of orange juice work very well. Sometimes you need a second treatment. Approximately 20 minutes after you try one of these solutions, measure your blood glucose to find out whether your level has risen enough.

Because your mental state may be mildly confused when you have hypoglycaemia, you need to make sure that your friends or relatives know in advance what hypoglycaemia is and what to do about it. Inform people about your diabetes and about how to recognise hypoglycaemia. Don't keep your diabetes a secret. The people close to you will be glad to know how to help you.

If you can't sit up and swallow properly when you have hypoglycaemia, people shouldn't try to feed you. Obviously you won't be able to swallow when you're unconscious, but you may not be able to swallow effectively if you're very drowsy, either. Anyone who is trying to treat your condition can:

✔ **Use an emergency kit, such as a glucagon injection set.** This kit includes a syringe with 1 milligram of glucagon, one of the main hormones that raises glucose, which your helper should inject into your muscle. The injection of glucagon raises your blood glucose so that you regain consciousness within 20 minutes.

You need to get a prescription from your doctor for this type of glucagon kit. Also make sure that the kit doesn't become out of date if you haven't used it for a long time. Glucagon corrects your hypoglycaemic condition for about an hour after you receive an injection.

✔ **Make an emergency call to 999 if there is no glucagon available, if your hypoglycaemia recurs shortly after you receive glucagon, or if your symptoms don't improve with glucagon.** (Sulphonylurea drugs most often cause such a severe case of hypoglycaemia.) The ambulance crew checks your blood glucose and gives you an intravenous (IV) dose of high-concentration glucose. Most likely, you will continue the IV in the Accident and Emergency department until you show stable and normal blood glucose levels.

Combating Ketoacidosis

Chapter 3 talks about the tendency of people with type 1 diabetes to suffer from a severe diabetic complication called *ketoacidosis,* which is very high blood glucose with large amounts of acid in the blood. The prefix *keto* refers to *ketones* – substances that your body makes as fat breaks down during ketoacidosis. *Acid* is part of the name because your blood becomes acidic from the presence of ketones.

Although ketoacidosis occurs mostly in people with type 1 diabetes (who develop diabetes at an early age), ketoacidosis usually begins only when you are 40 or more years old. Occasionally, ketoacidosis is the symptom that alerts doctors that you have type 1 diabetes, but more often than not, ketoacidosis occurs only after you already know that you have diabetes.

Ketoacidosis occurs mostly in people with type 1 diabetes because they have no insulin in their bodies except what they inject as medication. Those with type 2 diabetes (or with other forms of the disease) rarely get ketoacidosis because they have some insulin in their bodies, even though the insulin usually isn't fully active due to insulin resistance. People with type 2 diabetes get ketoacidosis mainly when they have severe infections or traumas that put their bodies under great physical stress.

The following sections explain the symptoms, causes, and treatments of ketoacidosis.

Symptoms of ketoacidosis

The symptoms of ketoacidosis regularly alert doctors to type 1 diabetes in children. But ketoacidosis more often occurs in adults with type 1 diabetes, so you should keep an eye out for the following symptoms:

- **Nausea and vomiting:** You experience these symptoms because of the build-up of acids and the loss of important body substances.

- **Rapid breathing:** (This is also known as *Kussmaul breathing,* after the man who first described it.) You experience rapid breathing when your blood is so acidic that your body attempts to blow off some of the acid through the lungs. Your breath has a fruity smell due to acetone.

- **Extreme tiredness and drowsiness:** You're tired because your brain is bathed in very thick blood, like syrup, and is missing the essential substances that get passed out in your urine when you suffer from ketoacidosis.

✔ **Weakness:** You become weak because your muscle tissue is unable to get its fuel, namely glucose.

In this age of self-monitoring for blood glucose levels, ketoacidosis is becoming more rare, but it still occurs. (See Chapter 7 for more on self-monitoring.) If you use a source of insulin that can be interrupted, you may unexpectedly develop ketoacidosis. For example, if you rely on an insulin pump, which pushes insulin under your skin automatically (as we describe in Chapter 10), the pump may stop for some reason; then, your insulin delivery will cease, your glucose level will rise, and ketoacidosis will develop if you don't notice the interruption soon enough.

You may notice that you have some symptoms of ketoacidosis and begin to suspect that you have this complication. But that diagnosis is best made by a doctor – preferably in the hospital, where you can begin treatment at once. Doctors make a diagnosis of ketoacidosis when they see the following abnormalities:

✔ High blood glucose, usually more than 16.6 mmol/l

✔ Acid condition of your blood

✔ Excessive levels of ketones in your blood and urine

✔ Dry skin and tongue, indicating dehydration

✔ Deficiency of potassium in your body

✔ An acetone smell on your breath

When your doctor finds these abnormalities, he will want to begin treatment immediately.

Causes of ketoacidosis

The most common causes of ketoacidosis are interruption of your insulin treatment or any kind of infection. Your body can't go for many hours without insulin activity before it begins to burn fat for energy and begins to make extra glucose that it can't use. The process of burning fat creates ketones in your blood, which are responsible for your ketoacidosis.

If you go on a strict diet to lose weight, your body burns some of its fat stores and produces ketones, in much the same way as it burns fat when you lack insulin. But in this case, your glucose remains low and (unless you have type 1 diabetes) you have sufficient insulin to prevent excessive production of new glucose or release of large amounts of glucose from your liver. So a strict diet doesn't generally lead to ketoacidosis.

Treatment of ketoacidosis

Ketoacidosis is a serious condition that requires professional treatment. But even though you leave the treatment to a professional rather than trying to manage it yourself, you should know the treatment processes so that you understand what's happening to you or to your loved one.

The basis of ketoacidosis treatment is to restore the proper amount of water to your body, reduce the acid condition of your blood by getting rid of the ketones, restore substances such as potassium that you've lost, and return your blood glucose to its normal level of around 4.4 to 6.5 mmol/l. All of these improvements should happen simultaneously after you begin treatment.

Your doctor sets up a flowchart to keep track of your levels of glucose, acid, potassium, and ketones, along with other parameters. Although you've lost a lot of potassium, for example, the initial blood reading of potassium on your flowchart may look normal or high. As your treatment progresses, more potassium goes into your cells to replenish losses there, so your blood potassium may fall. If that happens, the doctor administers more potassium to sort out the problem.

Because your lack of insulin gets you into this situation, your doctor gives you insulin intravenously to restore your insulin level and reverse the abnormalities in your body. At some point, your blood glucose may fall towards a hypoglycaemic level. If it does, your doctor gives you another IV made up of glucose and a solution of salt, potassium, and water.

After you receive insulin, your body stops breaking down fat for energy because your cells can use glucose for energy as they're supposed to. Soon, your body rids itself of the ketones in your bloodstream that caused your complication, and your body takes on a more normal condition.

Your doctor gives you large volumes of a saltwater solution intravenously to replace the six or more litres of fluids that you lose during ketoacidosis. Replenishing your body's fluids relieves the nausea and vomiting that you've endured, and you're now able to keep down liquid and solid foods again. Hopefully, you notice your normal mental functioning returning, which means that you're soon ready to resume self-administering your insulin and controlling your own diet. By this time, the doctor has probably found and corrected a malfunctioning insulin pump or an infection that was a factor in causing your ketoacidosis.

Ketoacidosis may not sound like a walk in the park, but you may think that your doctor can control it with little or no risk to you. For the most part, that's true, but be aware that ketoacidosis is fatal for 10 per cent of people with diabetes who get it – mostly elderly people with diabetes and those with other illnesses that complicate treatment. Recognising the symptoms early and seeking treatment quickly greatly enhance your chances of an uneventful recovery from ketoacidosis.

Managing the Hyperosmolar Syndrome

The highest blood glucose condition that you may find yourself in is called the *hyperosmolar syndrome*. Like ketoacidosis, the hyperosmolar syndrome is a medical emergency that needs to be treated in a hospital.

The hyperosmolar syndrome is also like ketoacidosis in its effects on your body. The hyperosmolar syndrome creates ketones in your blood, but it doesn't make your blood as acidic as ketoacidosis does. It also raises your blood glucose levels considerably higher than ketoacidosis does. (See the 'Combating Ketoacidosis' section for more information.)

The name *hyperosmolar syndrome* refers to the excessive levels of glucose in the blood. *Hyper* means 'larger than normal', and *osmolar* has to do with concentrations of substances in the blood. So hyperosmolar, in this situation, means that the blood is simply too concentrated with glucose. Other hyperosmolar syndromes occur when other substances are at fault.

The following sections explain the hyperosmolar syndrome's symptoms, causes, and treatments.

Symptoms of the hyperosmolar syndrome

Because the hyperosmolar syndrome complication is so similar to ketoacidosis, it has many of the same symptoms as ketoacidosis. The main difference is that with hyperosmolar syndrome, you don't experience the rapid Kussmaul breathing (see 'Symptoms of ketoacidosis' earlier in this chapter), because your blood isn't overly acidic as a part of this complication. Also, the symptoms of the hyperosmolar syndrome develop over many days or weeks, unlike ketoacidosis's quick and acute development in your body.

If you measure your blood glucose on a daily basis, you should never develop the hyperosmolar syndrome. This is because you notice if your blood glucose is getting high before it reaches the critical complication level.

The most important signs and symptoms of the hyperosmolar syndrome are as follows:

- Frequent urination
- Thirst
- Weakness
- Leg cramps
- Sunken eyeballs and rapid pulse, due to dehydration
- Decreased mental awareness or coma
- Blood glucose of 33 mmol/l or higher (if you wait longer to see your doctor)

You may also develop more threatening symptoms with this complication. Your blood pressure may be low. Your nervous system may be affected with paralysis of the arms and legs, although this paralysis responds to treatment. You may have high counts of potassium, sodium, and other blood constituents (such as white blood cells and red blood cells), but these counts usually fall rapidly and your doctor replaces these elements in your blood as water is restored to your body.

Causes of the hyperosmolar syndrome

The hyperosmolar syndrome afflicts mostly the elderly with diabetes who live alone or in nursing homes where they're not carefully monitored. Age and neglect combine to increase the likelihood of a person with diabetes losing large quantities of fluids through vomiting or diarrhoea and then not replacing those fluids. These people tend to have mild type 2 diabetes, and sometimes their diabetes is undiagnosed and untreated.

Age is also a contributing cause of the hyperosmolar syndrome because your kidneys gradually become less efficient as you age. When your kidneys are in their prime, your blood glucose level needs to reach only about 10 mmol/l before your kidneys begin to remove some excess glucose through your urine. But as your kidneys grow older and slower, they require a gradually higher blood glucose level before they start to send excess glucose to your urine. If you're at an age when your kidneys are really labouring to remove the excess glucose from your body (usually 70 or older for people in average health), and you happen to lose a large amount of fluids from sickness or neglect, your blood volume decreases, making it even harder for your kidneys to remove glucose. At this point, your blood glucose level begins to rocket. If you don't replace some of the lost fluids soon, your glucose rises even higher.

If you allow your blood glucose to rise and don't get the fluids that you need, your blood pressure starts to fall, and you get weaker and weaker. As the concentration of glucose in your blood continues to rise, you become increasingly confused, and your mental state diminishes as the glucose concentration rises, until you eventually fall into a coma.

Other factors – such as infection, failure to take your insulin, and taking certain medications – can raise your blood glucose to the hyperosmolar syndrome levels, but not replacing lost body fluids is the most frequent cause.

Treatment of the hyperosmolar syndrome

Even more so than ketoacidosis (see 'Treatment of ketoacidosis' earlier in this chapter), the hyperosmolar syndrome requires immediate and skilled treatment from a doctor.

By no means should you try to treat the hyperosmolar syndrome yourself. In fact, you should avoid doctors who are not experienced in treatment of this condition. You need the proper treatment from an experienced doctor – and you need it fast. The death rate for the hyperosmolar syndrome is high because most people who suffer from it are elderly and often have other serious illnesses that complicate treatment. When you arrive at the Accident and Emergency department with the hyperosmolar syndrome, your doctor must accomplish the following tasks fairly rapidly:

✔ Restore large volumes of water to your body

✔ Lower your blood glucose level

✔ Restore other substances that your body has lost, such as potassium, sodium, and chloride

Your doctor creates a chart to monitor your levels of glucose, blood concentration (*osmolarity*), potassium, sodium, and other tests, which are measured hourly in some cases. You may think that you need to receive large amounts of insulin to lower your high glucose level, but the large doses of fluids that your doctor gives you to replenish your body fluids do so much to lower your glucose that you need only smaller doses of insulin. As your body fluids return to normal, your kidneys begin to receive much more of the blood that they need in order to rid your body of the excess glucose.

Chapter 5

Preventing Long-Term Complications

*Y*ou may think that diabetes has made your life more complicated. But you'll long for those good old days when you 'just' had diabetes if you ever develop one of the severe complications that we describe in this chapter. The complications in this chapter are the problems that occur if you let your blood glucose rise and remain high over many years. The point that we stress throughout this book is that you have a choice. Working with your doctor and other helpers, you can keep your blood glucose near normal, and you shouldn't have to deal with the long-term complications covered in this chapter.

How Long-Term Complications Develop

For most long-term complications, such as kidney disease, eye disease, and nerve disease, doctors believe that years of high blood glucose levels initiate the complications. However, there's some emerging evidence that raised cholesterol and raised blood pressure can also play a part.

In the case of heart disease, raised cholesterol and blood pressure levels are mainly to blame, although high blood glucose levels may make the disease worse or more complicated. And since four out of five people with diabetes die of heart disease or stroke, you can see why we stress the essential requirement to take care of your blood pressure and cholesterol, as well as your blood glucose. Fortunately, you're in possession of a book that helps you to do just that!

Often the long-term complication itself (rather than a high blood glucose level) is the clue that leads a doctor to diagnose diabetes in a patient. In one study, for instance, doctors checked patients coming into hospital with a heart attack to see if they had diabetes. Of those who said that they didn't have diabetes, one third turned out to have undiagnosed diabetes and another third proved to have impaired glucose tolerance (a precursor of diabetes that we discuss in Chapters 2 and 3). Therefore, doctors need to look for long-term complications immediately after diagnosing diabetes, because the diabetes and any long-term complications may have been with the patient for quite some time already. (Most long-term complications require ten or more years to develop, which seems like a long time, until you consider that many people with type 2 diabetes have their diabetes for five or more years before a doctor diagnoses it.)

Kidney Disease or Nephropathy

Your kidneys rid your body of many harmful chemicals and other compounds produced during the process of normal metabolism. They act like filters through which your blood pours, trapping the waste and sending it out in your urine, while transmitting the normal contents of the blood back into your bloodstream. Your kidneys also regulate the salt and water content of your body. When kidney disease (also known as *nephropathy*) causes your kidneys to fail, you must either use artificial means, called *dialysis,* to cleanse your blood and control the salt and water, or you must receive a new working donor kidney, called a *transplant*.

More than a third of people with type 2 diabetes tend to develop some degree of kidney damage. In the United Kingdom, diabetic kidney disease accounts for more than a third of the people on dialysis, and it's reckoned to be the single biggest cause of severe kidney failure in the western world. Although kidney failure used to be thought of as a bigger problem in people with type 1 rather than type 2 diabetes, now we're discovering that the risk of kidney damage is about the same in both conditions.

Diabetic kidney disease is closely linked with heart disease and diabetic blood vessel disease away from the heart (you can find out more about these diseases later in this chapter). High blood pressure, which is a common problem in diabetics, can also damage your kidneys. If you have both high blood pressure and diabetes, the two conditions raise your risk of kidney disease much more than one would on its own. That's why we've explained in excruciating detail how to keep your blood pressure under control (later in this chapter). The good news, of course, is that by controlling both your diabetes and your blood pressure tightly, you can improve the outlook for your kidneys enormously.

What's more, as we explain in the section 'ACE inhibitors and AIIRAs to the rescue', later in this chapter, some medicines originally used to help bring high blood pressure down can actually protect your kidneys independently of their effect on your blood pressure. That's why under the General Practitioner Contract, there's a reminder to all general practitioners to make sure that you're taking an ACE inhibitor or AIIRA if you have any evidence of kidney damage, called microalbuminuria (see the section 'Time course: From minor problems to kidney failure').

Diabetes and your kidneys

Your kidneys contain a structure called the *glomerulus,* which is responsible for filtering and cleansing your blood (see Figure 5-1). Each kidney has hundreds of thousands of glomeruli. Your blood passes through the tiny glomerular capillaries, which are in intimate contact with tubules through which your filtered blood travels. As the filtered blood passes through the tubules, most of the water and the normal contents of the blood are reabsorbed and sent back into your body, while a small amount of water and waste passes from the kidney into the ureter and then into the bladder and out through the urethra.

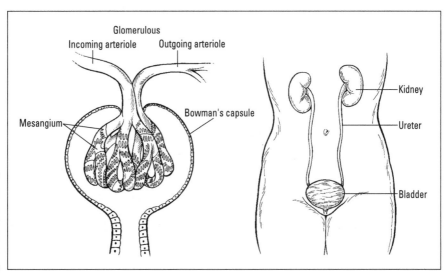

Figure 5-1:
The kidney,
internally
and
externally.

Early in the development of your diabetes, the membrane surrounding your glomeruli, called the *glomerular basement membrane,* thickens, as do other nearby structures. These expanding membranes and structures begin to take up the space occupied by the capillaries inside the glomeruli, so that the capillaries are unable to filter as much blood. Fortunately, you have many more glomeruli than you really need. In fact, you can lose a whole kidney and still have plenty of reserve to clean your blood.

If your kidney disease goes undetected for about 15 years, damage may become so severe that your blood shows measurable signs of the beginning of kidney failure, called *azotemia.* If the neglect of the disease reaches 20 years, your kidneys may fail entirely. (For more on the timing of kidney failure, see 'Time course: From minor problems to kidney failure'.)

Time course: From minor problems to kidney failure

Nephropathy progresses in a predictable fashion, going from relatively minor to very serious. Each stage has its treatment options, but, as you can imagine, the treatment becomes more drastic in the later stages. The following sections explain the various stages of the disease – what's happening and what the treatment plan may be.

Stage 1: Hyperfiltration

When you first get diabetes, your kidneys are enlarged and seem to function abnormally well, judging by how fast they clear wastes from your body. They appear to function so well because a large amount of glucose is entering them, which draws a lot of water with it. The flow of blood through the glomeruli increases and the kidneys become enlarged. This stage is known as *hyperfiltration.*

This stage can progress very quickly to microalbuminuria. In fact, many type 2 diabetics will already have microalbuminuria by the time they are diagnosed as having diabetes.

Stage 2: Microalbuminuria

In this stage, the rate of filtration stays high, and the glomeruli start to show signs of damage. This damage allows small amounts of *albumin,* a protein in the blood, to leak into the urine. In the early stages, the amount of albumin in the urine is less than that required to trigger a positive test when the traditional urine dipstick is used. Therefore, a more sophisticated test for microalbuminuria must be performed. See the sidebar 'Testing for microalbuminuria: A better dipstick' for details.

Testing for microalbuminuria: A better dipstick

General practitioners used to check for protein (or *macroalbuminuria*) in the urine using a dipstick test. Once macroalbuminuria is found, kidney disease can be slowed but not stopped.

Microalbuminuria is found about five years before the urine becomes dipstick positive for protein. At this earlier stage, treatment can reverse the kidney disease. This test is now offered to all patients with diabetes once a year.

The new General Practitioner Contract has lots of targets for high-quality care. One of them is that, if you have diabetes, you should have your urine checked for microalbumin at least once a year. Ask your practice nurse or general practitioner whether they perform the check annually. If they don't, you can ask to be checked for microalbuminuria.

Once microalbuminuria is present, 25 to 50 per cent of patients will go on to get proteinuria, the next stage of kidney disease, within 5 to 10 years. Taking certain medications, and keeping your blood pressure, cholesterol, and blood sugar under tight control, can delay this progression significantly. You can find out more in the section on treatment below.

Stage 3: Proteinuria

In this stage, the glomeruli get more and more damaged, which reduces their ability to filter waste out of the system. This leads to raised blood levels of two components of the blood called creatinine and urea.

When a patient with type 2 diabetes gets proteinuria, their kidney function inevitably worsens. They are likely to reach stage 5 (kidney failure) and need dialysis or a kidney transplant within seven years.

Kidney failure is not always inevitable

In June 2003 in the *New England Journal of Medicine*, researchers showed that microalbuminuria does not lead inexorably to kidney failure. A decline in microalbuminuria (and therefore kidney damage) in type 1 diabetes was noted when patients kept their readings to:

✔ Haemoglobin A1c under 8 per cent (see Chapter 7)

✔ Systolic (the upper reading) blood pressure under 115 mmHg (see Chapter 7)

✔ Cholesterol below 5.12 mmol/l

✔ Triglycerides below 1.64 mmol/l (see Chapter 7)

Stage 4: Advanced clinical nephropathy

The damaged kidneys cannot filter as much blood. Large amounts of protein leak into the urine, and creatinine and urea in the blood get higher. Hypertension almost always accompanies this stage.

Stage 5: End-stage renal failure

Once kidney function has dropped to 5 to 10 per cent of its ideal level, signs and symptoms of kidney failure start to show. This cannot be cured, and dialysis or kidney transplant are the only options.

Risk factors and other stuff to know

Not every person with diabetes is at equal risk for kidney disease and kidney failure. Kidney disease seems to be more common in certain families and among certain racial groups, especially Afro-Caribbeans and Asians. It is certainly more common when high blood pressure is present. Although we believe that high blood glucose is the major factor leading to nephropathy, only half of the people whose blood glucose has been poorly controlled go on to develop nephropathy.

Other factors besides high blood glucose contribute to the continuing destruction of the kidneys. They include

- **High blood pressure.** This may be as important as the glucose level. If your blood pressure is controlled by drugs, the damage to your kidneys slows very significantly.

- **Factors of inheritance.** Certain families and ethnic groups have a higher incidence of diabetic nephropathy.

- **Abnormal blood fats.** It has been shown that elevated levels of certain cholesterol-containing fats promotes enlargement of the mesangium (the cells between the tiny blood vessels in your kidneys).

- **Cigarette smoking.** Heart disease is greatly increased in diabetic nephropathy. Cigarettes are clearly linked to increased occurrence of heart disease.

Diabetic nephropathy doesn't occur alone. Other complications develop at a faster or slower rate. They include

- **Diabetic eye disease:** At the time of complete failure of the kidneys, called *end-stage renal disease,* diabetic *retinopathy* (eye disease) is always present (see the section 'Eye Disease', later in this chapter). As kidney disease gets worse, retinopathy accelerates. But only half the people with retinopathy also have nephropathy. Once microalbuminuria is present, all patients also have some retinopathy. Therefore, if you have diabetes and microalbuminuria and retinopathy isn't present, your doctor should look for another cause of kidney disease besides diabetes.

✔ **Diabetic nerve disease, or *neuropathy*:** The association between nephropathy and neuropathy is not as close. Fewer than 50 per cent of patients with nephropathy will have neuropathy. Neuropathy gets worse as kidney disease gets worse, but once dialysis is started, some of the neuropathy disappears so that part of the neuropathy may be due to wastes that are retained because of the failing kidney rather than true damage to the nervous system. (For more on this condition, see the section 'Nerve Disease or Neuropathy' later in this chapter.)

✔ **Hypertension:** Hypertension plays an important role in accelerating the kidney damage. Once there is macroalbuminuria, most patients have high blood pressure. As the blood tests for kidney failure begin to rise, virtually all patients are hypertensive. With end-stage renal disease, all have high blood pressure.

✔ **Ooedema:** *Ooedema,* or water accumulation, in the feet and legs occurs as the amount of protein in the urine exceeds 1 or 2 grams a day.

Treatment

Happily, you can avoid all the inconvenience and discomfort associated with diabetic nephropathy. Following are a few key treatments that can prevent the disease or significantly slow it down once it begins:

✔ **Control your blood glucose:** Controlling your blood glucose has been shown to delay the onset of nephropathy and slow it down once it starts. (For information on controlling your blood glucose, see Part III.) One of the best findings from the Diabetes Control and Complications Trial is that even eight years after the trial ended, benefits of reduced blood pressure and reduced albumin excretion (a marker for kidney damage) persisted. Controlling blood glucose will pay off years in the future.

✔ **Control your blood pressure:** By controlling your blood pressure, you protect your kidneys from rapid deterioration. Treatment begins with a low-salt diet, but drugs are usually needed. Two classes of drugs that seem particularly valuable in nephropathy are the *angiotensin-converting enzyme inhibitors,* or ACE inhibitors, and the *angiotensin II receptor antagonists,* or AIIRAs. (For more on ACE inhibitors and AIIRAs, see the sidebar 'ACE inhibitors and AIIRAs to the rescue'.)

✔ **Control the blood fats:** Because abnormalities of blood fats seem to make the kidney disease worse, you need to lower the bad, or LDL, cholesterol and raise the good, or HDL, cholesterol at the same time that you lower the other damaging fat, namely, the triglycerides. A number of excellent drugs, in a class called *statins,* can do this. The ACE inhibitors also seem to help the levels of fats. (See the sidebar 'ACE inhibitors and AIIRAs to the rescue' for more information.)

✔ **Avoid other damage to the kidneys:** People with diabetes tend to have more urinary tract infections, which damage the kidneys. People with diabetes also have nerve damage to the nerves that control the bladder, producing a neurogenic bladder. (See the section 'Disorders of automatic (autonomic) nerves' later in this chapter.) When the nerves that detect a full bladder fail, proper emptying of the bladder is inhibited, which can lead to infections.

When there is disease in the urinary system, doctors often do an *intravenous urogram* (IVU), a study to observe the appearance and function of the kidney and the rest of the urinary tract. People with diabetes and some kidney failure are at high risk for complete failure of the kidneys as a result of an IVU. Other types of studies that do not put the kidneys at risk should be used.

✔ **Consider the protein in your diet.** People with diabetic kidney damage are often advised not to eat more than 0.6–0.7 grams per kilogram of protein per day (that's 42–49 grams per day for someone weighing 70 kilograms). Doctors disagree, though, on whether this helps. We recommend that you look at your diet (see Chapter 8 for information on proteins in the diet) and just be aware of the amount of protein you're eating.

Haemodialysis versus peritoneal dialysis

With *haemodialysis*, the patient's artery is hooked into a tube that runs through a filtering machine that cleanses the blood and then sends it back into the patient's bloodstream. This treatment requires an operation to be performed initially, which usually involves making a connection between a vein and an artery for the blood to come out of and go back into. When the patient is moderately well, haemodialysis is done three times a week in a hospital-like setting. However, the potential exists for many complications, including infection and low blood pressure. In addition, with failure of the kidneys, a main source for the breakdown of insulin is gone, and the patient requires much less or no insulin, so control of the blood glucose may actually get easier.

Peritoneal dialysis consists of the insertion of a tube into the body cavity that contains the stomach, liver, and intestines, called the *peritoneal cavity.* A large quantity of fluid is dripped into the cavity, and it draws out the wastes, which are then removed as the fluid drains out of the cavity. Peritoneal dialysis is done at home, often on a daily basis. It requires the use of sugar in the fluid, so people with diabetes may have very high blood glucose levels unless insulin is added to the bags of dialysis fluid. Peritoneal dialysis is also associated with a high rate of infection where the tube enters the peritoneal cavity.

ACE inhibitors and AIIRAs to the rescue

Angiotensin-converting enzyme inhibitors (ACE inhibitors) and angiotensin II receptor antagonists (AIIRAs) are two groups of drugs developed in recent years to treat hypertension.

ACE inhibitors have long been known to lower blood pressure, but recent studies show that they lower the pressure inside the glomerulus. The result is a 50 per cent reduction in death due to diabetic nephropathy and an equal reduction in the need for dialysis or transplantation. More recently, studies have suggested that AIIRAs produce similar benefits.

Within the last couple of years, more exciting evidence of the benefits of ACE inhibitors and AIIRAs has emerged. For instance, they can

✔ Reduce the likelihood of non-diabetics going on to get type 2 diabetes

✔ Slow down the progress of diabetic kidney disease

✔ Cut death rates in people with heart failure

✔ Reduce complication rates in people with enlarged hearts (*left ventricular hypertrophy*)

The various national guidelines for people with diabetes or who are at high risk of cardiovascular disease all agree on what to do:

✔ If you have microalbuminuria, even if your blood pressure is not raised, you should now be started on an ACE inhibitor (or AIIRA).

✔ If your blood pressure is above 140/80 mmHg, your other risk factors for cardiovascular disease should be assessed. For diabetics, the target blood pressure is at or below 135/75 mmHg if you have microalbuminuria, or 140/80 mmHg if you don't.

✔ If your overall risk is high or your risk of having a heart problem in the next ten years is over 15 per cent, you should be offered treatment with an ACE inhibitor.

Until the last couple of years, most guidelines suggested ACE inhibitors, rather than AIIRAs, as first-line treatment because most of the studies showing the benefits of AIIRAs were published after the guidelines came out. Most guidelines now offer a choice of ACE inhibitor or AIIRA.

ACE inhibitors are not a perfect treatment because an incidence of cough exists, which some people find hard to tolerate, but the choice of a particular ACE inhibitor may solve this problem. If you can't tolerate the dry cough caused by an ACE inhibitor, talk to your doctor about changing to an AIIRA, which doesn't cause the same side effect. In addition, ACE inhibitors and AIIRAs tend to raise the potassium in the blood. This is already a problem with failing kidneys, so a higher potassium level may add to the problem. A very high potassium level can cause abnormalities in the heart.

✔ **Conduct dialysis if preventive treatment fails:** If dialysis is done, two techniques are currently in use: *haemodialysis* and *peritoneal dialysis*. The long-term survival of patients treated with haemodialysis compared with peritoneal dialysis is about the same, so the choice becomes one of convenience and the alternatives offered by your local hospitals. People with diabetes do not tolerate kidney failure well, so dialysis tends to be done earlier in them than in people without diabetes. For information on these dialysis procedures, see the sidebar 'Haemodialysis versus peritoneal dialysis'.

✔ **Receive a kidney transplant if preventive treatment fails:** Patients who receive a kidney transplant do seem to do better than dialysis patients, but in the United Kingdom, as in so many other countries, suitable kidneys are in short supply. The transplant is foreign to the person who receives it, and the person's body tries to reject it. This requires the use of anti-rejection drugs, some of which make diabetic control more complicated. Once a healthy kidney enters the body of a person with diabetes, it is subject to the damage done by elevated glucose levels, so that control of the glucose becomes even more important.

Eye Disease

The eyes are the second major organ of the body affected by diabetes over the long term. Some eye diseases, such as glaucoma and cataracts, also occur in the non-diabetic population, though they appear at a higher rate and earlier in people with diabetes. Glaucoma and cataracts respond to treatment very well. Diabetic retinopathy, however, is limited to the diabetic population and may lead to blindness. In the past, blindness was inevitable, but this result is far from the case today. (***Note:*** Because retinopathy is much more complicated and less treatable than the other two conditions, we discuss it in much more detail in the next sections.)

If you have diabetes, you must get an annual eye examination to preserve your vision. If you go to the hospital for your annual check, the eye check should be done there. More and more people with diabetes are now having their annual eye checks transferred into the community, either with their general practitioner or with another community clinic. Don't worry, you still get the same high-quality care from either clinic. If you haven't been doing so already, you need to get an eye examination at the time your type 2 diabetes is diagnosed. People with type 1 diabetes should have an eye check-up five years after their diagnosis and every year after that.

Here are some suggestions you can follow to ensure that you get the necessary care:

✔ The new General Practitioner Contract has lots of targets for high-quality care. One of these is that if you have diabetes, you should have your retina (the back of your eye) checked at least once a year. Check to make sure that your general practitioner is following the guidelines set out by the National Institute for Health and Clinical Excellence (NICE) about review and referral.

✔ Even if you are getting your eyes checked regularly by your doctor, we recommend that you visit your high-street optician at least once a year. Opticians have equipment that lets them perform the necessary checks, and they're highly trained to pick up early changes, even before you get any symptoms. If they have any anxieties, they give you a letter to hand in to your general practitioner, who can then organise a specialist referral.

If you have your eyes checked at hospital or in some community clinics, you probably have photographs taken of your retina. These can be compared with later photographs, and provide a very accurate picture of how any diabetic retinopathy is progressing. Retinal photography is fast becoming the investigation of choice for monitoring diabetic eye disease.

Cataracts

Cataracts are opaque areas of the lens and can block vision if they're large enough. Cataracts tend to be more common in people with diabetes, even at a young age. Cataracts can be surgically removed by a fairly routine operation in which the whole lens is removed and an artificial lens is put in its place. With removal, you have an excellent chance for your vision to be restored.

Glaucoma

Glaucoma is a disease of the eye marked by increased pressure inside the eye. This high pressure is enough to do damage to the optic nerve. Glaucoma is found more often in people with diabetes than in those without diabetes. If unchecked, the high pressure can destroy the optic nerve and your vision. Fortunately, medical treatment can lower the eye pressure and save the eye. Eye tests, either by an eye doctor or by a high-street optician, check for glaucoma on a routine basis.

Retinopathy

Diabetic retinopathy refers to a number of changes that are seen on the retina of the eye. These changes indicate that the patient has been exposed to high levels of blood glucose over time. If untreated at the appropriate time, retinopathy can lead to blindness. The first changes are seen after ten years of diabetes in both types 1 and 2.

How diabetes affects the eye

To understand how diabetes affects the eye, you need to have a basic understanding of the different parts of the eye and how the eye works.

Light enters the eye through the lens, where it is bent and focused on the retina. The place in the retina where the lens focuses is called the *macula*. The retina collects an image and transfers it to the optic nerve, which carries it to the brain where the image is interpreted. Between the lens and the retina is a transparent material called the *vitreous body*. Many more structures are within the eye, but they aren't important for the purposes of this chapter. The eye muscles surround the eye on all sides and are attached to it. These muscles allow you to look up, down, and sideways without moving your head. These eye muscles are important in the discussion of diabetic nerve damage, called *neuropathy*. (For more on this condition, see the section 'Nerve Disease or Neuropathy', later in this chapter.)

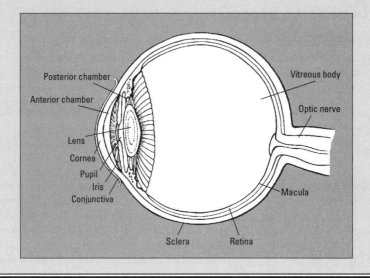

Types of retinopathy

Doctors break down retinopathy into two major types, according to their potential to cause visual loss:

> ✔ *Background retinopathy* is usually benign but can be a predictor of worse problems. Following are some of the problems caused by background retinopathy:
>
> • **Retinal aneurysms.** These are the first changes that your ophthalmologist is likely to notice. Retinal aneurysms are the result of

weakening of the capillaries of the eye. These aneurysms appear as small red dots on the back of the eye. They are benign and disappear over time.

- **Retinal haemorrhages and hard exudates.** If the weakened capillaries rupture and release blood, *retinal haemorrhages* and *hard exudates* are formed. The hard exudates, which are yellowish and appear round and sharp, are scars from the haemorrhage and fat deposits in the retina. If they extend into the macular area (the area marked on the figure), they reduce vision. These exudates and haemorrhages can last for years.

- **Macular oedema.** If the weakened capillaries in the retina allow fluid and other things to flow into the *macula* (the central part of the retina), you get *macular oedema* (swelling) and loss of vision.

- **Cotton wool spots or soft exudates.** As the capillaries close, you have a decreased blood supply to the retina, and *cotton wool spots* or *soft exudates* appear. These areas of discoloration represent destruction of the nerve fibre layer because of the lack of blood.

These changes usually do not cause loss of vision, but in about 50 per cent of cases they go on to the more serious proliferative retinopathy.

✔ *Proliferative retinopathy* ends up with vision loss if untreated. Just as in many other parts of the body, when the blood supply is reduced, new blood vessels form to carry more blood to the retina. When this happens, the patient enters the stage of proliferative retinopathy, when some visual loss becomes more certain. The growth of blood vessels takes place in the *vitreous* (the transparent material between the lens and the retina). Haemorrhaging into the vitreous blocks vision. As the haemorrhage forms a clot and contracts, it may pull up the retina to produce *retinal detachment.* Because the lens can no longer focus the light on to the macula, you have a complete loss of vision.

Other things you need to know about retinopathy

Retinopathy has a number of important associations. You are at higher risk of developing retinopathy if you

✔ **Are of South Asian origin:** Certain ethnic groups are at very high risk of retinopathy. These include people of South Asian origin. At the moment, researchers are uncertain whether Afro-Caribbeans are at higher risk.

✔ **Have a specific genetic material, in addition to your diabetes.** The combination of diabetes and this genetic material may increase the incidence of retinopathy. At the moment, the evidence for this is shaky. This genetic material can be found by doing a chemical analysis of a person's chromosomes, the material in each cell that holds the genes.

In addition, the eye disease can be made worse in the following situations:

- ✔ You have high blood pressure.
- ✔ Your diabetes has gone on for a while (greater duration of diabetes results in more eye disease).
- ✔ You smoke or drink alcohol (just one more reason for quitting).

If all this isn't bad enough, if you have diabetic retinopathy, you're at increased risk of heart attacks. In addition, nephropathy (diabetic kidney disease; see the section 'Kidney Disease' earlier in this chapter) occurs along with the eye disease.

Treatment

No drugs are currently available to treat retinopathy, but laser surgery is an excellent treatment option. The use of laser surgery to create many burns in the retina has been shown to save many eyes. The original studies used one eye as the untreated or control eye and the other as the treated eye. Only 5 per cent of diabetics with proliferative retinopathy who undergo laser treatment develop severe visual loss. The results of laser surgery include the following:

- ✔ The risk of severe visual loss is reduced to less than half.
- ✔ Because the retina is being burned, you have some minor loss of vision.
- ✔ You also have a mild decrease in night vision and a minor decrease in the size of the field that your eye can take in at one time.

The procedure is performed outside the hospital. Doctors use it to treat macular oedema as well.

Laser surgery cannot treat a detachment that has already occurred. To do so, a surgical procedure called *vitrectomy* is used. This operation, done under general anaesthesia, involves the removal of the vitreous body and its replacement with a sterile solution. Attachments to the retina are cut, and the retina returns to its place. Any haemorrhages in the vitreous are removed at the same time. Vitrectomy is successful in restoring some vision about 80 to 90 per cent of the time. If retinal detachment is also present, the amount of improvement depends on the extent and duration of the retinal detachment, with restoration of vision occurring about 50 to 60 per cent of the time.

If you are blind or visually impaired

Being registered blind or partially sighted entitles you to some financial benefits. You should be able to get support from your local social services department as well. Diabetes UK, the Royal National Institute for the Blind, or your local Citizens' Advice Bureau clinic (the number is in the phone book) can all help you with these claims.

Determining blindness or the degree of impairment

The most common measurement of your eyesight is a test of visual acuity, which looks at the letters you can read on a Snellen chart. If your visual acuity is measured at 6/60 or worse, you can be registered as partially sighted. If your visual acuity is measured as 3/60 or worse, you can be registered blind.

Resources available to you

You have no reason to feel alone with your visual problem. Many resources are available to you. If you are visually impaired, your general practitioner may be able to give you details about local resources. Alternatively, your local diabetic specialist nurse can be an invaluable source of information and advice. The eye clinic at your local hospital should be able to help you with visual aids, and its staff may refer you on to the occupational therapy department to get practical devices. Other resources include the Royal National Institute for the Blind (RNIB) and Diabetes UK. You can find details about them in Appendix C.

The World Wide Web is also an enormous resource for the visually handicapped. (If you are visually impaired and have difficulty reading things on the computer screen, you may be able to get screen magnification.)

Nerve Disease or Neuropathy

The third major organ system of the body that is attacked by poorly controlled diabetes is the nervous system. Around 60 per cent of people with diabetes are shown to have some abnormality of the nervous system, and the disease is found most often in the people who have diabetes the longest. Those who develop *neuropathy* usually have poor glucose control, smoke, and are over 40. Unfortunately, many patients usually don't realise they have neuropathy because the disease doesn't have any early symptoms.

The major problem with respect to diabetic neuropathy is the high frequency of foot infections, foot ulcerations, and amputation – complications that are all entirely preventable. (See the section on 'Diabetic Foot Disease', later in this chapter.)

What causes neuropathy?

Diabetic neuropathy occurs in any situation where the blood glucose is abnormally elevated for ten years or more, so it's not limited to type 1 or type 2 diabetes, although these are the most common diseases where it is found. When the elevated blood glucose is brought down to normal, the signs and symptoms improve. In some cases, the neuropathy disappears.

In addition to a persistently high blood glucose, the following conditions make neuropathy worse:

- ✔ **Age** is important because neuropathy is most common over the age of 40.
- ✔ **Height** is a consideration. Neuropathy is more common in taller individuals, who have longer nerve fibres to damage.
- ✔ **Alcohol consumption** is especially important because even small quantities of alcohol can make neuropathy worse.

Diagnosing neuropathy

The speed with which a nervous impulse travels down a nerve fibre is called the *nerve conduction velocity* (NCV). In diabetic neuropathy, the NCV is slowed. This slowing may not be accompanied by any symptoms at first, providing a way of diagnosing neuropathy in people without symptoms. Sensitive tests, called nerve conduction studies, can pick up these very early changes. If patients have very mild symptoms, the improvement that follows medication may be hard to detect except by doing a nerve conduction velocity study. A medication that helps the neuropathy would be expected to speed up the NCV.

Doctors can test nerve function in a variety of ways because different nerve fibres seem to be responsible for different kinds of sensation, such as light touch, vibration, and temperature. The connection between the kind of test and the fibre it tests for is as follows:

- ✔ **Vibration testing,** using a tuning fork for example, can bring out abnormalities of large nerve fibres.
- ✔ **Temperature testing,** using a warm or cold item, tests for damage to small fibres, which are very important in diabetes. When small fibres are damaged, the patient can, for example, lose the ability to feel that she is entering a burning hot bath.
- ✔ **Light touch testing** reflects the large fibres, which sense anything touching our skin. This test is done using a filament that looks like a hair. The thickness of the filament determines how much force is needed to bend the filament so that the patient feels it. For example, normal feet can feel a filament that bends with 1 gram of force. If a patient cannot feel a filament that bends with 10 grams of force, this person is likely to suffer damage to the foot without feeling it. If the patient cannot feel any sensation with a filament that requires 75 grams of force to bend, that area is considered to have lost all sensation.

 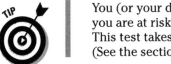 You (or your doctor) can use the 10-gram filament to discover whether you are at risk for damage to your feet because you cannot feel the pain. This test takes a minute to do and can save your feet from amputation. (See the section on 'Diabetic Foot Disease', later in this chapter.)

Symptoms of neuropathy

The various disorders of the nervous system are broken down into the following categories:

- ✔ Disorders associated with loss of sensation, where the sensory nerves are damaged
- ✔ Disorders due to loss of motor nerves, which carry the impulses to muscles to make them move
- ✔ Disorders due to loss of automatic (known as *autonomic)* nerves, which control muscles we do not have to think about, such as the heart muscles, the intestinal muscles, and the bladder muscles.

The following sections describe the various conditions associated with these disorders.

Disorders of sensation

Disorders of sensation are the most common and bothersome disorders of nerves in diabetes. There are a number of different conditions, which break down into *diffuse neuropathies* involving many nerves and *focal neuropathies* involving one or several nerves. This section is about the diffuse neuropathies affecting sensation.

Distal polyneuropathy

Distal polyneuropathy is the most frequent form of diabetic neuropathy. *Distal* means far away from the centre of the body – in other words, the feet and hands. *Poly* means many, and *neuropathy* is disease in nerves. So this is a disease of many nerves, which is noticed in the feet and hands. Physicians believe that distal polyneuropathy is a metabolic disease (too much glucose in the blood, specifically).

The signs and symptoms of distal polyneuropathy are:

- ✔ Diminished ability to feel light touch or to feel the position of a foot, whether bent backwards or forwards, resulting from the loss of the large fibres
- ✔ Diminished ability to feel pain and temperature from the loss of the small fibres
- ✔ Minor weakness
- ✔ Tingling and burning
- ✔ Unpleasant sensations, often described as being like walking on pebbles
- ✔ Extreme sensitivity to touch

✔ Loss of balance or coordination

✔ Worsening of symptoms at night

The danger of this kind of neuropathy is that the patient doesn't know, without looking, whether she has trauma to her feet, such as a burn or stepping on a tack.

The complications of this loss of sensation are preventable. If you cannot feel your feet, you must look at them. In the section 'Diabetic Foot Disease', later in this chapter, we offer specific techniques to preserve your feet when neuropathy is present.

The following are serious complications associated with distal polyneuropathy:

✔ **Neuropathic foot ulcer:** This is the most serious complication of loss of sensation in the feet. As pressure mounts on an area of the foot, the pressure is felt because of pain. However, in diabetic neuropathy, this pressure is not felt. A callus forms and, with continued pressure, the callus softens and liquifies, finally falling off to leave an ulcer. This ulcer becomes infected. If the ulcer isn't promptly treated it spreads, and amputation may be the only way of saving the patient.

✔ **Neuroarthropathy, or Charcot's joint:** Although a less common complication in distal polyneuropathy, this condition occurs when a trauma, which isn't felt, occurs to the joints of the foot or ankle. The bones in the foot get out of line, and many painless fractures may occur. The patient has redness and painless swelling of the foot and ankle. The foot becomes unusable and is described as a bag of bones. Treatment of distal polyneuropathy starts with the best glucose control possible and extremely good foot care.

Your doctor should look at your feet on every visit, particularly if you have any evidence of loss of feeling. Even more importantly, you should check your feet every day. After all, you're around your feet all the time, and your doctor sees them only every few months. Chapter 7 gives you more details on how to do this.

Your doctor may also prescribe medication, either drugs or creams, to help with the pain. See the sidebar 'Drugs for distal polyneuropathy' for details about the available medications.

Radiculopathy – nerve root involvement

Sometimes a severe pain in a particular area suggests that the root of the nerve, as it leaves the spinal column, is damaged. The pain can be so severe that doctors mistake it for an internal abdominal emergency. Fortunately, the pain goes away after a variable period of time – anywhere from 6 to 24 months. In the meantime, your doctor may be able to prescribe treatment to help.

Drugs for distal polyneuropathy

Some simple painkilling drugs like paracetamol can help with the pain. You may need stronger painkillers, like codeine or dihydrocodeine. Non-steroidal anti-inflammatory drugs, like ibuprofen and diclofenac, often don't help much. They can also be dangerous if you have diabetic kidney disease. Other drugs, such as the antidepressants amitriptylene or imipramine, reduce the pain and other discomfort. A cream called capsacin, which is applied to the skin, reduces pain as well. The results of these treatments are variable and seem to work about 60 per cent of the time. However, the longer the pain has been present and the worse the pain, the less likely that these drugs will work.

Some anti-epilepsy drugs have been found to help with the nerve pain of diabetic neuropathy.

Carbamazepine, for instance, can help with shooting pains. A newer drug called gabapentin has been found to work more often than many of the older drugs, but it causes dizziness and sleepiness, which may make treatment more complicated.

A promising study in *Diabetes Care* in October 2002 described the use of a spray of isosorbide dinitrate for the treatment of painful diabetic neuropathy. It was effective in half of the patients treated. Another large trial, this time using alpha lipoic acid, which has to be injected into your vein, was very successful in improving pain and other symptoms. It was reported in *Diabetes Care* in March 2003. Since painful neuropathy is often difficult to treat, these new methods are certainly worth trying.

Polyradiculopathy-diabetic amyotrophy

Polyradiculopathy-diabetic amyotrophy, is a mixture of pain and loss of muscle strength in the muscles of the upper leg, so that the patient cannot straighten the knee. Pain extends down from the hip to the thigh. Polyradiculopathy-diabetic amyotrophy generally has a short course, but may continue for years and doesn't particularly improve with better diabetic control.

Disorders of movement

Neuropathy can affect the nerves to various muscles. The result is a sudden inability to move or use those muscles. Researchers think that these disorders originate as a result of sudden closing of a blood vessel supplying the nerve. What muscles become unusable depends on which nerve (or nerves) is affected. If one of the nerves to the eyeball is damaged, the patient cannot turn her eye to the side that nerve is on. If the nerve to the face is affected, the eyelid may droop or the smile on one side of the face may be flat. The patient can have trouble with vision or problems with hearing. Focusing the eye may not be possible. No treatment really exists, but fortunately the disorder goes away on its own within about three months.

Disorders of automatic (autonomic) nerves

Many movements of muscles are going on all of the time, but we're unaware of them. The heart muscle is squeezing down and relaxing. The diaphragm is rising up to empty the lungs of air and relaxing to draw air in. The oesophagus is carrying food down from the mouth to the stomach. The stomach then pushes it into the small intestine, which pushes it into the large intestine. All these functions of muscles are under the control of nerves from the brain, and diabetic neuropathy can affect all of them. These automatic functions are called the *autonomic nerves*. When sensitive tests are done, as many as 40 per cent of people with diabetes have some form of autonomic neuropathy. Where the problem appears depends on the nerve involved. Some of the areas are

- **Bladder abnormalities, starting with a loss of the sensation of bladder fullness.** The urine is not eliminated, and urinary tract infections result. After a while, loss of bladder contraction occurs, and the patient has to strain to urinate or loses urine by dribbling. The doctor can easily diagnose this abnormality by finding out how much urine is left in the bladder after urinating. The treatment is to remember to urinate every four hours or take a drug that increases the force of bladder contraction.

- **Sexual dysfunction in 50 per cent of males with diabetes and 30 per cent of females with diabetes.** Males cannot sustain an erection, and females have trouble lubricating the vagina for intercourse (see Chapter 6 for more information on these problems).

- **Intestinal abnormalities of various kinds.** The most common abnormality is constipation. If nerves to the stomach are involved, the stomach does not empty on time. Intestinal abnormalities affect a quarter of all patients with diabetes. This can lead to 'brittle' diabetes because the insulin is active when there is no food. Fortunately, a drug called metocloprimide helps to empty the stomach.

- **Involvement of the gall bladder leads to gallstones because it does not empty.** Normally, the gall bladder empties each time you eat, especially if you eat a fatty meal, because the substances in the bile (within the gall bladder) help to break down fat. If disease of the nerve to the gall bladder prevents it from emptying, these same substances form stones.

- **Involvement of the large intestine that can result in diabetic diarrhoea, with as many as ten or more bowel movements in a day.** Accidental loss of bowel contents can occur, and bacteria can grow abnormally in the intestine. This problem responds to antibiotic treatment. Diarrhoea is treated with one of several drugs, which quiets the large intestine.

- **Heart abnormalities from loss of nerves to the heart.** The heart may not respond to exercise by speeding up as it should. The force of the heart may not increase when the patient stands, and the patient then becomes light-headed. A fast, fixed heart rate also may occur, and the rhythm of the heart may not be normal. Such patients are at risk of sudden death.

- **Sweating problems, especially in the feet.** The body may try to compensate for the lack of sweating in the feet by sweating excessively on the face or trunk. Heavy sweating can occur when the patient eats certain foods, such as cheese.

✔ **Abnormalities of the pupil of the eye.** The pupil determines the amount of light that is let in. As a result of the neuropathy, the pupil is small and does not open up in a dark room.

You can see that you can run into all kinds of problems if you develop diabetic neuropathy. None of them need ever bother you, though, if you follow the recommendations in Part III – and the closest you will ever get to a nerve problem will be when you try to get a date with that cute next-door neighbour.

Heart Disease

In this section, you find out about the special problems that diabetes brings to the heart.

Coronary heart disease is the term for the progressive closure of the arteries, which supply blood to the heart muscle. When one or more of your arteries closes completely, the result is a heart attack (*myocardial infarction*). In diabetes, the incidence of coronary heart disease (CHD) is increased even in the young type 1 patient. The length of time with the diabetes promotes CHD in type 1 patients. CHD affects males and females equally.

Type 2 diabetes is different. CHD is the most common reason for death in type 2 patients. In non-diabetics, women are at lower risk of CHD than men before the menopause. This protection against CHD doesn't apply if you are a type 2 diabetic woman. Many other risk factors promote CHD in the type 2 patient. Among them are

✔ High glucose levels (poor glycaemic control)

✔ Hypertension (high blood pressure)

✔ Abnormal blood fats, especially reduced HDL cholesterol and increased triglycerides; The abnormal fats may persist even when blood glucose is well controlled

✔ Increased production of insulin because of the insulin resistance

✔ Obesity

✔ Central adiposity, which refers to the distribution of fat, particularly in your waist area (see the section on 'The metabolic syndrome and CHD' later in this chapter)

✔ Smoking

As with kidney disease and some of the other long-term complications discussed earlier in this chapter, several factors can affect your risk of CHD if you are a type 2 diabetic. The more risk factors you have, the greater your risk of CHD. On the other hand, tackling more than one of your risk factors also cuts your risks much more than tackling just one, so there are greater benefits to be had, too.

The national guidelines in the UK, such as the National Service Frameworks for Coronary Heart Disease and Diabetes, set standards and targets for people at high risk. These are the people who are likely to benefit most from treatments such as tight blood pressure control and lowering of cholesterol. Even if you are otherwise healthy, having diabetes puts you into a high-risk category for CHD. This means that you have various treatments that can cut your risks of CHD dramatically. They include statins and other drugs to reduce your cholesterol; aspirin to cut your risk of heart attack; and blood pressure-reducing drugs, including ACE inhibitors and AIIRAs (see the side-bar 'ACE inhibitors and AIIRAs to the rescue' for details).

If you have diabetes, you are two to four times more likely to get CHD than a person who doesn't have diabetes. Between 2 and 5 per cent of people with type 2 diabetes are diagnosed with CHD every year. To put this risk into per-spective, one study in Finland found that otherwise healthy people with diabetes were just as likely to have a heart attack over a seven-year period as people without diabetes who had already had a heart attack. About half of people with diabetes who have had a heart attack and who do not get treat-ment to cut their risks afterwards, have another heart attack within five years.

The picture is not a pretty one for the person with diabetes who has coro-nary artery disease. If a heart attack occurs, the risk of death is much greater for the person with diabetes. If non-diabetics have a heart attack, they die 15 per cent of the time, but people with diabetes die 40 per cent of the time. The death rate is worse for the person with diabetes who was in poor glucose control before the heart attack. That same poorly controlled person has more complications, such as shock and heart failure, from a heart attack than the person without diabetes. Once a heart attack occurs, the outlook is much worse for the person with diabetes. A second heart attack occurs in 50 per cent (25 per cent without diabetes), and the death rate in five years is much worse (80 per cent versus 25 per cent).

The treatment for CHD is the same for the person with diabetes as it is for the person without diabetes. Therapy can be used to dissolve the clot of blood that is obstructing the coronary artery, but people with diabetes do not do as well with angioplasty, the technique by which a tube is placed into the artery to clean it out and open it up.

People with diabetes do as well with surgery to bypass the obstruction (called bypass surgery) as do those without diabetes, but the long-term prog-nosis for keeping the graft open is not as good.

If you have type 2 diabetes, you are more likely to die from CHD than from any other condition. Cerebrovascular disease (such as strokes and transient ischaemic attacks, or TIAs, which produce the same symptoms as strokes but where the symptoms and signs recover within 24 hours) is the second commonest cause of death. Although you can reduce your risks of getting these conditions by tight glucose control, the benefits from keeping hypertension and raised cholesterol tightly controlled are even greater.

If having diabetes increases your risks of CHD more than the risk of someone who doesn't have diabetes, reducing your risks means that you can cut your absolute risk of CHD much more than someone without diabetes, too. The latest Joint British Societies guidance on reducing cholesterol, which came out in December 2005, suggests that you should be taking a statin to improve your cholesterol if you have diabetes and:

- ✔ you're over 40
- ✔ you're 18–39 years old and you have any other risk factor, including:

  - features of the metabolic syndrome (see the section below)

  - cholesterol over 6.0 mmol/l

  - raised blood pressure needing treatment with medication

  - retinopathy (see earlier in this chapter)

  - nephropathy (including microalbuminuria; see earlier in this chapter)

  - haemoglobin A1c over 9 per cent or

  - a family history of premature CHD or stroke

The metabolic syndrome and CHD

The earliest abnormality in type 2 diabetes is insulin resistance, which is found in people even before diabetes can be diagnosed. Basically, it means that your body becomes resistant to the effects of insulin, and finds it increasingly difficult over time to keep your blood sugar down to a normal level. When insulin resistance is found in combination with other risk factors, it's called the metabolic syndrome. The same combination used to be known as insulin resistance syndrome. About 1 in 4 adults in the UK has the metabolic syndrome, and while not all of them have diabetes now, many or even most of them will go on to develop it unless they do some serious work to improve their lifestyle.

The International Diabetes Federation has come up with a definition of the metabolic syndrome that involves having at least three of the risk factors in Table 5-1. Each of them on their own increases the risk of CHD; add them together, and they more than triple your risk of CHD compared to someone who doesn't have them.

Table 5-1	Definition of the Metabolic Syndrome
Abdominal obesity (waist >90 centimetres in males, >84 centimetres in females if European, less if Asian)	
Together with at least two of:	
raised triglycerides ≥1.7 mmol/l	
low HDL cholesterol, <1.04 mmol/l in males and <1.29 mmol/l in females	
blood pressure ≥130/85 mmHg	
fasting hyperglycaemia (fasting glucose ≥5.6 mmol/l) or previous diagnosis of diabetes or impaired glucose tolerance	

Source: International Diabetes Federation, 2005

Why do these factors add up to such a potentially lethal combination? Well, the problem is largely down to abdominal obesity, that big midriff, or being an 'apple' rather than a 'pear' shape. The 'visceral fat' that accumulates inside your abdomen is far more than merely unsightly, it's actually metabolically active, changing the proportions of cholesterol and clotting factors circulating in your system. It's different from subcutanous fat (the kind of fat under the skin – the kind where you 'pinch an inch'). Fortunately, by losing just 10 per cent of your body weight, you can cut this visceral fat by a massive 30 per cent.

Consider the following:

✔ **Hypertension:** This problem may be caused by the increased insulin required to keep the glucose normal when there is insulin resistance. When people are given insulin to control the glucose, a rise in blood pressure often occurs. You can find out more about hypertension in Chapter 7.

✔ **Abnormalities of blood fats:** Metabolic syndrome is associated with an increase in triglycerides, a type of fat that makes it easier for your arteries to get completely clogged; and a decline in the amount of *HDL (high-density lipoprotein),* the 'good' cholesterol particle that helps to clean out the arteries.

People who have metabolic syndrome often also have other indications that they're at higher risk of CHD:

✔ **Increased plasminogen activator inhibitor-1:** This chemical, which blocks the activity of plasminogen activator, prevents the breakdown of blood clots that form in the arteries of the heart and other areas.

✔ **Microalbuminuria:** This strongly correlates with the development of coronary artery disease.

✔ **C-reactive protein:** This marker for inflammation in the body (easily obtained by a blood test) rises as the severity of the metabolic syndrome increases. It indicates that inflammation plays an important role. The presence of inflammatory factors in the blood that come from fat tissue and increase production of fats while they block glucose metabolism confirms the significant role of inflammation, as do inflammatory cells that promote atherosclerosis in the arteries.

Each of the risk factors in the metabolic syndrome increases your risk of CHD. If you have several of these risk factors, keep in mind that they may act synergistically. This means that the size of your risk if you have several risk factors is greater than you can expect by just adding the individual risk factors up. That makes it all the more important to look at tackling all of these risk factors at the same time.

A number of treatments are available for the metabolic syndrome. If you are obese and have a sedentary lifestyle, you can make a huge difference by working on these problems. It does not take a lot of weight loss or exercise to make a major contribution towards cutting the risk of a heart attack.

You can treat raised triglyceride and reduced HDL cholesterol with drugs such as statins. The thiazolidendione drugs (glitazones) – a new class of drugs of which rosiglitazone and pioglitazone are the only ones currently available in the United Kingdom (see Chapter 10) – directly attack insulin resistance. People with diabetes and non-diabetics with the features of the metabolic syndrome may find these drugs useful in the future.

Cardiac autonomic neuropathy

We discuss cardiac autonomic neuropathy briefly in the section on neuropathy, earlier in this chapter. Basically, the heart is under the control of nerves, and high glucose levels can damage these nerves. There are a number of ways to test for this:

✔ **Measure the resting heart rate.** It may be abnormally high (greater than 100).

✔ **Measure the standing blood pressure.** It may fall abnormally low (a decrease of 20 mmHg, or millimetres of mercury, which is the measure used in blood pressure machines, sustained for three minutes).

✔ **Measure the variation in heart rate when the patient breathes in compared to breathing out.** It may be abnormally low (under 10).

The presence of cardiac autonomic neuropathy makes survival rates worse even when no coronary artery disease is present.

Cardiomyopathy

Cardiomyopathy refers to an enlarged heart and scarring of the heart muscle in the absence of CHD. The heart does not pump enough blood with each stroke. The patient may be able to compensate by a more rapid heart rate, but if hypertension is present, a stable condition can deteriorate.

The key treatment in this condition is control of the blood pressure as well as control of the blood glucose. Studies in animals have shown healing with control of the blood glucose.

Diabetic Blood Vessel Disease Away from the Heart

The same processes that affect the coronary arteries can affect the arteries to the brain, producing *cerebrovascular disease*. The same applies to the arteries that supply blood to the rest of the body, producing *peripheral arterial disease*.

Peripheral arterial disease

Peripheral arterial disease (PAD) occurs much earlier in people with diabetes and proceeds more rapidly than it does in non-diabetic people. The clogging of the arteries results in loss of pulses in the feet so that, after ten years of diabetes, a third of men and women no longer feel a pulse in their feet. The most common symptom is intermittent pain in the calves, thighs, or buttocks that begins after some walking and ends with rest. The distance you can walk before the pain comes on is usually fairly predictable for you, although it's likely to be shorter if you're walking uphill or into the wind. People with PAD also have a reduction in life expectancy. When PAD occurs, it is much worse in people with diabetes who have much greater involvement of arteries, just as in the heart. Many risk factors increase the severity of PAD. The following risk factors are unavoidable:

- ✔ **Genetic factors:** PAD is more common in some families and certain ethnic groups.
- ✔ **Age:** The risk of PAD increases as you age.
- ✔ **Diabetes:** The condition certainly makes PAD much worse.

You can address the following risk factors with some success:

- ✔ **Smoking,** which is the single biggest risk factor for PAD. It clearly promotes early amputation, but you *can* stop if you really want to! See the section on smoking at the end of this chapter.

- ✔ **High cholesterol,** which makes PAD worse, and which can be treated with diet and statins, or other drugs.

- ✔ **High glucose,** which you can control.

- ✔ **Hypertension,** which you can control with pills if necessary.

- ✔ **Obesity,** which you can control.

Besides controlling the preceding factors as much as possible, some drugs help prevent closure of the artery and loss of blood supply. Aspirin, which inhibits clotting, is among the most useful. In addition, exercise improves blood flow and promotes the development of blood vessels around an obstruction. When none of this reverses the symptoms, some form of surgery that opens or bypasses the blocked arteries may be necessary.

Cerebrovascular disease

Cerebrovascular disease (CVD) is disease of the arteries that supply the brain with oxygen and nutrients. The risk factors and the approach to treatment of CVD are similar to those used for PAD (peripheral arterial disease, explained in the preceding section). However, the symptoms are very different because the clogged arteries in CVD supply the brain. If a temporary reduction in blood supply to the brain occurs, the person suffers from a *transient ischaemic attack,* or TIA. This temporary loss of brain function may present itself as slurring of speech, weakness on one side of the body, or numbness. TIA may disappear after a few minutes, but may come back again some hours to days later. If a major artery to the brain completely closes, the person suffers a stroke. Fortunately, stroke victims who are seen soon enough after the stroke can take advantage of clot-dissolving materials.

People with diabetes are at increased risk for CVD just as they are for PAD. Their disease tends to be worse than it is for the non-diabetic, and they can have blockages in many small blood vessels in the brain. These multiple blockages lead to loss of intellectual function, which is similar to Alzheimer's disease.

The treatable risk factors for CVD are the same as those for PAD (see the preceding section). You should make attempts to improve them.

Diabetic Foot Disease

If we ever have an opportunity to save people from the consequences of diabetes, that opportunity lies in this section of the book. Without careful foot care and diabetic control, diabetics are between 15 and 70 times more likely than non-diabetics to need an amputation. But if you learn to take good care of your feet, you should be able to cut your risks of amputation by an astonishing 85 per cent. Of course, this care requires lots of commitment and attention to the other risk factors that cause diabetic foot problems in the first place. But the risk factors for diabetic foot disease are, on the whole, the same as the risk factors for other complications of diabetes. That means that by taking care of your feet, you can benefit the rest of your body as well.

Look through the list of risk factors below, for instance, and see how many of them you recognise:

- ✔ **Poor glycaemic control:** High blood sugar over a long period can affect your feet in a number of ways. It reduces the mobility of your joints; it leads to abnormal pressures on your feet, which in turn cause foot ulcers; it increases the formation of hard skin, or callus, which can also lead to ulcers; and it increases your risk of neuropathy.

- ✔ **Smoking:** Smoking dramatically increases your risk of peripheral arterial disease, which affects the blood circulation to your feet before affecting you anywhere else.

- ✔ **Hypertension:** Hypertension increases your risk of peripheral arterial disease by 500 per cent.

- ✔ **Raised cholesterol:** Raised levels of 'bad' cholesterol in your blood clog up your arteries, leading to peripheral arterial disease.

- ✔ **Lack of exercise:** Exercise helps the blood in your legs circulate and can stimulate your body to produce new blood vessels if old ones are clogged by peripheral arterial disease. Of course, you need to protect your feet while you are exercising, especially if your sensation is reduced. You can read more about this in this section and in Chapter 7.

Staving off problems: Preventive measures

Your doctor should check your feet every time you see her, which should be about every three to six months. You, on the other hand, have a chance to check your feet every single day. That puts you in a perfect position to spot and deal with changes before they become problems. Talk to your GP or practice nurse about the chiropody service in your area. You do have a right to regular chiropody if you have problems looking after your own feet. If you are housebound, you can use a home visiting service, which is available all over the country. Some areas also have a direct-access chiropody service, where you can refer yourself if you notice a new change.

Even if you don't have any evidence of neuropathy or peripheral arterial disease, still get into the habit of checking your feet daily. That way, you're able to stop problems before they start. Besides, being in the habit of checking your feet daily makes it that much easier to remember to check your feet carefully if you do get problems.

If you have diminished sensation, some of the following ideas may save your feet:

- ✔ Change your shoes about every five hours. If your shoes are new, change them every two hours at first. Consider getting cushioned shoes – such as a decent pair of trainers.

- ✔ Pay attention to how your shoes fit. Your shoes shouldn't be too tight or too loose.

  Talk to your general practitioner, nurse, or chiropodist about specially fitted footwear. You may be able to get a referral to a hospital *orthotist* (a specialist fitter) who can make specially fitted shoes for you if you're at high risk.

- ✔ Never walk barefoot, and shake out your shoes before you put them on.

- ✔ Inspect your feet daily, and get medical help straight away if you notice an ulcer forming.

- ✔ Do not use a heating pad on your feet.

- ✔ Stop smoking. If you smoke, you're just asking for an amputation.

Insist on seeing a healthcare professional without delay if you have any anxieties. Don't risk going to the bottom of a six-month waiting list. If you don't have an immediate self-access chiropody clinic, talk to your general practitioner or practice nurse.

Amputations in diabetics are more amenable to preventive treatment than any other diabetic complication. Best of all, much of the prevention doesn't need tablets or blood tests. It just needs you to be aware of the disastrous results of ignoring your feet, and to think about foot care every day.

Remedies and treatments

If your feet are dry, you may have loss of sweating. Loss of sweating is usually accompanied by loss of touch sensation and development of ulcers. You need to moisturise your feet, first by soaking them in water, which you test with your hand for its temperature, and then by drying them with a towel and applying a moisturiser.

Ulcers of the foot can develop in a number of ways:

✔ Constant pressure

✔ Sudden higher pressure

✔ Constantly repeated moderate pressure

It takes very little pressure constantly applied to damage the skin. If you do develop an ulcer, the treatment is to take pressure off the site by resting the foot and elevating it. Once the infection is localised in a foot with adequate blood supply, a plaster cast is applied to overcome the natural tendency of everyone to stand or do some other walking. The cast protects the ulcer from the slight trauma necessary to prevent healing.

District nurses carry out most ulcer treatment in the United Kingdom, often at specialist ulcer clinics. If you can't get to them, they can visit you regularly at home to dress your ulcer.

Skin Disease in Diabetes

Many conditions involve the skin and are unique to the person with diabetes because of the treatment and complications of the disease. The most common and important complications include the following:

✔ Bruises due to cutting of blood vessels by the insulin needle.

✔ *Vitiligo* (loss of skin pigmentation) is part of the autoimmune aspect of type 1 diabetes and can't be prevented.

✔ In *necrobiosis lipoidica,* you have patches of reddish-brown skin on the shins or ankles, and the skin becomes thin and can ulcerate. Females tend to have this condition more often than males. Steroid injections are used, and the areas eventually become depressed and brown.

✔ *Xanthelasma,* which are small yellow flat areas called *plaques* on the eyelids, and can occur even when cholesterol is not raised.

✔ For unknown reasons, *alopecia,* or loss of hair, can occur in type 1 diabetes.

✔ *Insulin hypertrophy* is the accumulation of fatty tissue where insulin is injected. This normal action of insulin is prevented by moving the injection site around.

✔ *Insulin lipoatrophy* is loss of fat where the insulin is injected. Although the cause is unknown, the condition is rarely seen now that human insulin has replaced beef and pork insulin.

✔ Dry skin, which is a consequence of diabetic neuropathy, leads to a lack of sweating.

✔ Fungal infections can occur under the nails or between the toes. Fungus likes moisture and elevated glucose. Lowering the glucose and keeping the toes dry prevents these infections. Medication may cure this problem, but it recurs if you don't continue to manage your glucose and moisture.

✔ *Acanthosis nigricans,* a velvety-feeling increase in pigmentation on the back of the neck and the armpits, causes no problems and needs no treatment. It is usually found when hyperinsulinaemia (high circulating levels of insulin in the blood) and insulin resistance exist. It is seen in children with type 2 diabetes.

✔ Diabetic thick skin, which is thicker than normal skin, occurs in those who have had diabetes for more than ten years.

How high glucose leads to complications

Although doctors aren't certain about the causes of most long-term complications, we mention the current theories about the causes of the problems as we explain each complication in the following sections of this chapter. But all long-term complications share several common characteristics, described in the following list:

✔ Advanced glycated end products (AGEs) are one of the substances that damage tissues. AGEs can damage the eyes, the kidneys, the nervous system, and other organs in your body. You always have glucose in your blood, and some of that glucose attaches to other substances in your bloodstream to form glycated (glucose-attached) products. In this way, haemoglobin, which carries oxygen through your blood to cells and tissues throughout your body, attaches to glucose to form haemoglobin A1c. Albumin, a protein in blood, forms glycated albumin. Glucose can attach to red blood cells and white blood cells as well as to other cells and molecules in the bloodstream. When these normal body substances attach to glucose, they no longer work normally.

✔ When glucose attaches to other substances and cells, it alters their functions, usually in a negative fashion. For example, haemoglobin A1c holds on to oxygen more strongly than haemoglobin, so the cells that need oxygen don't get it as easily. Red blood cells that are glycated do not last as long in your blood circulation. Glycated white blood cells can't fight infection as well as unglycated white cells can.

✔ Your body handles a certain level of glycated substances. But when your blood glucose is elevated for prolonged periods of time, the level of glycated cells and substances becomes excessive, and the complications we describe in this chapter result.

✔ The polyol pathway is another major source of damage to the body in diabetes. The polyol pathway refers to one direction, or pathway, that glucose can take as it is metabolised (broken down). For example, the common pathway is to form carbon dioxide and water as energy is produced. When you have a lot of glucose in your blood, an abnormal amount is metabolised to become a product called sorbitol. Sorbitol is a member of a class of substances called polyols. Sorbitol accumulates in many tissues, where it can damage them by swelling or by chemical reactions.

Smoking and diabetes

Smoking has a number of effects on people without diabetes, but the effects have been found to be even worse in people with diabetes. Among other things, smoking

✔ Reduces blood flow in arteries and blocks increased flow when it is needed

✔ Increases pain in the legs in people with PAD and in the heart in people with coronary artery disease

✔ Increases *atheromatous plaques,* the changes in arteries in the heart and other areas like the brain and the legs that precede closing of the blood vessels

✔ Increases clustering of platelets, the blood elements that form a plug or clot that blocks the artery

✔ Increases blood pressure, which also worsens atheromatous plaques

These problems don't even take into account the effects of smoking on the lungs, the bladder, and the rest of the body.

One of the targets of the National Service Framework for Coronary Heart Disease was that all areas of the country should set up specialised smoking-cessation clinics. Your general practitioner or practice nurse can give you the details of how to refer yourself to your local clinic. Here you can get advice, support from trained professionals, and nicotine replacement therapies (patches, gum, etc.) to help overcome your cravings. You'll be able to take part in regular self-help groups with other would-be quitters. The evidence is that even if you have failed before in your attempts to quit, the support these clinics offer can greatly improve your chances of stopping, and of staying an ex-smoker. What are you waiting for?

Chapter 6

Diabetes, Sexual Function, and Pregnancy

In This Chapter

▶ Coping with diabetes in pregnancy

▶ The baby in a diabetic pregnancy

▶ Treating impotence

▶ Dealing with female sexual problems

*N*othing is quite so pleasant as walking into the hospital room of a mother with diabetes who is holding her healthy newborn. Perhaps even slightly more pleasant is the knowledge that you have contributed in some way to this outcome. Pregnancy associated with diabetes used to be a disaster for the baby and the mother – no longer. With the proper precautions, the diabetic pregnancy can proceed like a pregnancy without diabetes. This chapter describes everything you need to know to enjoy a healthy pregnancy and deliver a healthy baby.

And, of course, sexual intercourse remains the starting point for most babies. People with diabetes – both male and female – have some problems with this part of the experience of having a baby. This chapter also covers these problems.

Pregnancy and Diabetes

Pregnancy in a mother with diabetes is definitely more complicated than in a mother without. For this reason, specialist centres around the country employ the latest techniques and equipment, and knowledgeable healthcare workers are available.

If you have diabetes and want to become pregnant, you need to confer with your general practitioner, or with an expert in pregnancy and diabetes, before you conceive.

About 0.35 per cent of pregnancies occur in women with pre-existing diabetes, called *pre-gestational diabetes*. An additional 2 to 4 per cent occur in women who develop diabetes some time in the second half of the pregnancy. This type of diabetes is called *gestational diabetes.* About 365,000 births occur every year in the United Kingdom, and 7,500–15,000 women will be affected by diabetes during their pregnancy. So you're not alone.

Which kind of diabetes do you have? You can find this out in Chapter 3. The sort of treatment you need depends partly on what kind of diabetes you have and partly on how well controlled your diabetes is:

- ✔ **If you have type 1 diabetes,** you need to carry on taking insulin, although the amount you need may change during pregnancy.

- ✔ **If you have type 2 diabetes** (and had it before you became pregnant), you need to stop taking tablets and change to insulin treatment as soon as you find out you're pregnant. However, you should be able to go back to using tablets after you have your baby and finish breastfeeding.

- ✔ **If you have gestational diabetes** (which develops in the later part of your pregnancy), you may need to make changes to your diet. If you need drug treatment as well, you start on insulin injections (your general practitioner or specialist can advise on this). You should be able to stop these almost immediately after you have your baby.

Preventing problems when you have pre-gestational diabetes

If you were diagnosed as diabetic before you became pregnant, you can take a number of steps to prevent problems arising during your pregnancy.

Mums-to-be with type 1 diabetes

In a non-diabetic pregnancy, the body makes enough insulin to overcome the effect of pregnancy hormones (which block insulin action), and the blood glucose stays normal. If you have type 1 diabetes, you can't make more insulin and need two or three times the usual dose. The increasing need for insulin usually stabilises in the last several weeks of the pregnancy, and by the last one or two weeks, you may begin to have hypoglycaemia (see Chapter 4). Once you have delivered the baby, your insulin needs plummet immediately.

If you have type 1 diabetes, you may have retinopathy before you get pregnant (see Chapter 5). If the condition is severe, your eyesight may deteriorate during the pregnancy. This deterioration is probably the result of rapid improvement of the blood glucose after less than ideal blood glucose levels before pregnancy. Once you have delivered the baby, your eyes return to their previous state.

Children of mothers who smoke during their pregnancy are at much greater risk of developing obesity and diabetes in later life. However, a study in *Diabetes Care* in November 2003 did not find an increase in gestational diabetes or pre-gestational diabetes among women who smoked.

Nephropathy (another name for kidney disease; see Chapter 5) increases the risks during pregnancy for both you and your baby. Severe, permanent worsening of nephropathy is unusual, but a temporary decline in kidney function may occur.

If you have type 1 diabetes, you must take action in advance to avoid problems during your pregnancy, by controlling your glucose before conception (see Part III for more on how to manage your diabetes). In addition, you need to monitor your diet after you become pregnant. See the section 'Coping with diabetes and pregnancy' later in this chapter for more information.

Mums-to-be with type 2 diabetes

If you have type 2 diabetes, you, like women with type 1 diabetes, need to take precautions to control your glucose before you conceive.

If you are on oral agents to lower glucose, you will need to stop them and use insulin to control the glucose instead. In addition, obesity, a frequent finding in type 2 diabetes, puts you at greater risk for high blood pressure during the pregnancy. If you have type 2 diabetes, just as if you have type 1 diabetes, you must talk to your doctor before you get pregnant. You want to work with your doctor to make sure your diabetes is as well controlled as it possibly can be, before you start trying to get pregnant. You also have to be monitored more closely during your pregnancy than you would be if you didn't have diabetes.

Most type 2 pregnancies can be allowed to go to term at 39 weeks, but if you have a history of hypertension or a previous history of delivery that wasn't normal, you may be advised to have an earlier delivery (your general practitioner or specialist should be able to advise you on this).

Diagnosing gestational diabetes

Deciding which women have gestational diabetes is not as simple as you may expect. This is because in a normal, non-diabetic pregnancy, the fasting plasma glucose level falls, while the level two hours after an oral glucose tolerance test rises. The normal levels also change during pregnancy, so the same woman, who doesn't have diabetes, might have different results in different trimesters.

As a result, there is no absolute consensus on what level of glucose you need to have for your doctor to make a diagnosis of gestational diabetes. When doubt exists, the final decision is left to the doctor. The World Health

Organisation's values are fairly widely accepted in the United Kingdom. According to this organisation, gestational diabetes should include all women who would previously have been diagnosed as having gestational impaired glucose tolerance, as well as gestational diabetes. This is tested with a 75 gram dose of oral glucose. Impaired glucose tolerance is diagnosed if the blood glucose two hours later is over 7.8 mmol/l, but below 11.1 mmol/l. Diabetes is diagnosed if the blood glucose level two hours later is over 11.1 mmol/l. You can find out more details about this in Chapter 2.

Should all pregnant women who don't already have diabetes be checked for it? Some experts advocate selective screening, suggesting that a thin pregnant woman with no family history of diabetes who is physically active is an unlikely candidate for diabetes. At the moment, however, most healthcare professionals providing antenatal care in the United Kingdom check your urine for glucose at every antenatal appointment. If sugar is found in your urine, your doctor checks your plasma glucose. Some hospitals routinely do a glucose tolerance test at about 28 weeks. (If gestational diabetes was present in a previous pregnancy, the screening test is done as early as the 13th week.) If you have had gestational diabetes in a previous pregnancy, you are treated as if you have gestational diabetes in all future pregnancies. If you haven't had any kind of diabetes diagnosed in the past, everyone agrees that if the glucose tolerance is normal in weeks 27 to 31 of the pregnancy, you don't need to do more screening.

If the newborn's father is the one with diabetes, the newborn develops normally. The potential for the baby to develop later problems, such as congenital deformities or even stillbirth, only apply if the mother has diabetes. The environment in which the foetus is developing is responsible for the potential abnormalities in the baby. Elevated blood glucose, along with abnormalities of proteins and fats that result from the elevated glucose, and the loss of sensitivity to insulin, explain the problems.

Glucose levels during pregnancy

In addition to controlling your glucose levels before conceiving, a pre-gestational woman with diabetes needs to

- ✔ Discontinue prescription drugs that harm a foetus
- ✔ Have her eyes and kidneys evaluated to establish a baseline for future damage control
- ✔ Stop tobacco and alcohol use

If you are a pre-gestational woman with diabetes, you need to achieve a stricter level of control during pregnancy than when you aren't pregnant. Your foetus is removing glucose from you at a rapid rate, so your blood glucose level is lower than usual. In addition, your body turns to fat for fuel much sooner, so you produce ketones (the breakdown products of fat – refer to Chapter 4 for more details) earlier. Too many ketones can damage the foetus as well. The fact that you break down fat so early is termed *accelerated starvation.*

In order to maintain your blood glucose at the proper level, you must measure it more frequently. Measure it before meals, at bedtime, and occasionally one hour after eating. Your goal is to achieve the levels of blood glucose listed in the following:

Fasting and Pre-meal	*1 Hour After*	*2 Hours After*
4–6 mmol/l	Under 8.3 mmol/l	Under 7 mmol/l

Studies have shown recently that the one-hour-after-meal glucose level may be the most important to keep under control. Although you can deliver insulin in other ways besides a syringe and needle (see Chapter 10), several studies indicate that the syringe-and-needle method is as effective as any other for the pregnant woman with diabetes.

You also need to check for ketones in the urine before breakfast and before supper. You can do so by placing a test strip in the stream of urine. The strip indicates whether ketones are present. If the test strip is positive, you are not eating enough carbohydrates, and your body is going into accelerated starvation. Too much of this condition is not good for the growing foetus.

Weight and diet during pregnancy

Your appropriate amount of weight gain depends on your weight at the time you become pregnant. Your BMI determines your weight gain. You need to work out your BMI (see Chapter 3 if you're not sure how to do this calculation). If your BMI is normal, you should gain 25 to 35 pounds (11.5–16 kilograms) during the pregnancy. However, if you are overweight, then you need to gain less weight through the pregnancy. You can work out your recommended weight gain in pregnancy by plugging your BMI into Table 6-1.

Table 6-1	Recommended Weight Gain in Pregnancy
BMI (kg/m²)	*Recommended Weight Gain (kg)*
20–26	11.5–16
26–29	7.0–11.5
Over 29	Less than 6

Chapter 8 tells you what you need to know about diet and diabetes, but pregnant women with diabetes have some special requirements:

- ✔ **Your daily food intake should be 35 to 38 kilocalories (rather than calories, which is an incorrect term) per kilogram of ideal body weight (IBW).** You can use your height to determine your ideal body weight. As a woman, you should weigh 7 stone if you are 5 feet tall and add 5 pounds for every inch over 5 feet you are. For example, a 5-foot, 4-inch woman should weigh 8 stone 8 pounds, ideally (and approximately because we are really talking about a range, not a single weight). You then change that figure to kilograms by dividing the pounds by 2.2. Then multiply that number by 35 to get the low end of the daily calorie intake and by 38 to get the high end. So, if you weigh 8 stone 8 pounds, you weigh 54.6 kilograms. Your daily food intake should then be between 1,900 and 2,100 kilocalories.

- ✔ **Your protein intake should be 1.5 to 2 grams per kilogram of IBW.** The woman with an IBW of 54.6 should eat about 110 grams of protein daily. Because each gram of protein contains four kilocalories, protein takes up about 440 of the 2,100 daily kilocalories.

- ✔ **Your carbohydrate intake should be 50 to 55 per cent of the approximately 2,000 daily kilocalories, which works out to be about 1,000 kilocalories of carbohydrate.** Because each gram of carbohydrate has 4 kilocalories, just like protein, this amounts to 250 grams of carbohydrate.

- ✔ **Your fat intake should be less than 30 per cent of the total daily 2,000 kilocalories, which amounts to 630 kilocalories of fat.** Because fat contains 9 kilocalories per gram, this equals 70 grams of fat a day.

- ✔ **You should eat three meals a day plus a bedtime snack.** This meal schedule helps prevent the accelerated starvation that results from a prolonged fast between supper and breakfast.

- ✔ **You should maintain your fasting and pre-meal glucose between 4 and 6 mmol/l.** Your glucose should be less than 7.7–8.3 mmol/l one hour after meals.

Why macrosomia occurs

Macrosomia, or an abnormally large foetus, has to do with the elevated glucose, fat, and amino acid levels in the mother in the second half of pregnancy. If these levels aren't lowered, the foetus is exposed to high levels. This stimulates the foetal pancreas to begin to make insulin earlier and to store these extra nutrients. The foetus becomes large wherever fat is stored, such as the shoulders, chest, abdomen, and arms and legs. Because they are large, these macrosomic babies are delivered early in order to make the delivery easier and avoid birth trauma. However, though they are large, they are not fully mature. This puts them at risk of problems with their breathing.

We know that these calculations are very detailed, and that you (like us!) may find them a bit complicated. Head to Chapter 8 for some simple, practical tips on how to eat healthily with diabetes.

In addition, you can use a good multivitamin and mineral preparation. A moderate amount of exercise is also very helpful in controlling the blood glucose and keeping you in top shape during your pregnancy.

Coping with diabetes and pregnancy

If you develop gestational diabetes or already have pre-gestational diabetes, a whole new group of important considerations arises that you need to be aware of in order to deliver a healthy baby and maintain your health.

Early pregnancy problems

If you already have diabetes before you conceive, your major concern is to be under good blood glucose control when you do get pregnant. Both miscarriages and congenital malformations are a result of poor glucose control at conception and shortly thereafter. Most of the congenital abnormalities happen in the very early stages of pregnancy, between five and nine weeks, sometimes before the woman even knows she is pregnant. This is why it is so important to be in the best possible shape before you even try to conceive. (For more on managing diabetes, see Part III.)

When you try to get really tight control of your blood glucose, you may be at slightly higher risk of hypoglycaemic episodes, or 'hypos' (see Chapter 4 for more about hypoglycaemia). This is especially likely in the early stages of your pregnancy. Most hypos won't do your baby any harm.

Folic acid tablets and blood tests

Taking a single tablet of folic acid (400 micrograms) a day from a month before you intend to conceive until 12 weeks into your pregnancy can reduce your risk of having a baby with spina bifida (a spinal cord abnormality) by up to 75 per cent. You also want to have a blood test before you get pregnant to check whether you're immune to rubella (German measles).

This condition is relatively harmless if you aren't pregnant, but it can cause very severe deformities in your baby if you catch rubella in the early weeks of pregnancy. Even if you've already had rubella or have been vaccinated against it, get a blood test anyway. A few women aren't fully protected against the disease even though they've been vaccinated.

If you have gestational diabetes, you don't have to worry about your baby having congenital malformations more often than babies whose mothers don't have diabetes. This is because your blood glucose did not start to rise until halfway through the pregnancy, long after the baby's important body structures were formed. (Another major reason that more babies aren't born with congenital malformations may be that a woman in poor control of her diabetes has more trouble conceiving a baby than does a woman whose diabetes is well controlled.)

Late pregnancy problems

Both the pre-gestational and gestational woman with diabetes needs to be concerned about a large baby. A baby is considered large if it weighs more than 4.5 kilograms or 9.9 pounds at birth. In large babies born to women without diabetes, the growth is proportional throughout the pregnancy, so that the baby's shoulders aren't out of proportion to their heads, and delivery is not complicated. But in children born to women who have diabetes, this largeness is not proportional. The areas that are most responsive to insulin, where fat is stored in the baby, are the ones that enlarge the most.

A high blood glucose left untreated has major consequences for you and your baby. If present early in the pregnancy, the result may be congenital malformations (physical abnormalities that may be life threatening) in the foetus. In the third trimester, the growing foetus may exhibit macrosomia (abnormal largeness) that can lead to a too early delivery or damage to the baby or mother during delivery.

After the pregnancy

Gestational diabetes usually disappears with the end of the pregnancy. However, if you develop gestational diabetes during pregnancy, you are at much higher risk for later development of diabetes. If your fasting blood glucose is greater than 7 mmol/l during the pregnancy, the risk of developing diabetes later in life is as much as 75 to 90 per cent. You need to have a test for glucose tolerance between 6 and 12 weeks after the pregnancy and annually after that if diabetes is not found.

If you have had gestational diabetes, several factors predispose you to develop diabetes later on. Some factors cannot be changed and include

- ✔ **Ethnic origin:** Certain ethnic groups, such as South Asians and Afro-Caribbeans, are at a higher risk.
- ✔ **Pre-pregnancy weight:** Those with a higher pre-pregnancy weight are at a greater risk.

- ✔ **Age:** Pregnancies later in life triple the risk of permanent diabetes.

- ✔ **Number of pregnancies:** The more pregnancies you have, the higher your risk.

- ✔ **Family history of diabetes:** If a family history is present, you are at a higher risk.

- ✔ **Severity of blood glucose during pregnancy:** Higher blood glucose levels mean a higher risk.

On the other hand, you can change or modify several factors to decrease your chances of developing diabetes later:

- ✔ **Future weight gain:** Gain less weight in future pregnancies.

- ✔ **Future pregnancies:** Have fewer children.

- ✔ **Physical activity:** Increase your activity.

- ✔ **Dietary fat:** Limit the fat in your diet.

- ✔ **Smoking and certain drugs:** Stop smoking and using drugs.

Women who have had gestational diabetes can use oral contraceptives with low levels of oestrogen and progesterone to prevent conception. These drugs, along with hormonal replacement therapy after menopause, do not increase your risk of later diabetes. They may, in fact, decrease the risk and decrease blood glucose levels in those who have diabetes already. Women with both type 1 and type 2 diabetes can use the same preparations.

The story is similar for postmenopausal women. A recent study in *Diabetes Care* in October 2003 showed that use of oestrogen by women with diabetes – with or without progesterone – resulted in a decrease in coronary heart disease in these patients. Oestrogen and progesterone are the hormones used in hormone replacement therapy, or HRT. Since women with diabetes are at very high risk for coronary heart disease, this is an important finding. However, other health risks (such as a possible rise in breast cancer) associated with HRT exist, especially when HRT is taken for more than 2 or 3 years. Talk to your doctor about the relative risks and benefits for you.

Another large study reported that women on hormone replacement therapy have better control of their blood glucose than those not on such treatment. This was reported in *Diabetes Care* in July 2001.

If you are breastfeeding, you need about 300 extra kilocalories above your usual needs. You cannot take oral agents for diabetes because these pass through the milk into the baby.

Measuring the risks

The haemoglobin A1c is an excellent measurement of overall glucose control and provides a good indicator of the risk of miscarriage. If it is high, it indicates that the diabetic woman was in poor control at conception, and the likelihood of a miscarriage is greater. If overall glucose control is normal, a woman with diabetes is no more likely to miscarry than a woman without diabetes.

The situation for congenital malformations is a little more complicated. These malformations increase with increasing glucose levels, as well as with the level of *ketones,* the breakdown product of fats. Measuring the ketones, however, doesn't tell you whether malformations will definitely occur.

The baby in a diabetic pregnancy

Research into diabetes during pregnancy has resulted in a great reduction in malformations in babies, as well as the macrosomia (abnormal largeness) that leads to complications at delivery. Unfortunately, many diabetic women do not have control of their diabetes at conception, so malformations still occur. If an obvious malformation is present at birth, it is important to search for other malformations.

The foetus produces a lot of insulin to handle all the maternal glucose entering through the placenta. Maternal glucose is cut off suddenly at delivery, but the high level of foetal insulin continues for a while. The danger of hypoglycaemia (explained in Chapter 4) exists in the first four to six hours after delivery. The baby may be sweaty and appear nervous or even have a seizure. It is necessary to do a blood glucose test on the baby hourly until it is stable, and at intervals for the first 24 hours.

Besides hypoglycaemia, the baby may have several other complications right after birth:

- **Respiratory distress syndrome:** This breathing problem occurs when the baby is delivered early, but it responds to treatment. Respiratory distress syndrome is rare with good prenatal care.

- **Low calcium with jitteriness and possibly seizures:** Calcium needs to be given to the baby until its own body can take over. Low calcium is usually a result of prematurity.

- **Low magnesium:** This produces the same symptoms as low calcium and is also a result of prematurity.

- **Polycythaemia:** This condition, where too many red blood cells exist, occurs for unknown reasons. Blood is removed from the baby. How much blood is removed depends on how much extra blood is present.

✔ **Hyperbilirubinaemia:** This condition is the product of too much breakdown of red blood cells. It is treated by placing your baby under a special kind of light for a few hours at a time.

✔ **Lazy left colon:** Occurring for unknown reasons, this condition may look like an obstruction of the bowel but clears up on its own.

If the baby was exposed to high glucose and ketones during the pregnancy, it may show diminished intelligence. This is not obvious at birth but is discovered later, as the baby develops.

A large baby with a poorly controlled diabetic mother usually loses its fat during the first year of life. Starting at ages six to eight, however, the child has a greater tendency to be obese. Controlling the blood glucose in the mother may prevent later obesity and even diabetes in the offspring.

When a Man Can't Get an Erection

If carefully questioned, more than 50 per cent of all males with diabetes admit to difficulty with sexual function. In diabetic men over the age of 70, the figure rises to more than 75 per cent. This difficulty usually takes the form of *erectile dysfunction,* the inability to have or sustain an erection sufficient for intercourse.

Although the problem is still something of a social taboo, about one man in ten over the age of 40 has erectile dysfunction, whether they have diabetes or not. The figure goes up steadily with increasing age. Many reasons besides diabetes cause this problem, and you should rule them out before blaming diabetes. Even if diabetes is partly at fault, other factors can contribute. Some other possibilities include the following:

✔ Smoking, drinking, or taking illegal drugs

✔ Trauma to the penis

✔ Medications such as certain antihypertensives and antidepressants

✔ Hormonal abnormalities (such as insufficient production of the male hormone testosterone or overproduction of a hormone from the brain, called *prolactin*)

✔ Operations on the bowel, prostate gland, or bladder, which can damage the nerves connected to the penis

✔ Poor blood supply to the penis due to blockage of the artery by peripheral arterial disease (see Chapter 5)

✔ Spinal cord damage

✔ *Psychogenic impotence* (see the sidebar 'Psychogenic versus physical impotence')

Psychogenic versus physical impotence

Anxiety, stress, depression, and conflict with your partner can all cause psychogenic impotence – an inability to have an erection for psychological rather than physical reasons. This type of impotence differs from organic (physical) impotence in a number of ways. Psychogenic impotence is often specific to a particular sexual partner and comes on very suddenly. Erections occur during sleep and in the morning, but not when the man attempts sexual intercourse with that partner.

Differentiating physical from psychological impotence may require a few nights in a sleep lab, where a device that detects erections during sleep is placed around the penis. Men without physical impotence normally have three or more erections during sleep, while their eyes are going through a state of rapid eye movement (REM). (Who knows what they are looking at!) Doctors can measure both the erections and the REM. If erections occur at various times of day or night, the impotence is psychological and not physical.

Some doctors have suggested a 'home test' using postage stamps, which are placed around the penis at night. If the stamps break, then an erection has occurred. However, this method is associated with problems such as the stickiness of the stamps and the tendency of a male to try to remove a foreign body on the penis.

Alternatively, you may be able to work out for yourself if the problem is psychogenic. Don't forget, though, that even if a physical problem exists, psychological factors can often co-exist. The sort of things that suggest a psychogenic rather than a physical cause include:

- ✔ Getting early-morning erections

- ✔ Being able to sustain an erection during masturbation, but not during sexual intercourse with your partner

- ✔ Getting an erection unexpectedly in certain arousing situations

Psychological impotence is very responsive to a kind of therapy called psychosexual therapy. The results are much better if you are in a relationship and have therapy with your partner. Your general practitioner can advise where you can get psychosexual therapy.

After you eliminate all the possibilities for erectile dysfunction, then you can consider diabetes to be the source of the problem. In order to understand how diabetes affects an erection, a brief understanding of the normal production of an erection is necessary.

The erection process

As a result of some form of stimulation, whether by touch, sight, sound, or something else, the brain activates nerves in the parasympathetic nervous system, part of the autonomic nervous system. These nerves cause muscles to relax so that blood flow into the penis greatly increases. As blood flow increases, the veins through which blood leaves the penis compress, and the penis becomes erect. When the penis is erect, it contains about 11 times as much blood as when it's flaccid. With sufficient stimulation, muscles contract, propelling semen through the urethra, the tube in the penis that normally carries urine from the bladder, to the outside of the body. The pleasant sensation that occurs along with the muscle contractions (ejaculation) is called *orgasm*.

Orgasm and ejaculation are the result of stimulation by the other side of the autonomic nervous system, the sympathetic nervous system. As the stimulation causes contraction of the muscles, it closes the muscle over the bladder so that urine does not normally accompany expulsion of semen, and the semen does not go back into the bladder.

The effect of diabetes on erections

Diabetes can damage the parasympathetic nervous system so that the male cannot get enough of an erection for sexual intercourse. The sympathetic nervous system is spared, so that ejaculation and orgasm can occur. Of course, intercourse may be unpleasant for the partner because the inability of the male to provide a firm erection has psychological consequences.

The following factors determine the onset of erection failure:

- ✔ **Degree of control of the blood glucose.** Better control is associated with fewer problems.
- ✔ **Duration of the diabetes.** The longer you have diabetes, the more likely you are to be unable to have an erection.
- ✔ **Interaction with the partner.** A positive relationship is important.
- ✔ **Use of drugs or alcohol.** Both may prevent erection.
- ✔ **State of mind.** A positive frame of mind is associated with more successful erections.

Treatment of erection problems

Fortunately for the diabetic male with erectile dysfunction, numerous approaches to treatment exist, beginning with drugs, continuing with external devices to create an erection, and ending with implantable devices that provide a very satisfactory erection. Treatment is successful in 90 per cent or more of men, but only 5 per cent ever discuss the problem with their doctor. Following are treatment options:

- ✔ **Viagra et al.:** Viagra, also called sildenafil, has been specifically studied in diabetic males and is successful in 70 per cent of patients compared to 10 per cent of men who received a pill that contained no active ingredient. (For information on how Viagra works, see the sidebar 'How Viagra, Levitra, and Cialis work'.)

However, Viagra is not free of side effects. Some men experience headaches, facial flushing, or indigestion, which generally decline with continued use of the drug. Viagra does not seem to affect diabetic control. It has also been found to cause a temporary colour tinge to a man's vision as well as increased sensitivity to light and blurred vision. These side effects do decline with continued use of Viagra.

Viagra is taken no more than once a day about an hour before sexual activity. While the starting dose is 50 milligrams for men, when diabetes is present, 100 milligrams are often required. An erection only occurs if there is some kind of sexual stimulation. Viagra does not bring on an erection, it prevents it from subsiding so that it lasts longer. You can expect the effect to be present up to 4–6 hours after taking the drug.

The pharmaceutical company that makes Viagra could not expect to have the playing field to itself for very long, when the game is something that most men want to play. Two newer alternatives include:

- Vardenafil (brand name Levitra). Its characteristics are very similar to Viagra but the dosage is 10 milligrams, which probably means 20 milligrams for men with diabetes.

- Tadalafil (brand name Cialis). It works like the other two pills above, but it stays active for 36 hours. In addition, its onset of action is 20 minutes, half the time of Viagra or Levitra. It has been named the 'weekender pill', since it permits spontaneous sexual activity from Friday to Sunday. The starting dose for Cialis is 20 milligrams, but, again, the male with diabetes may need to start at twice that.

One important group of men must not take Viagra or the other two drugs. Men who have chest pain often take nitrate drugs, the most common of which is nitroglycerine. The combination of Viagra and nitrates may cause a significant and possibly fatal drop in blood pressure.

✔ **Uprima:** Uprima, also known by the rather user-unfriendly name of apomorphine hydrochloride, is another tablet that can help with erectile dysfunction. Luckily, the tablet is easier to get your tongue around than the name – it dissolves under the tongue and produces an erection within 20 minutes in most men. However, its side effects include nausea, headache, dizziness, yawning, sleepiness, flushing, sweats, and altered taste.

Like with Viagra, men with severe unstable angina, low blood pressure, or heart failure, or who have had a recent heart attack or are taking nitrate drugs, shouldn't use Uprima.

✔ **Injection into the penis:** The patient himself can use two different kinds of injections to create an erection. The first one, a mixture of drugs called papaverine and phentolamine, has now been replaced for the most part by alprostadil (Caverject or Viridal Duo), which is another chemical that relaxes the blood vessels in the penis to allow more flow. The drug is injected about 30 minutes before intercourse, and no more than once in 24 hours and 2–3 times per week. An injection of either preparation gives a full erection lasting about an hour in 85 to 95 per cent of men, except for those who have the most severe loss of blood flow to the penis. Alprostadil does not require sexual stimulation in order to work. Complications of injections are rare but include bruising, pain, and the formation of nodules at the injection site.

A very rare complication of injection is *priapism,* where the penis maintains its erection for many hours. If the erection lasts more than four hours, the patient must see his doctor to get an injection of a *vasoconstrictor,* a drug that squeezes down the arteries into the penis so that blood flow is interrupted.

✔ **Suppository in the penis:** Alprostadil (see the preceding bullet) also comes in a suppository form. The patient inserts a tube containing this small pill into the opening of the penis after urination. Once the tube is fully in the opening, the top is squeezed so that the pill exits from the tube. This preparation, called MUSE, comes in several different strengths so that patients can use a higher dose if the lower dose does not result in a satisfactory erection. It may safely be used twice in 24 hours. It is also associated with some pain in a few men. Again, sexual stimulation is unnecessary.

✔ **Vacuum constriction devices:** These tubes, which fit over the penis, create a closed space when pressed against the patient's body. A pump draws out the air in the tube, and blood rushes into the penis to replace the air. Once the penis is erect, a rubber band is placed around the base of the penis to keep the blood inside it. Sometimes pain and numbness of the penis occur. Because a rubber band is constricting the penis, semen does not get through, so conception cannot take place. The rubber band may be kept on for up to 30 minutes.

✔ **Implanted penile prostheses:** If the patient doesn't like the idea of injecting himself in his penis or using a vacuum device, and Viagra or one of the other medications doesn't work, a *prosthesis* (an artificial substitute) can be implanted in the penis to give a very satisfactory erection. These come in several varieties. A semi-rigid type produces a permanent erection, but some men do not like the inconvenience of a permanent erection. An inflatable prosthesis involves a pump in the scrotal sac that contains fluid. The pump can be squeezed to transfer the fluid into balloons in the penis to stiffen it. When not pumped up, the penis appears normally soft. In the past few years, the surgery to insert these prostheses has become very effective.

There has been a lot of publicity in recent years about which of these preparations are available on National Health Service prescription, and for whom. If you have diabetes, you are eligible for any of these on prescription. If your doctor writes 'SLS' on the prescription, they are issued to you free. However, some of these treatments are only prescribed initially by a specialist clinic, such as a sexual dysfunction clinic. Talk to your general practitioner about the options and whether or not you may benefit from a referral to a specialist clinic.

How Viagra, Levitra, and Cialis work

Certain muscles need to relax for blood to flow into the penis (see the section 'The erection process' earlier in this chapter). A certain chemical in the penis permits this to happen. Another chemical breaks down the first one so that the erection ends. Viagra, Levitra, and Cialis block the action of this second chemical so that the erection can continue. Therefore, they depend on some stimulation to get the first chemical flowing and don't work in the absence of stimulation.

Impotence is a remarkably common problem, and there is a great deal of help available if you ask for it. If you want to find out more about the various treatments available, you can contact the Sexual Dysfunction Association, Windmill Place Business Centre, 2–4 Windmill Lane, Southall, Middlesex UB2 4NJ, Helpline 0870-774-3571, Web site: www.impotence.org.uk, e-mail info@sda.uk.net.

Female Sexual Problems

Because women do not have a penis that has to enlarge during sex, sexual complications caused by diabetes are not as visually obvious. However, problems can occur and can be just as difficult for women. Several of these problems are also seen in menopause, particularly a dry vagina and irregular menstrual function, so menopause must be ruled out as the culprit. The following problems are associated with diabetes:

- You may have a dry mouth and dry vagina because of the high blood glucose.
- Your menstrual function may be irregular when your diabetes is out of control.
- You may develop yeast infections of the vagina that make intercourse unpleasant.
- Because type 2 diabetes is usually associated with obesity, you may feel fat and unattractive.
- You may feel uncomfortable discussing the problem with your partner or your doctor.
- You may have loss of bladder control due to a neurogenic bladder (see Chapter 5).
- Your increasing age may predispose you to a reduction in oestrogen secretion and the vaginal thinning and dryness associated with that.

A female with long-standing diabetes may have several other problems that are specific to her sexual organs. These problems include

- ✔ **Reduced lubrication because of parasympathetic nerve involvement:** Lubrication serves to permit easier entry of the penis, but it also increases the sensitivity of the vagina to touch, thus increasing pleasant sensations.

- ✔ **Reduced blood flow because of diabetic blood vessel disease:** Some of the lubrication comes from fluid within the blood vessels.

- ✔ **Loss of skin sensation around the vaginal area:** This loss of sensation reduces pleasure.

Most women who have problems with lubrication medicate themselves with over-the-counter preparations. These preparations fall into three categories:

- ✔ Water-based lubricants, like K-Y jelly and In Pursuit of Passion

- ✔ Oil-based lubricants, like vegetable oils

- ✔ Petroleum-based lubricants, (although these aren't recommended for women because of the possibility of bacterial infection)

Use of these products is a matter of choice, although water-based products are probably the easiest to use and clean up.

If you are using condoms or a diaphragm (cap) for contraception, you should avoid oil-based lubricants. These can perish the rubber, which rather defeats the object of the contraceptive!

When psychological or interpersonal issues exist, a discussion with a therapist, the use of antidepressant medications (some of which can dry the vagina, by the way), and sex therapy with your partner are important steps to take to improve sexual pleasure.

As with all of the diabetic problems you read about in this book, maximum control of the blood glucose prevents or slows down a lot of these complications.

The Sexual Dysfunction Association can help women with sexual problems, as well as men. You can contact the Sexual Dysfunction Association at Windmill Place Business Centre, 2–4 Windmill Lane, Southall, Middlesex UB2 4NJ, Helpline 0870-774-3571, Web site: www.impotence.org.uk, e-mail info@sda.uk.net.

Part III

Managing Diabetes: The 'Thriving with Diabetes' Lifestyle Plan

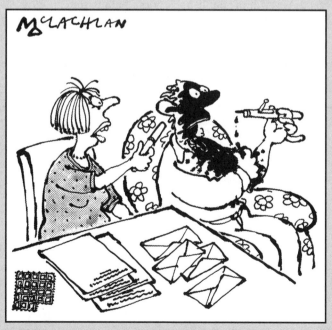

'Oops – I've got your insulin pen
– You've got my fountain pen.'

In this part . . .

Is it possible for you to be healthier with diabetes than your friends who do not have diabetes? This part shows that the answer to that question is yes. While other people continue their bad habits, leading to illness and perhaps premature death, you can find out exactly what you have to do not just to live with diabetes but to thrive with diabetes. The steps you need to take are simple and basic. You will probably ask yourself many times: 'Why didn't I think of that?'

Another function of this part is to show you that lots of people – some of whom you may not have thought of – are around to provide the information that you need to know.

Chapter 7

Glucose Monitoring and Other Tests

· ·

· ·

*I*f you read Part II, you know all the bad things that can happen to you, but you're not panicking because you know they won't happen to you. Why? Because you're going to practise all the important recommendations in this and the next five chapters. True, it's a bit of a bother and will cost a few quid, but you're worth it.

Not only that, but you're among the most fortunate people with diabetes who have ever lived. Most of the products and treatments we cover in this part were not available just 20 years ago. And the new products coming along will knock your socks off (but put them back on because you shouldn't go barefoot!).

In this chapter, you discover all you need to know to put your diabetes in its proper place. You find out how well you're currently controlling your blood glucose, whether complications are beginning to show up, and what changes you need to make in your therapy to reverse or slow the progression of these complications.

Tests You Need to Stay Healthy

Your doctor (and you, if feasible) should perform the 'every visit' tests below on at least four visits a year if you take insulin or if your blood and other measurements are less than ideal. If you don't take insulin or if your measurements are good, your doctor should perform these tests on at least two visits a year:

'Every visit' tests

- ✔ Evaluate your blood glucose measurements each visit. (See the section 'Monitoring Your Blood Glucose: It's a Must', later in this chapter.)
- ✔ Obtain haemoglobin A1c two to four times a year. (See the section 'Tracking your glucose over time: Haemoglobin A1c', later in this chapter.)
- ✔ Examine your bare feet at each visit. (See the section 'Examining Your Feet', later in this chapter.)
- ✔ Measure blood pressure at each visit. (See the section 'Measuring Blood Pressure', later in this chapter.)
- ✔ Measure weight at each visit. (See the section 'Checking Your Weight', later in this chapter.)

Annual tests

Your doctor should perform these tests at least once a year, usually at your annual check-up:

- ✔ Check for microalbuminuria once a year. (See the section 'Testing for Kidney Damage: Microalbuminuria', later in this chapter.)
- ✔ Have a dilated eye examination by a doctor once a year. (See the section 'Checking for Eye Problems', later in this chapter.)
- ✔ Check your blood lipids once a year. (See the section 'Tracking Cholesterol and Other Fats', later in this chapter.)

These tests are the minimum standards for proper care of diabetes. Once your doctor finds an abnormality, the frequency of testing increases to check on your response to treatment.

A progress report on doctors

How are doctors actually doing in medical care for a person with diabetes? Several recent studies have been eye-openers. The results were (sadly) as follows:

- Only 3 per cent of insulin users and 1 per cent of non-insulin users met all the standards for routine testing.

- Three out of four people with diabetes have never heard of haemoglobin A1c.

- One in four people with diabetes does not even make an annual visit to the doctor.

- Two in five have never had their feet examined or had a dilated eye examination.

- Fewer than half of diabetics realise that diabetes can cause heart disease.

- Ninety-six per cent of general practices have a diabetic register, where they keep an accurate list of all patients with diabetes. That sounds impressive, until you realise it means that 4 per cent of practices fall at this most basic of hurdles!

- Seventy-one per cent of general practices run a diabetic clinic, which means that 29 per cent of practices don't have a dedicated clinic. Fortunately, the new General Practitioner Contract (you can find out more about this in Chapter 2) includes lots of criteria for measuring the care of patients with diabetes. That means that most general practice surgeries now offer formal call and recall for ongoing monitoring of patients with diabetes, and those that don't have a formal diabetic clinic are gradually developing them.

- Only 1 in 10 general practices has a diabetes education programme, although the number is increasing fast.

- Only one in three people with type 2 diabetes takes all of their tablets. The more tablets they have been prescribed, the less likely they are to take them all. You can find out more about tablets for diabetes in Chapter 10.

Together, these studies show how much work there is to be done to get the message across about the importance of taking diabetes seriously. It also shows how much you deserve a hearty hurray for taking your condition seriously enough to be reading this book!

Monitoring Your Blood Glucose: It's a Must

Insulin was extracted and used for the first time over 75 years ago. Since then, nothing has improved the life of people with diabetes as much as the ability to measure their own blood glucose with a drop of blood.

The occasional blood glucose test done in your doctor's surgery is of little or no value in understanding the big picture of your glucose control. It is exactly like trying to visualise an entire painting by Seurat, who painted with dots, by looking at one dot on the canvas. For this reason, you need to monitor your glucose regularly yourself.

Whatever happened to testing urine for glucose?

Prior to blood glucose self-monitoring, testing the urine for glucose was the only way to determine whether your blood glucose was high, but urine testing could not tell at all whether the glucose was low. These days, the European Non-Insulin-Dependent Diabetes Mellitus Policy Group and the American Diabetes Association recommend blood glucose rather than urine testing. The European consensus guide does give advice on urine testing, but only recommends it when blood testing is not possible. Testing the urine for other things such as ketones and protein can be of value.

Keeping your blood glucose under tight control undoubtedly reduces the chance of developing complications of diabetes. Obviously, you can't keep your glucose under tight control unless you check it. But if you don't act when your blood glucose measurements are out of the ideal range, little point exists in doing the tests in the first place. If you want to translate regular measurements of glucose into good diabetic control, you need to know what to do if your blood glucose is higher than ideal. Talk to your general practitioner or diabetic nurse about what to do about different glucose levels.

Knowing how often to test

One of the first things that doctors learned when frequent testing of blood glucose became feasible was that, in a person with diabetes, even a fairly stable one, tremendous variation in the glucose occurs in a relatively short time, especially in association with food, but even in the fasting state before breakfast. This is why multiple tests may be needed. How often you test is determined by the kind of diabetes you have, the kind of treatment you're using, and the level of stability of your blood glucose:

- **If you have type 1 diabetes or type 2 diabetes and you're taking insulin, you may need to test before each meal and at bedtime**. This is especially important if you adjust your insulin dose for each meal, depending on your blood glucose level. A glucose profile, where you carry out a random selection of blood glucose tests at different times of the day, can be very useful as well. If you find it impractical to test that often, don't beat yourself up. Missing the odd measurement isn't going to do any major damage. However, you should try to work regular blood testing into your daily routine as often as you can. If you have type 2 diabetes and you're taking insulin, it is important to take some measurements of fasting glucose first thing in the morning. You can also take an occasional measurement in the middle of the night, to check whether your glucose is going too low.

The tighter your blood glucose control on insulin, the more likely you are to get hypoglycaemic episodes. If you feel unwell, check your blood glucose to see if you're hypoglycaemic. This check is especially important when your dose of insulin has been changed, or if you're pregnant or unwell for another reason.

✔ **If you have type 2 diabetes and you're on pills or just diet and exercise,** you may want to check your blood glucose twice a day before breakfast and dinner. If your haemoglobin A1c is very good (more about this in the section 'Tracking your glucose over time: Haemoglobin A1c' later in this chapter), your doctor may recommend that regular blood glucose monitoring isn't necessary. If you're taking tablets or just diet and exercise to control your diabetes, testing your blood glucose regularly doesn't make that much difference to your diabetic control. For some people testing is very helpful, because it gives you an indication of how your blood sugar changes with your lifestyle. However, some people find it frustrating if they can't adjust their medication when their blood sugar is high (you can do this if you take insulin, but not on a day-to-day basis if you take tablets). Talk to your doctor or diabetic specialist nurse about what works best for you.

For some diabetics, frequent checking of blood glucose may have disadvantages. In one study, diabetics not treated with insulin showed higher levels of distress, worry, and depressive symptoms if they were self-monitoring very frequently. The same was not true of diabetics treated with insulin, who adjusted their dose in response to their test results. The moral of this particular story seems to be that monitoring your glucose helps you feel in control if you can do something about it, but may serve to worry you if you can't.

✔ **If you're pregnant, see the testing guidelines outlined in Chapter 6.** Our guess is that you're probably willing to test numerous times a day to keep your developing foetus as healthy as possible.

While your diabetes treatment is first being stabilised, you will probably be asked to check your glucose several times a day. Once your control is good, you may be able to test less often. How often you test depends on how regular your routine and lifestyle are. However, there are some situations when testing more frequently can help you enormously:

✔ If your mealtimes vary a great deal

✔ If your levels of exercise vary

✔ While you are menstruating

✔ Before and during a long journey if you are driving (you can find much more about diabetes and driving in Chapter 15)

There are three other situations where checking your blood glucose regularly is absolutely essential:

- ✔ If you're planning a pregnancy

- ✔ If you suspect you are getting hypoglycaemic episodes, especially if you drive, handle machinery, or take part in potentially dangerous sports

- ✔ If you are unwell for another reason (you can find out more about what to do if you're feeling unwell in the section 'Under-the-weather tips if you're on insulin' later in this chapter)

The blood glucose test can be useful at many other times of day. If you eat something off your diet and want to test its effect on your glucose, do a test. If you're about to exercise, a blood glucose test can tell you whether you need to eat before starting the exercise or can use the exercise to bring your glucose down.

You're not being graded on your glucose test results. The human body has too much variation in it to expect that each time you take the same medication, do the same exercise, eat the same way, and feel the same emotionally, you will necessarily get the same test result. If the person who reviews your results with you sees your abnormal results as bad, she does not understand this point. You may want to consider finding someone who does.

Under-the-weather tips if you're on insulin

If you're unwell for any reason, from a cold to a tummy bug, your blood sugar is likely to go up. One of your body's natural responses to being ill is to make more glucose. That means that even if you have a tummy bug that makes you vomit, or if you're not feeling well enough to eat, you need to carry on taking your insulin. In fact, you may even need to take more insulin, despite the fact that you're not eating much or keeping much food down. If you don't, your blood sugar can rise. If you have type 1 diabetes, this rise can be enough to cause a complication called diabetic ketoacidosis, which you can find out more about in Chapter 4.

Never stop taking your insulin when you're unwell, even if you're not eating.

If you're poorly, following a few simple rules can help prevent your blood sugar rising too much. If you don't feel up to checking your sugar and ketones for yourself, ask a carer to do it for you.

- ✔ Check your blood sugar every 2–4 hours and adjust your insulin dose accordingly. If you're not sure how to do this, you can talk to your general practitioner or diabetic nurse.

- ✔ If you have type 1 diabetes, check your urine or blood for ketones every 2–4 hours.

✔ Drink at least five pints of sugar-free liquids every day while you're ill. If you can't manage large quantities of fluid, sip small amounts often.

✔ Try to eat your normal diet. If you can't, you can replace your meals with liquid carbohydrates. Table 7-1 gives you some fluids with 10 grams of carbohydrate in a serving. Try to take about 10 grams of carbohydrate an hour.

Table 7-1	10 Grams of Carbohydrates in a Serving
Unsweetened fruit juice	100 ml
Non-diet cola/lemonade	150 ml
Lucozade	50 ml
Milk	200 ml

✔ Contact your diabetic team or general practitioner if your symptoms don't improve after 24–48 hours, if you carry on vomiting, if your blood sugar stays high despite increasing your insulin, or if you develop symptoms of diabetic ketoacidosis (see Chapter 4).

Performing the test

Two kinds of test strip for testing your blood glucose are available today. Both require that glucose in a drop of your blood reacts with an enzyme. In one strip, the reaction produces a colour. You read your glucose measurements by comparing the colour of your strip with a standard chart. You can also use these strips with a meter, in which case the meter reads the amount of colour to give a glucose reading. With the other type of strip, the reaction produces electrons, and a meter then converts the amount of electrons into a glucose reading.

If you're colour blind or have problems with your vision, you may not be able to read colour strips by eye. If this applies to you, you obviously need a meter that reads the measurement for you.

If you don't already have a meter, be sure to check out the following section, 'Choosing a blood glucose meter'. All meters require a drop of blood, usually from the finger. You place the blood on a specific part of a test strip and allow enough time, 20 seconds to one minute, for a reaction to occur. Some strips allow you to add more blood within 30 seconds if the quantity is insufficient. In less than a minute, the meter reads the product of that reaction, which is determined by the amount of glucose in the original blood sample.

Keep the following tips in mind when you're testing your glucose:

- **If you have trouble getting blood, you can use a rubber band at the point where your finger joins your hand.** You may be amazed at the flow of blood. Take off the rubber band before a major haemorrhage occurs (just joking).

- **Keep in mind that some meters use whole blood and some use the liquid part of the blood, called the *plasma*.** A lab glucose tests the plasma. The blood value is about 12 per cent less than the plasma value, so knowing which you're measuring is important. The various recommendations for appropriate levels of glucose are plasma values.

- **Studies have shown that the qualities of test strips, which are loose in a vial, deteriorate rapidly if the vial is left open.** Be sure to put the lid on the vial. Two hours of exposure to air may ruin the strips. Strips that are individually foil wrapped don't have this problem.

Choosing a blood glucose meter

So many meters are on the market that you may be confused about which one to use. Which meter you opt for depends on many factors that are personal to you. For instance, if you work away from home a lot, you may be particularly keen to have a small, easily portable meter. If you have problems with your manual dexterity, you may prefer a bigger meter with fewer small, fiddly buttons. If eyesight is an issue, you probably want to opt for a monitor that gives a printed readout of your glucose level, rather than one that involves comparing colours on a chart.

Ask yourself the following questions when choosing a meter:

- If a small child is to use it, can the child easily use the meter and strips?

- Are the batteries common ones, or hard to get and expensive?

- Does the meter have a memory that you and your doctor can check?

- Is the meter downloadable to a computer program that can manipulate the data?

- If I can't use the meter myself for any reason, can a relative or carer use it properly?

- Is it simple and straightforward to use?

- Can I read the measurements easily?

Following are two considerations that shouldn't play any part in your decision:

- ✔ **The cost of the meter:** Blood glucose meters aren't available on the National Health Service, but the test strips you use in them are. Although meters cost up to about £60, the bulk of the cost of glucose monitoring, with blood monitoring strips costing 20 to 30p each, is borne by the National Health Service.

- ✔ **The accuracy of the various machines:** All are accurate to a degree acceptable for managing your diabetes. Keep in mind, though, that they do not have the accuracy of a laboratory. They are probably about plus or minus 10 per cent compared to the lab.

Ask your practice nurse, diabetic specialist nurse, or doctor her advice about the meter she uses in your diabetic clinic and why. Lots of people find it easier to go with the machine their own diabetic clinic uses regularly. (***Note:*** Your doctor may have a meter that she prefers to work with because a computer program can download the test results from the meter and display them in a certain way. This analysis can be enormously helpful in deciding how to alter your therapy for the best control of your glucose.)

Minimally- and non-invasive blood glucose monitoring devices

To get a drop of blood for a glucose meter test, you need to get through the tough protective outer layer of skin to the soft, fleshy tissue underneath. As well as containing blood, this tissue also contains pain sensors that are designed to alert you to damage to the body tissues. Without pain sensors, you don't take steps to protect yourself against damage. The fact that pain is there to protect you is, frankly, precious little comfort when you're stabbing yourself for the fourth time in a day. That's why there has been so much research into blood glucose monitoring devices that don't require you to use a lancet every time. Models that are being looked into include the following:

- ✔ A needle left under the skin for up to three days at a time

- ✔ Patches worn on the skin

- ✔ Infra-red or laser devices that use light to measure glucose levels

At present, none of these devices is available on the National Health Service. However, GlucoWatch Biographer was approved in the United States in 2001. It's worn like a wristwatch and measures blood glucose via the *interstitial fluid* (the fluid that fills up a blister when you burn yourself), which the meter can read without using a lancet. There are definite disadvantages, though. Both the meter and the sensors are very expensive (over £400 for the meter and about £50 for a box of ten AutoSensors, which aren't available on prescription), and the results differ by more than 30 per cent from blood glucose readings up to 25 per cent of the time.

We don't recommend the GlucoWatch Biographer, or any other minimally or non-invasive meter, until more studies have been done. However, you can find out more about this product by phoning 0800-028-5256 from 3 p.m. to midnight, Monday to Saturday.

Blood glucose meters need to be checked regularly to see whether they're accurate. Even if you write down your blood glucose readings, rather than recording them on your meter, bring your meter with you every time you visit the diabetic clinic so that your nurse can check the accuracy of your readings.

Using your blood glucose results

The European Diabetes Policy Group has suggested figures for blood glucose that show you the effect your diabetes is likely to have on your body. Their low risk levels are the ones to aim for. If your blood sugars lie in the arterial risk range, you're at greater risk of developing problems with heart disease (see Chapter 5 for more about this). If your blood sugars are in the microvascular risk range, you need to be concerned about eye, nerve, and kidney problems (also covered in more detail in Chapter 5).

The fasting blood result you get from a skin-prick test is called a *fasting capillary blood glucose*. This level is about 1.0 mmol/l lower than *venous blood glucose,* which is the level your doctor gets when she sends a blood sample to the lab. After a meal, your capillary blood glucose will be about the same as a venous blood glucose level.

	Low risk	*Arterial risk*	*Microvascular risk*
Venous plasma glucose			
Fasting (mmol/l)	<6.6–6.9	7 or over	
Self-monitoring blood glucose			
Fasting (mmol/l)	up to 5.5	5.5–6	>6
Venous plasma glucose			
Post-prandial or peak (mmol/l)	up to 7.5	7.5–9	>9
Haemoglobin A1c (%)	up to 6.5	6.5–7.4	>7.5

If your doctor has the right computer programme, she may be able to download your blood glucose results to find patterns. If, for example, your blood glucose tends to be high before breakfast and you're using rapid-acting lispro insulin before meals, you may need to increase your pre-breakfast dose by 2 units.

Always take your blood glucose results with you when you go to the diabetic clinic. Even if your doctor does not have a computer programme to analyse your results, she can give you useful tips about how to manage low or high measurements. If you are using insulin, always ask your doctor for a personally tailored programme to tell you what to do in the event of certain blood test results.

Tracking your glucose over time: Haemoglobin A1c

Individual blood glucose tests are great for deciding how you're doing at that moment and what to do to make your glucose levels better, but they don't give the big picture. They show just a moment in time. Glucose can change a great deal even in an hour. What you need is a test that gives an integrated picture of many days or weeks or even months of blood glucose levels. The test that accomplishes this important task is called the *haemoglobin A1c*.

With the haemoglobin A1c test, you can look back over a period of time to see whether you were or were not in control of your blood glucose. This is a perfect test, for example, for the diabetic woman who wants to get pregnant. She can know whether her blood glucose has been well controlled before she tries to conceive. If not, she can wait until the test shows good control and then try to get pregnant. In this way, she reduces the possibility of foetal malformations (see Chapter 6 for more on pregnancy and diabetes). The haemoglobin A1c test is also a great way to follow the effects of treatment. If treatment is working, this test should show improvement.

The standard method of measuring the haemoglobin A1c is the way it was done in the Diabetes Control and Complications Trial, the study that showed that controlling the blood glucose prevents complications in type 1 diabetes. In that study, a normal level was about 6.05 per cent. Figure 7-1 shows you the correlation between haemoglobin A1c and blood glucose when this method is used.

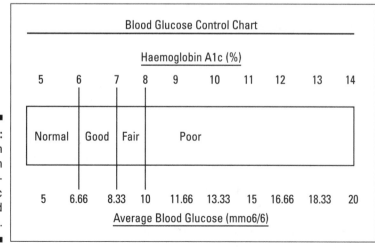

Figure 7-1:
Comparison
between
haemo-
globin A1c
and blood
glucose.

How haemoglobin A1c works

Haemoglobin is a protein that carries oxygen around the body and drops it off wherever it's needed to help in the chemical reactions that take place constantly. The haemoglobin is packaged within red blood cells, which live in the bloodstream for 60 to 90 days. As the blood circulates, glucose in the blood attaches to the haemoglobin and stays attached. It attaches in several different ways to the haemoglobin, and the total of all the haemoglobin attached to glucose is called *glycohaemoglobin*. Glycohaemoglobin normally makes up about 6 per cent of the haemoglobin in the blood. The largest fraction, two-thirds of the glycohaemoglobin, is in the form called haemoglobin A1c, making it easiest to measure. The rest of the haemoglobin is made up of haemoglobin A1a and A1b. The more glucose in the blood, the more glycohaemoglobins form. Because glycohaemoglobin remains in the blood for two to three months, it is a reflection of the glucose control over the entire time period and not just the second that a single glucose test reflects.

As you can see in the figure, a normal haemoglobin A1c of less than 6 per cent corresponds to a blood glucose of less than 7 mmol/l, while a fair haemoglobin A1c of 7 per cent reflects an average blood glucose of 9 mmol/l.

A good haemoglobin A1c is highly motivating to keep up good self-care, while a poor result gives immediate feedback as to the need for tighter control.

Testing for Kidney Damage: Microalbuminuria

The finding of very small but abnormal amounts of protein in the urine, called *microalbuminuria,* is the earliest sign that high glucose may be damaging the kidneys (see Chapter 5 for more on this condition, called *nephropathy*). Microalbuminuria is found when it is still early enough to reverse much of the damage.

When the diagnosis of type 2 diabetes is made, and within the fifth year after the diagnosis of type 1 diabetes, your doctor must order a urine test for microalbuminuria. If the test is negative, it must be repeated annually. If it's positive, a second test is performed to verify the result. If the test is positive again, your doctor should

  ✔ **Put you on a drug called an ACE inhibitor (or an AIIRA).** After you have been on this drug for some months, your doctor can repeat the test to see whether it has turned negative. You can find out more about these drugs and their benefits in Chapter 5.

✓ **Bring your blood glucose under the tightest control possible.** This helps to reverse the damaging process as well.

✓ **Normalise your body fats so that your cholesterol and triglycerides (see 'Tracking Cholesterol and Other Fats', later in this chapter) remain within target limits.** Elevated cholesterol and triglycerides have been found to damage the kidneys.

Doing this simple little test can protect your kidneys from damage. Ask your doctor if you think you've never received this test. Show your doctor this page if she is unclear why the test must be performed.

Checking for Eye Problems

All people with diabetes need to have a dilated eye exam done annually. A specially trained general practitioner at your surgery can do this. If no specially trained general practitioner is available, you can go to a local community clinic, where a specially trained doctor does the test, or to your high-street optician instead. For this exam, the high street optician instils drops into your eyes and uses various instruments to examine the pressure, the appearance of your lens, and, most importantly, the retina of your eye.

Through this exam, the optician can identify some of the changes that occur in diabetes. If she discovers changes, she gives you a form to take back to your general practitioner. This form tells your doctor why your optician thinks you should be referred to a specialist eye clinic at the hospital. Most doctors don't dream of disagreeing with an optician and refer their patients on immediately. If your general practitioner seems unwilling, you have a right to demand a second opinion.

All kinds of things can be done if abnormalities are found, but they must be discovered first. (See Chapter 5 for more information on eye problems.) Therefore, make sure that you receive this test at your annual check-up. More and more general practitioners are offering this service at the surgery, or at a local specialist clinic, either based at a hospital or at a community clinic. Many of these clinics can take photographs of your *retina* (the back of your eye), which makes their screening superior to the kind you get from your optician. Talk to your general practitioner about getting this screening. However, you should still see your optician regularly.

Examining Your Feet

Unfortunately, foot problems often result in an amputation. An amputation is really evidence of inadequate care. (For more on foot problems, see Chapter 5.)

The doctor is not necessarily at fault here. The doctor sees you once in a while; you're with yourself much more often.

If you have any problem sensing touch on your feet, you need to take the following precautions:

- ✔ You must use your eyes to examine your feet every day.

- ✔ You must use your hand to test hot water before you step into it so that you don't get burnt.

- ✔ You must shake out your shoes before you step into them to make sure no stone or other object is inside.

- ✔ You must not go barefoot.

- ✔ You must keep the skin of your feet moist by soaking them in water, drying them, and applying a moistening lotion.

Your doctor can test your ability to feel an injury by using a 10 gram filament, but, again, she does that only when you have an appointment. You are the best person to pick up early changes in your feet.

If you have any suggestion of a loss of sensation, at each visit to the doctor who takes care of your diabetes, take off your shoes and socks and have the doctor inspect your feet.

Tracking Cholesterol and Other Fats

Most people these days know the level of their cholesterol. What they actually know is the level of their *total* cholesterol. Cholesterol circulates in the blood in small packages called *lipoproteins.* These tiny round particles contain fat and protein.

A second kind of fat found in the lipoproteins is *triglyceride.* Triglyceride actually represents the form of most of the fat you eat each day. Although you eat only a gram or less of cholesterol (an egg yolk is one third of a gram of cholesterol), you eat up to 100 grams of triglyceride a day. (For more on the place of fats in your diet, see Chapter 8.) The fat in animal meats is mostly triglycerides.

To understand whether you have too much bad cholesterol (LDL) or a satisfactory level of good cholesterol (HDL), you need to know which particle the cholesterol comes from.

You don't need to fast to do a test for total cholesterol and HDL cholesterol. However, you do need to fast for eight hours to find out your LDL cholesterol – and some people may get an inaccurate triglyceride result if they have fasted for less than 12 hours before a test.

Types of fat particles

✔ **Chylomicrons,** the largest particles, which contain the fat that is absorbed from the intestine after a meal. They are usually cleared from the blood rapidly. Ordinarily, chylomicrons are not a concern with respect to causing *arteriosclerosis* (hardening of the arteries).

✔ **Very low-density lipoprotein (VLDL) particles,** which contain mostly triglyceride as the fat. These are smaller than chylomicrons.

✔ **High-density lipoprotein (HDL),** known as 'good' cholesterol, the next smallest in size. This particle functions to clean the arteries, helping to prevent coronary artery disease, peripheral vascular disease, and strokes.

✔ **Low-density lipoprotein (LDL),** known as 'bad' cholesterol. This particle seems to be the one that carries cholesterol to the arteries, where it's deposited and causes hardening of the arteries.

You should have a fasting blood lipid check at least once each year. Table 7-2 is based on the Joint British Societies' recommendations, published in 2005, for the best levels of these lipids in terms of keeping your risk of cardiovascular disease down.

Table 7-2	Ideal Levels of Fat and the Risk for Cardiovascular Disease
Serum total cholesterol (mmol/l)	<4.0
Serum LDL cholesterol (mmol/l)	<2.0
Serum HDL cholesterol (mmol/l)	>1.0 (male) or 1.2 (female)
Serum triglycerides (mmol/l)	<1.7

You can see from Table 7-2 that the risk goes up as the LDL cholesterol goes up and the HDL cholesterol goes down. You can get a good picture of the risk by dividing the total cholesterol by the HDL cholesterol.

The Joint British Societies' recommendations (at the time of writing) are that pretty much everyone who has diabetes should be taking a statin tablet to get their cholesterol levels to the targets in Table 7-2. More specifically, they recommend that you should be taking a statin to reduce your cholesterol if:

✔ You are over 40 and have diabetes.

✔ You are aged 18–39 and have diabetes and any other risk factor for cardiovascular disease, which includes

• retinopathy (see Chapter 5)

- nephropathy, including persistent microalbuminuria (see Chapter 5)

- poor glycaemic control (haemoglobin A1c over 9 per cent)

- raised blood pressure requiring antihypertensive treatment (see below)

- features of the metabolic syndrome (see Chapter 3)

- family history of cardiovascular disease in a first-degree relative (parent or sibling) under 55 years if they are male or under 65 years if they are female

With diabetes, defining your risk of heart disease gets a little more complicated because of the metabolic syndrome (explained in Chapter 3). In the metabolic syndrome, the total cholesterol may not be very high, but the HDL cholesterol is low and the triglycerides are elevated. These patients also have a lot of a dangerous form of LDL cholesterol, so they are also at higher risk for coronary artery disease. This increased risk must be taken into account in considering treatment for the fats.

Measuring Blood Pressure

Diabetics are more likely to suffer from high blood pressure than non-diabetics of the same age because diabetics

- Can get kidney disease

- Have increased sensitivity to salt, which raises blood pressure

- Lack the night-time fall in blood pressure that normally occurs in people without diabetes

High blood pressure in epidemic proportions

The United Kingdom is experiencing an epidemic of high blood pressure *(hypertension)* similar to the epidemic of diabetes. The reasons are the same:

- Britons are more sedentary than before and getting fatter.

- Britons are storing fat in the centre of the body, the so-called *abdominal visceral fat.*

- Britons are getting older as a population. The fastest-growing segment of the population is over 75 years of age. In the last 70 years, the number of people over 65 in the United Kingdom has doubled. In the 30 years between 1995 and 2025, we reckon the number of people over 80 will go up by 50 per cent, and the number of people over 90 will double.

That, coupled with the fact that raised blood pressure worsens all the complications of diabetes (especially diabetic kidney disease, but also eye disease, heart disease, nerve disease, peripheral arterial disease, and cerebrovascular disease), means that people who are diabetic absolutely must control their blood pressure.

Aiming for normal – for diabetics, that is

The fourth British Hypertension Society guidance, issued in 2004, recommends that patients with diabetes should have their blood pressure controlled to a level of below 130/80 mmHg. They should be started on medication to reduce their blood pressure if the systolic blood pressure (the upper reading, as you can see in the sidebar 'The meaning of your blood pressure') is persistently at least 140 mmHg, or the diastolic blood pressure (the lower reading; see sidebar) is at least 90 mmHg. You can remind yourself what these figures mean in terms of long-term effect by looking in Chapter 5. For years, doctors considered a high diastolic blood pressure more damaging, and an elevation in that pressure was treated with greater importance than an elevation in the systolic blood pressure (the upper reading). Recent studies have shown that the systolic blood pressure is just as important as the diastolic blood pressure.

Why controlling blood pressure is important

The most recent evidence of the importance of controlling blood pressure in diabetes comes from the United Kingdom Prospective Diabetes Study (UKPDS), published in late 1998. This study found that a lowering of blood pressure by 10 mm systolic and 5 mm diastolic resulted in a 24 per cent reduction in any diabetic complication and a 32 per cent reduction in death related to diabetes.

The meaning of your blood pressure

What does the blood pressure measurement mean, and what is high blood pressure? When you get a reading, it usually looks something like 120/70, an upper reading and a lower reading:

✔ The upper reading, called the *systolic pressure*, is the amount of force exerted by the heart when it contracts to push blood around the body.

✔ The lower reading, called the *diastolic blood pressure*, is the pressure in the artery when the heart is at rest.

The UKPDS showed that keeping your blood pressure under tight control is even more important for diabetics than for non-diabetics. To keep complications to a minimum, you need to look at all the lifestyle measures that can keep your blood pressure, as well as your blood glucose, down. The good news is that lots of the measures that help control your glucose, like exercise, avoiding obesity, and a healthy diet, help your blood pressure, too.

Checking Your Weight

Determining your weight is one of the easiest measurements in medicine. Your doctor should measure your weight at every visit.

Knowing what you should weigh

To give you a general idea of how much you ought to weigh, you can use the following formula:

- ✔ If you're a woman, give yourself 100 pounds for being 5 feet tall and add 5 pounds for each inch over 5 feet. For example, if you're 5 feet 3 inches, your appropriate weight is 115 pounds.

- ✔ If you're a man, give yourself 106 pounds for being 5 feet tall and add 6 pounds for each inch over 5 feet. A 5 foot 6 inch male should weigh 142 pounds.

Working out your weight in pounds is easier than in stone. To convert your weight from stone to pounds, multiply each stone by 14 and then add on the extra number of pounds. That means, for instance, that 10 stone is 140 pounds, and 10 stone 7 is 140 + 7 = 147 pounds.

Figuring in your BMI

Body Mass Index (BMI) relates the weight to the height, so a tall person has a lower BMI than a short person of the same weight (see Chapter 3 for more on BMI). A person with a BMI under 20 is considered slim. A person with a BMI from 20 to 25 is normal. A person with a BMI from 25 to 29.9 is overweight, and a person with a BMI over 30 is obese. By this definition, more than half the people in the United Kingdom are overweight or obese.

To save you some time in figuring out your BMI, Table 7-3 shows your height in inches and in metres and your weight in pounds. If you know your weight in kilograms, convert it to pounds by multiplying by 2.2. Find your height in the left-hand column. Move your finger across that row until you come to your weight in pounds. Look at the top of that column to find your BMI. For example, if your height is 66 inches and your weight is 161 pounds (or 11 stone 7 pounds), your BMI is 26 kilograms per metre squared. Alternately, you can calculate your BMI as shown in Chapter 3.

Table 7-3	Body Mass Index Chart												
	Body Mass Index (kg/m²)												
	19	20	21	22	23	24	25	26	27	28	29	30	35	40
Height (inches/ metres)	**Body Weight (pounds)**												
58/1.47	91	96	100	105	110	115	119	124	129	134	138	143	167	191
59/1.50	94	99	104	109	114	119	124	128	133	138	143	148	173	198
60/1.52	97	102	107	112	118	123	128	133	138	143	148	15	179	204
61/1.55	100	106	111	116	122	127	132	137	143	148	153	158	185	211
62/1.57	104	109	115	120	126	131	136	142	147	153	158	164	191	218
63/1.60	107	113	118	124	130	135	141	146	152	158	163	169	197	225
64/1.63	110	116	122	128	134	140	145	151	157	163	169	174	204	232
65/1.65	114	120	126	132	138	144	150	156	162	168	174	180	210	240
66/1.68	118	124	130	136	142	148	155	161	167	173	179	186	216	247
67/1.70	121	127	134	140	146	153	159	166	172	178	185	191	233	255
68/1.73	125	131	138	144	151	158	164	171	177	184	190	197	230	262
69/1.75	128	135	142	149	155	162	169	176	182	189	196	203	236	270
70/1.78	132	139	146	153	160	167	174	181	188	195	202	207	243	278
71/1.80	136	143	150	157	165	172	179	186	193	200	208	215	250	286
72/1.83	140	147	154	162	169	177	184	191	199	206	213	221	258	294
73/1.85	144	151	159	166	174	182	189	197	204	212	219	227	265	302
74/1.88	148	155	163	171	179	186	194	202	210	218	225	233	272	311
75/1.90	152	160	168	176	184	192	200	208	216	224	232	240	279	319
76/1.93	156	164	172	180	189	197	205	213	221	230	238	246	287	328

Maintaining a BMI in the normal range makes controlling your diabetes and blood pressure easier. You need to eliminate obesity as a risk factor for coronary artery disease.

Testing for Ketones

You can get ketone sticks to check your urine from your general practitioner on prescription. Check for ketones if

- Your blood glucose rises above 13.9 mmol/l and you have type 1 diabetes
- You're pregnant, have diabetes, and your blood glucose is below 3.3 mmol/l

Finding ketones means that your body has turned to fat for energy. With a high glucose, it may mean you need more insulin. With a low glucose in pregnancy, it may mean the need for more carbohydrates in your diet.

To test for ketones, insert a test strip into your urine and observe a purple colour. The deeper the colour, the greater the ketone level. If you find a large amount of ketones, contact your doctor.

Checking the C-reactive Protein

C-reactive protein is a substance in the blood that is produced by the liver when there is infection or inflammation. You can measure it with a simple blood test. Diabetes is associated with several features that suggest that inflammation plays an important role in the disease. People who develop diabetes have higher C-reactive protein than those who don't. Other substances associated with inflammation are also found to be elevated in diabetes.

Drugs that improve your diabetes and cholesterol also lower the amount of C-reactive protein, which is also considered a marker for coronary artery disease.

On the whole, C-reactive protein isn't routinely measured at present as part of your diabetes screening in the United Kingdom. That's not a concern as long as you're having other indicators of diabetes and cholesterol control, like haemoglobin A1c and full lipid profile, measured regularly. However, C-reactive protein is becoming more accepted as an indicator of inflammation and coronary artery disease risk, so don't be surprised if your doctor starts to include it in your blood screening tests within the next couple of years.

Chapter 8

Diabetes Diet Plan

. . . .

In This Chapter

▶ Concentrating on diet – total calories

▶ Knowing how much you need of certain types of foods: carbohydrates, proteins, fats, and more

▶ Understanding the role that vitamins, minerals, and water play in your diet

▶ Recognising how alcohol and substitute sweeteners affect your diet

▶ Considering the dietary needs of type 1 and type 2 diabetes

▶ Putting together a plan for losing weight

▶ Coping with eating disorders and diabetes

. . . .

*A*re you watching your weight go higher and higher? Do you think that low calorie means the food on the bottom shelf of the supermarket? Language specialists claim that the five sweetest phrases in the English language are:

- ✔ I love you.
- ✔ Dinner is served.
- ✔ All is forgiven.
- ✔ Sleep until noon.
- ✔ Keep the change.

To that, most people would certainly add, 'You've lost weight.'

About four out of five type 2 diabetics in the United Kingdom are overweight when they're diagnosed. If you have diabetes and your body mass index (BMI) is over the ideal maximum of 25, your risks of dying prematurely are dramatically increased. (If you're not sure what BMI is, head over to Chapter 7 for more details.) The more overweight you are, the more at risk you are. But the good news is that losing weight cuts your risks, too – a fact that makes appropriate nutrition and weight loss more of a necessity than an option.

The Diabetes Control and Complications Trial clearly shows that if you're diabetic, following a careful nutrition programme can reduce your haemoglobin A1c (discussed in Chapter 7) by as much as 1 per cent compared to the person with diabetes who is careless about diet. The consequence of that lowering is a very significant reduction in both the short- and long-term complications of diabetes. In this chapter, you find out all you need to know to make your diet work for you, not only to improve your diabetes and control your blood glucose, but to improve your overall quality of life.

Considering Total Calories First

Wanda B. Thinner, age 46, was a new type 2 diabetic patient who came to me because of high blood glucose levels, some blurring of her vision, and some numbness in her toes. She was 5 feet 5 inches tall and weighed 12 stone. She was taking pills for the diabetes, but they weren't helping. Another doctor had told her she needed to lose weight but gave no further instructions. I started her on a diet based on the principles in this chapter. She was willing to follow the diet and lost 1 ½ stone, which she has kept off. Her blood glucose is now about 6 most of the time. She no longer has blurring of vision, and her toes are beginning to improve. She's off the diabetes medication and feels much better.

No matter how you slice it, your weight is determined by the number of calories you take in, minus the number of calories you use up by exercise or lose in the urine or bowel movement. If you take in an excess of calories and have insulin with which to store them, you gain weight. If you take in fewer calories than you use up, you lose weight. (See Chapter 7 if you're not sure how much you should weigh.)

Reducing your weight by even a little reduces your risk factors for complications dramatically. For instance, losing 10 per cent of your weight:

- Cuts your total cholesterol by about 10 per cent
- Cuts your LDL (bad) cholesterol by about 15 per cent
- Increases your HDL (good) cholesterol by about 8 per cent
- Cuts your blood pressure by about 10/5 mmHg
- Halves your average fasting glucose if you have diabetes

In addition, by losing weight, you:

✔ Markedly reduce your risk of developing type 2 diabetes

✔ Prevent impaired glucose tolerance from progressing into type 2 diabetes

✔ Can potentially make your diabetes respond to drugs that, although initially effective, no longer work (Chapter 10 has more details on this)

✔ Reduce your likelihood of needing insulin therapy if you are a type 2 diabetic

✔ Reduce your risk of dying from diabetes

✔ Increase your life expectancy if you have type 2 diabetes

A study of portion size between 1977 and 1998 (published in the *Journal of the American Medical Association* in January 2003) showed that portion sizes in the United States have increased dramatically, especially in fast-food restaurants and at home. Sadly, to judge from the proliferation of 'super-size-me' adverts from fast food outlets in the United Kingdom, we're just as bad. One simple and effective way to cut your calories is to eat ½ to ⅔ of what you are served and save the rest for another time.

How much energy you use up depends on how active you are and your basal metabolic rate (BMR). Energy is measured in kilocalories (kcal). Kilocalories are also used to measure the amount of energy you need to expend to use up a given amount of food. When most people talk about the calorie content of food or energy expenditure, they're actually talking about the kilocalorie content. For the purposes of this chapter, we use the term 'calories' to talk about kilocalories.

Your weight (more specifically, your lean body mass) and how fast your organs 'tick over' determines your BMR. Physical exertion accounts for between 10 and 50 per cent of your total energy expenditure. The heavier you are, the more energy physical exertion uses up. If you've ever been on a diet, you've probably experienced that irritating 'sticking point' where you stop losing weight after a while, even though you're not eating any more. That's because keeping a heavy body going takes more energy than keeping a lighter one going. But even though that seems unfair, you don't help yourself if you use it as an excuse to give up on your diet.

To work out your energy needs without taking exercise into account, you need to know your desirable weight in pounds. You can use the table in Chapter 7 to figure out your ideal weight, and you can follow this formula to calculate your energy needs:

1. **Multiply your weight in pounds by 10 to get an idea of your basic energy requirements.**

   If you are a male and your desirable weight is 140 pounds (10 stone), for example, your basic energy needs will be about 1,400 calories.

2. **Depending on how active you are, add a percentage of calories to that number.**

   Of course, everyone does some exercise, even if you're only reaching for the television control! Use the following as a guide to see what percentage of your calories you need to add:

   • If you're a sedentary male, add about an extra 10 per cent of your basic energy needs in 'exercise'.

   • If you're a moderately active male, add 20 per cent.

   • If you're a very active male, add 40 per cent or more, depending on the length and the degree of exercise.

These formulas are true for women as well, but women usually require fewer calories to maintain the same weight as men.

Do be aware, though, that these measures are only approximate. They vary not only between people, but also in the same person on different days. Your calorie needs also vary at different stages in your life. As you get older, your calorie needs tend to go down. If you are pregnant or breastfeeding, for example, you need more calories. Even this varies, though, depending on your weight – see Chapter 6 for more details.

This calculation gives you a rough idea of the number of calories you need to maintain your weight. You can then base your diet on this total calorie need. Of course, if you take in fewer calories than you use up in energy, you lose weight (explained in the later section, 'Reducing Your Weight').

Once you determine the total calories, the question becomes how to divide the calories among the various foods. Basically, three foods contain calories: Carbohydrates, proteins, and fats. Within these foods, you have many variables, which we explain in the following sections.

Making up your diet

You can divide your diet up into the proportions of your total energy (or kcal) intake that should come from each food category. Table 8-1 gives the recommended dietary composition of the various food groups, according to the European Diabetes Policy Group. To determine the total amounts of each component you should be eating, multiply the percentage figure by your personal calorie need.

Table 8-1	Recommended Dietary Composition
Food Group	*Percentage of Your Calorie Needs*
Carbohydrate*	More than 50–55%
Added sugar	Under 25 g/day
Total sugar	Under 50 g/day
Fat	Under 25–30%
Saturated	Under 10%
Mono-unsaturated	10–15%
Polyunsaturated	Under 10%
Protein	10–15%
Fibre	Over 30 g/day
Salt**	Under 6 g/day
Cholesterol	Under 300 mg/day
Alcohol***	Under 30 g/day

*Carbohydrate should be mainly fibre rich and 'complex' rather than 'refined', with little (under 50 g/day) as simple sugars (you can find out more in the section 'Counting carbohydrates', later in this chapter).

**Salt intake should be under 3 g/day if you have hypertension.

***Alcohol should be under 20 g/day for women, and only taken with meals.

Keeping track of the number of calories, grams, and percentages of different foods can be really difficult, so use a healthy eating pyramid. The healthy eating pyramid, shown in Figure 8-1, is based on an intake of about 2,000 kcal/day, so you can work out your own pyramid according to your own calorie needs. That way, you have a ready reckoner of the number of servings of each food you need a day. Keep your pyramid pinned to the fridge to remind you and the cook (if that's not you!).

Counting carbohydrates

If a more controversial area exists in nutrition for the diabetic person than carbohydrate, we'd like to know about it. Until the 1970s, doctors told diabetics to limit their carbohydrate intake drastically to keep their blood sugar under good control. In fact, a diet low in carbohydrate is likely to be higher in fat, which is the last thing you need if you're at high risk of cardiovascular disease. The European Diabetes Policy Group now recommends that 50–55 per cent of your total calorie content should come from carbohydrate.

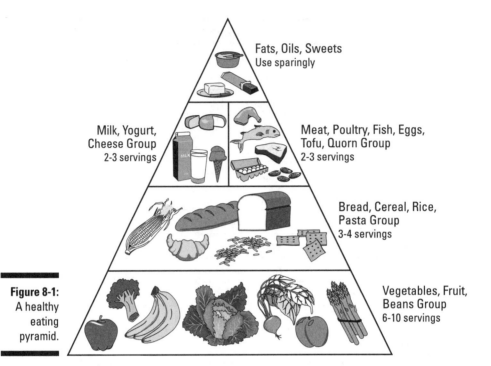

Figure 8-1:
A healthy
eating
pyramid.

But, of course, diet is not as simple as that. It seems likely that much of the confusion about carbohydrates has arisen because experts haven't differentiated between different types of carbohydrate. To understand more, you have to go back to basics.

Carbohydrates are the source of energy that starts with glucose, the sugar in your bloodstream that is one sugar molecule, and include substances containing many sugar molecules called complex carbohydrates, starches, cellulose, and gums. Some of the common sources of carbohydrate are bread, potatoes, grain, cereals, and rice. The forms of carbohydrate like glucose, which are made up of simple molecules, are called *refined carbohydrates*. The ones made up of lots of molecules are called *complex carbohydrates*. Many of the complex carbohydrates are high in fibre, too. As explained in the section 'Knowing the glycaemic index (GI) of carbohydrates', these are broadly the same as low glycaemic index carbohydrates.

Physicians know a lot of information about carbohydrate in the body:

- Carbohydrate is the primary source of energy for muscles.

- Glucose is the carbohydrate that causes the pancreas to release insulin.

- Carbohydrate causes the triglyceride (fat) level to rise in the blood. However, this usually only happens if the carbohydrate in your diet is largely refined, where your total calorie intake is high, or where your blood sugar control is poor.

✔ When insulin is not present or is ineffective, more carbohydrate raises the blood glucose higher.

You need to choose your type of carbohydrate carefully. If you have too much refined carbohydrate and not enough complex carbohydrate, your triglycerides can rise.

The way to eat the right amount of carbohydrate without increasing your blood glucose or triglycerides is to eat low glycaemic index (GI), high-fibre carbohydrate. Foods that are both low GI and high fibre include oats, legumes, and fruit. The following sections tell you more.

Knowing the glycaemic index (GI) of carbohydrates

All carbohydrates are not alike in the degree to which they raise the blood glucose. This is because it takes different times to digest different carbohydrates into absorbable sugar. Experts recognised this fact some years ago, and created a measurement called the *glycaemic index* to quantify it. The glycaemic index of a food is determined by how fast your body absorbs the carbohydrate in the food.

The *glycaemic index* (GI) uses white bread as the indicator food and assigns it a value of 100. Another carbohydrate of equal calories is compared to white bread in its ability to raise the blood glucose and assigned a value in comparison to white bread. A food that raises glucose half as much as white bread has a GI of 50, while a food that raises glucose 1½ times as much has a GI of 150.

A glycaemic index of 70 or more is high, 56–69 is medium, and 55 or below is low. GI has problems that have caused it to be under-utilised:

✔ The GI of a carbohydrate may be different depending on whether you eat it alone or as part of a mixed meal.

✔ The GI of a carbohydrate can also be influenced by protein or fat that you eat at the same time.

✔ The GI of a food may differ if it's processed and prepared differently.

✔ Some low GI foods, like chocolate, contain a lot of fat.

✔ Diabetes educators have been reluctant to teach the concept of the glycaemic index because they believe it's hard to understand and will create confusion.

However, good clinical studies have shown that knowledge of the glycaemic index of food sources can be very valuable. Looking at the diets of people who develop diabetes compared with the diets of those who don't shows that, all other things being equal, the people with the highest GI diet most often developed diabetes. Once diabetes is present, those who eat the lowest GI carbohydrates have the lowest levels of blood glucose. Patients in these studies have not had great difficulty changing to a low GI diet. The other thing that happens when low GI food is incorporated into a diet is that the levels of triglycerides and LDL (or 'bad') cholesterol fall in both type 1 and type 2 diabetes. In addition, many of the foods listed as having a low glycaemic index contain a lot of fibre, and that helps to reduce the blood glucose (see the section 'Understanding the type of fibre in your carbohydrates' for details).

A good case can be made for believing that switching to low GI carbohydrate is very beneficial for controlling glucose. You can easily make some simple substitutions in your diet, as shown in Table 8-2.

Table 8-2	Simple Diet Substitutions
High GI Food	*Low GI Food*
Bread (wholemeal or white)	Wholegrain bread
Corn or wheat-based cereals	Oat-based cereals, including porridge
Plain biscuits and crackers	Biscuits made with dried fruits or whole grains like oats
Cakes and muffins	Cakes and muffins made with fruit, oats, and whole grains
Cooked or over-ripe fruit	Raw, not over-ripe fruit
Fruit juice	Raw fruit
Tropical fruits like bananas	Temperate-climate fruits like apples and plums
Instant potato, old potatoes (especially if mashed)	New potatoes
Potatoes	Pasta or legumes (peas or beans)
Long-grain rice	Basmati rice

Because bread and breakfast cereal are major daily sources of carbohydrate, these simple changes can make a major difference in lowering your glycaemic index. Foods that are excellent sources of carbohydrate but have a low GI include legumes (such as peas or beans), pasta, grains like barley, parboiled rice and bulgar wheat, and wholegrain breads.

Even though a food has a low GI, it may not be appropriate because it's too high in fat. You need to evaluate each food's fat content before assuming that all low GI foods are good for a person with diabetes.

Understanding the type of fibre in your carbohydrates

Fibre is the part of the carbohydrate that isn't digestible and therefore adds no calories. Fibre is found in most fruits, grains, and vegetables. Fibre comes in two forms:

- ✔ **Soluble fibre:** This form of fibre can dissolve in water and can lower blood glucose and fat levels, particularly cholesterol.

  Soluble fibre improves glycaemic control by slowing absorption of glucose after a meal and smoothing out peaks and troughs in blood glucose. It may also have a small beneficial effect on lipids.

- ✔ **Insoluble fibre:** Also called *bulk fibre* or *roughage*, this form of fibre cannot dissolve in water and remains in the intestine. It absorbs water and stimulates movement in the intestine. Insoluble fibre also helps prevent constipation and possibly colon cancer.

  Although insoluble fibre, unlike soluble fibre, has little or no effect on blood glucose control or blood lipids, it still offers lots of benefits for non-diabetics as well as for diabetics. These benefits include reduced levels of constipation, piles, diverticular disease, cancer of the colon, and possibly other cancers.

Studies suggest that the Scots may have been onto a good thing for centuries! Eating 50–100 grams of oat bran every day can reduce your cholesterol by 2–3 per cent.

Before the current trend to refine foods, people ate many sources of carbohydrate that were high in fibre. These were all in plant foods, such as fruits, vegetables, and grains. Animal foods contain no fibre. To look at the effect of high-fibre foods on general health, contrast the average Western diet with the high-fibre diet of the average African. Malnutrition aside, Africans have far fewer problems with obesity, constipation, and other digestive problems.

Protein chemistry

Just as most carbohydrate contains no protein, most protein contains no carbohydrate. Therefore, protein does not raise blood glucose levels significantly under normal circumstances.

When the protein enters the small intestine, it is broken down into the smaller molecules of amino acids of which it is made. The amino acids are absorbed into the bloodstream and head for the liver, where some are converted into glucose. So dietary protein can raise glucose, but this takes place slowly and is not a major contributor to the blood glucose. Some of the amino acids are used to build new protein.

The recommendation for daily fibre is over 30 grams (or 20–25 grams if you are on a weight-reducing diet). Most Britons eat only about 15 grams daily.

Because too much fibre causes diarrhoea and gas, you need to increase the fibre level in your diet fairly slowly.

Proteins

Unless you're a vegetarian, protein in your diet is actually the muscle of other animals, such as chicken, turkey, beef, or lamb. For this reason, people used to think that you can build your own muscle by eating lots of another animal's muscle, but the truth is that you can build up the muscle only by exercising or weightlifting. You need little protein to maintain your current level of muscle.

Because of their relatively low intake of fat and sugar, many diabetics eat more protein in their diets than non-diabetics. There have been concerns that eating too much protein can increase your risk of diabetic kidney disease (Chapter 5 gives more details about this). Several studies have shown that a low-protein diet may slow down how quickly diabetic kidney problems progress at all stages, although a very large study in the *New England Journal of Medicine* in 1994 came to a different conclusion. It showed that a low-protein diet didn't preserve kidney function any better than a high-protein diet.

High-protein diets also tend to be high in saturated fats, which can damage your kidneys as well as your heart. Of course, you can get round this problem by sticking to non-animal versions of protein.

Having said that, not eating enough protein can cause breakdown of muscle, even if you are eating enough calories overall. Non-diabetics adapt to a low-protein diet and stop breaking down muscle, but diabetics don't seem to be able to adapt in the same way.

Weighing up all these factors, it is now recommended that you get 10–15 per cent of your daily calorie intake from protein. This is less than the British average.

With so much conflicting advice, knowing what to do about your protein intake can be hard. It's worth talking to your doctor, nurse, or dietician before you make any drastic changes, though, especially if you have kidney problems.

Your choice of protein is very important because some is very high in fat while some is relatively fat free. The following lists can give you an idea of the fat content of various sources of protein. (The next section explains how to integrate fat into your diet.)

Some sources of protein are very high in saturated fats, making them higher in calories but, more importantly, making them very bad for your heart. Animal sources of protein can be especially deceptive, with even relatively lean cuts containing hidden fats. White meat, such as chicken, turkey, and game, doesn't have nearly as much hidden fat. Frying rather than grilling just adds insult to injury!

One ounce of **very lean** meat, fish, or its equivalent (see Appendix B Exchange lists) has 7 grams of protein and 1 gram of fat. Here are some examples:

- Skinless white-meat chicken or turkey
- Cod, haddock, halibut, or tuna canned in water
- Fat-free cheese (cottage cheese or Quark)

An ounce of **lean** meat, fish, or equivalent has 7 grams of protein and 3 grams of fat. Here are some examples:

- Lean beef, lean pork, lamb, or veal
- Dark-meat chicken without skin or white-meat chicken with skin
- Sardines, salmon, or tuna canned in oil
- Other meats or cheeses with 3 grams of fat per ounce

An ounce of **medium-fat** meat, fish, or equivalent has 7 grams of protein plus 5 grams of fat. Examples include the following:

- Most beef products
- Medium cuts of pork, lamb, or veal
- Dark-meat chicken with skin or fried chicken
- Fried fish
- Cheeses with 5 grams of fat per ounce, such as Edam, feta, and mozzarella

High-fat meat, fish, or equivalent contains 8 grams of fat and 7 grams of protein per ounce. Consider these examples:

- Pork spare ribs or pork sausage
- Bacon
- Full-fat cheeses like Cheddar, Double Gloucester, Cheshire, and most soft French cheeses
- Processed sandwich meats

Eggs, cholesterol: Good, bad, or indifferent?

Eggs have long had a bad press healthwise because they contain high levels of cholesterol. However, they don't contain much in the way of saturated fat, and high saturated fat food that your body can convert to cholesterol is worse for your heart than cholesterol itself. A recent study looking at egg addicts concluded that eating an egg a day doesn't increase your chance of dying of heart disease. Most other foods that you eat regularly don't contain a lot of cholesterol, but whole milk and hard cheeses like Cheddar contain saturated fat, which raises the cholesterol in the body. Interestingly, changing to a low-cholesterol diet after you have a heart attack doesn't reduce your chance of getting another one. But changing to a Mediterranean diet, with less saturated fat, more fish, more olive oil, and more fruit and vegetables, does cut your risks significantly.

You can see the huge difference in calories between low-fat sources of protein and high-fat sources. An ounce of skinless white-meat chicken contains about 40 calories, while an ounce of pork spare ribs has 100 calories. Because most people eat a minimum of four ounces of meat at a meal, they're eating from 160 to 400 calories depending on the source.

Use the healthy eating pyramid (refer to Figure 8-1) to guide your protein intake. If your daily calorie allowance is 1,700 kilocalories, you can take up to 250 kilocalories as protein without exceeding the present European Diabetes Policy Group's guidelines. That's a healthy 16 ounces of tofu or 8 ounces of white chicken meat, but only 2 ½ ounces of pork spare ribs!

Fat

The amount of fat you need is a lot less controversial than the carbohydrate and protein in your diet. Everyone agrees that you should eat no more than 30 per cent of your diet as fats. (Currently, the British population eats over 35 per cent of its diet as fats.)

Keep in mind that some fats are more dangerous in their tendency to promote coronary heart disease than others. These fats should make up less of the dietary fat than the safer fats. Don't forget, though, that these 'less dangerous' forms of fat have just as many calories as the 'more dangerous' alternatives.

Cholesterol is the fat everyone knows. It's been shown to be the culprit in the development of coronary heart disease, as well as peripheral arterial disease and cerebrovascular disease (Chapter 5 tells you more about these diseases). The recommendation is that no more than 300 milligrams a day of fat come from cholesterol.

There are various types of fat:

- **Saturated fat** is the kind of fat that usually comes from animal sources. The streaks of fat in a steak are saturated fat. Butter is made up of saturated fat. Bacon, cream, and cream cheese are other examples. Currently, most British diabetics eat about 14–17 per cent of their daily calorie intake as saturated fats, which is about the same as their non-diabetic compatriots. It is recommended that the maximum amount of saturated fat in the diet be 10 per cent of your total calorie intake. Vegetable sources of saturated fat include coconut, palm, and palm kernel oils.

  Eating a lot of saturated fat increases your blood cholesterol level. It also increases your low-density lipoprotein (LDL) cholesterol, which is the kind that does most damage to your cardiovascular system.

  Keeping in mind that 30 per cent of total daily calories should come from fat; it is recommended that less than a third of that amount come from saturated fats.

- **Trans fatty acid** is produced when polyunsaturated fat, described below, is heated and hydrogen is bubbled through it. Fully hydrogenated, trans fatty acid becomes solid fat, but partially hydrogenated, it has a consistency like butter and can be used instead of butter. Trans fatty acids are used by food manufacturers to replace butter because they are cheaper, and are particularly widely used in shop-bought pastries and cakes. If they are present in food, you will see 'partly hydrogenated oil' in the list of ingredients. Trans fatty acids may contribute even more to the development of heart disease than saturated fats. Keep them out of your diet!

- **Unsaturated fat** comes from vegetable sources like olive oil, some nuts, and margarine. It comes in two forms:

  - **Monounsaturated fat** does not raise cholesterol. Avocado, olive oil, and rapeseed oil are examples. The oil in nuts like almonds and peanuts is monounsaturated. You should have 10–15 per cent of your total daily calorie intake as monounsaturated fat.

  - **Polyunsaturated fat** also does not raise cholesterol but causes a reduction in the good or HDL cholesterol. Examples of polyunsaturated fats are soft fats and oils such as corn oil, mayonnaise, and margarine. You should limit your intake of polyunsaturated fats to less than 10 per cent of your total daily calorie intake.

As you think about how you can reduce your fat intake, keep these tips and suggestions in mind:

✔ Lots of margarines contain olive oil or other monounsaturated fats. So consider changing from polyunsaturated to monounsaturated margarine, and from vegetable oil to rapeseed or olive oil for cooking.

You can't fill your chip pan with olive oil and stop worrying! Even monounsaturated fats, if heated and cooled repeatedly, can lose their beneficial properties and become just as harmful to your heart as the saturated version. Ideally, cut down the use of any oil in cooking to a minimum.

✔ Eskimos eat a lot of fat (more than is recommended), and yet they have a low incidence of coronary heart disease. Their protection comes from essential fatty acids. These acids are found in fish oils, which the Eskimos consume to a great extent. Essential fatty acids reduce triglycerides, lower blood pressure, and increase the time that it takes for blood to clot, which protects against a blood clot in the heart. You can have the benefits of fish oil by substituting fish for meat two or three times a week in your diet.

Fish oils had bad publicity in April 2006 after a study in the *British Medical Journal* suggested they could do more harm than good. In fact, the study had some major flaws, and the results should be taken with a pinch of salt (although not more than a pinch, because salt in excess is bad for you!) The vast majority of the evidence about omega 3 fatty acids, of which fish oils are one of the biggest sources, suggests that their benefits far outweigh any risks.

Although you can get omega 3 fatty acids from plant sources and fortified foods, your body can't process them as efficiently as the fish variety – so it's worth considering a fish oil supplement (containing about 450 mg of omega 3) every day if you don't like oily fish.

The flesh (as opposed to the liver) of non-oily fish (such as cod and halibut) only contains low levels of omega 3 fatty acids. You need to take oily fish (such as salmon, mackerel, and sardines) or fish liver oil to get the full benefits of omega 3 fatty acids.

✔ Reducing intake of saturated fats is almost as good for the non-diabetic heart as the diabetic one. So stop buying butter and cream for the rest of the family, and convert them all to healthier alternatives. An added benefit is that, if you don't have these high-fat items in the house at all, you won't be tempted by them, either!

Getting Enough Vitamins, Minerals, and Water

Your diet must contain sufficient vitamins and minerals, but the amount you need may be less than you think. If you eat a balanced diet that comes from the various food groups, you generally get enough vitamins for your daily needs. Table 8-3 lists the vitamins and their food sources.

Table 8-3	Vitamins You Need	
Vitamin	*Function*	*Food Source*
Vitamin A	Needed for healthy skin and bones	Liver, milk, green vegetables
Vitamin B1 (thiamin)	Converts carbohydrates into energy	Meat, wholegrain cereals
Vitamin B2 (riboflavin)	Needed to use food properly	Milk, cheese, fish, green vegetables
Vitamin B6 , (pyridoxine) pantothenic acid, and biotin	All needed for growth	Liver, yeast, many other foods
Vitamin B12	Keeps the red blood cells and the nervous system healthy	Animal foods (for example meat), Marmite
Folic acid	Keeps the red blood cells and the nervous system healthy	Potatoes, green leafy vegetables, wholegrain bread, fortified breakfast cereals
Niacin legumes	Helps release energy	Lean meat, fish, nuts,
Vitamin C	Helps maintain supportive tissues	Fruit, potatoes
Vitamin D	Helps with absorption of calcium	Dairy products, sunlight
Vitamin E	Helps maintain cells	Vegetable oils, wholegrain cereals
Vitamin K	Needed for proper clotting of the blood	Leafy vegetables, bacteria in your intestine

Vitamin A and pregnancy

During a particularly hard winter in the Arctic, an unusually large number of Eskimo women gave birth to blind babies. When researchers looked into the cause, it became apparent that because there were very few fish or other food sources, these women were eating large quantities of polar bear liver. Their husbands were saving this 'treat' for them, in the belief that it was full of vitamins and other nutrients they needed. It turns out that polar bear liver has particularly high levels of vitamin A, which can cause blindness in babies if taken in large quantities. This was one of the first warnings that vitamins may not always be good for you.

As you look through the vitamins in Table 8-3, you can see that most of them are easily available in the foods you eat every day.

In certain situations, such as if you're pregnant, you need to be sure that you're getting enough vitamins every day. You can find out more about one such vitamin, folic acid, in Chapter 6. But remember that some vitamins can actually be dangerous in excess, especially if you are pregnant, so check with your doctor before you take any vitamin supplements. Consider these examples:

✔ Vitamin A can damage your baby's eyes if you have too much of it while you're pregnant. Liver contains high levels of vitamin A, so we recommend that you avoid liver as much as possible during pregnancy.

✔ There has been a suggestion that large doses of vitamin C can protect against colds. However, even vitamin C can cause complications such as kidney stones if taken in huge doses.

As far as vitamins go, the proof just doesn't exist that large amounts of the vitamins are beneficial, and in some cases they may be harmful. So avoid taking megadoses of these vitamins.

Minerals are also key ingredients of a healthy diet. Most are needed in tiny amounts, which are easily consumed from a balanced diet, although there are a few exceptions:

✔ **Calcium, phosphorus, and magnesium build bones and teeth.** Milk and other dairy products provide plenty of these minerals, but evidence suggests that people aren't getting enough calcium. Adults should get 1,000 milligrams of calcium every day and 1,500 milligrams if you are growing up (adolescents) or growing out (pregnant women). Older people must be sure to eat 1,500 milligrams a day.

Magnesium deficiency can be a side effect of certain oral hypoglycaemic drugs, as well as ketoacidosis and certain heart arrhythmias. If any of these apply to you, have a chat with your doctor about the benefits of magnesium supplements.

✔ **Iron is essential for red blood cells and is found in meat, dark green leafy vegetables, beans, nuts, and wholemeal bread.** A menstruating woman tends to lose iron. Your body can usually accommodate this, but if you become anaemic because of very heavy periods, you may need to take iron supplements.

✔ **Sodium regulates body water.** You need only about 220 milligrams a day, but most people take in 20 to 40 times that much, which can make high blood pressure worse. Don't add salt to your food because it already contains plenty, and you're likely to enjoy the taste a lot more without added salt.

Do beware hidden salt in manufactured foods. Food manufacturers add salt to all sorts of unlikely foods, such as cornflakes, and the amount added by the same manufacturer for different countries varies according to the national taste for salt. Sadly, the amount added for the British market is more than for most other countries. About three-quarters of the average Briton's sodium intake comes from manufactured foods, including bread and ready meals. Most Britons eat about 50 per cent more sodium than they should – about 9 grams a day rather than the recommended 6 grams a day.

✔ **Chromium is needed in tiny amounts.** No scientific evidence shows that chromium is especially helpful to the person with diabetes in controlling blood glucose, despite reams of articles to the contrary in health-food magazines.

✔ **Iodine is essential for the production of thyroid hormones.** Iodine is added to salt in order to ensure that people get enough of it. In areas where iodine is not found in the soil, people suffer from very large thyroid glands known as *goitres*. These form a large lump in the front of your neck. Because goitres used to be a big problem in Derbyshire, 'Derbyshire neck' is a recognised medical term.

✔ **Various other minerals, like chlorine, cobalt, tin, and zinc, are found in many foods.** These minerals are rarely lacking in the human diet.

Water is the last important nutrient discussed in this section, but it is by no means the least important. Your body is made up of 60 per cent or more water. All the nutrients in the body are dissolved in water. You can live without food for some time, but you can't last long without water. Water can give you a feeling of fullness that reduces appetite. In general, people don't drink enough water.

You need to drink a minimum of 10 cups, or 5 pints, of water a day.

Adding Alcohol

Alcohol is a chemical that has calories but no particular nutritional value. You notice that we call alcohol a chemical – that's because alcohol is often taken to excess and does major damage to the body. It wrecks the liver and can lead to death.

Of course, this book isn't the place for a discussion of the social issues that surround the use of alcohol. Suffice it to say that drinking in excess destroys lives and families. This section focuses on the part that alcohol plays in the life of the person with diabetes.

Because alcohol has calories, if you drink some, you must account for it in your diet. In the United Kingdom, most alcohol is measured in percentages. Wine is mostly 12 per cent alcohol, beer 5 per cent, and spirits up to 40 per cent alcohol. To work out the number of calories in a drink, you can use the following formula:

Calories = 0.06 × percentage alcohol × ml

So, for example, using the formula for a 400 ml can of beer, you get this:

0.06 × 5 × 400 = 120 kilocalories

For a couple of 120 ml glasses of wine, you get

0.06 × 12 × 240 = 175 kcalories.

Alcohol stories and news coverage

The British media love any new study showing that alcohol in any form is good for you. Readers love to hear it, so the press loves to write about it. But don't believe everything you read. For instance, a lot of publicity has surrounded the protective effect of alcohol on your heart. What the media don't tell you, though, is that this protection doesn't apply to everyone. What's more, a single glass of wine a day does just as much good as larger amounts, without any of the dangers of excess alcohol.

If alcohol is so high in calories, why aren't more alcoholics fat?

Alcohol calories add up pretty quickly. You may even wonder why alcoholics are not often over-weight. The answer is that alcohol becomes their primary source of nutrition, and they develop wasting diseases associated with inadequate intake of protein, carbohydrate, fat, vitamins, and minerals.

The European Diabetes Policy group recommends that diabetics limit their alcohol intake to 30 grams of alcohol per day for men and 20 grams per day for women. That translates roughly to:

Drinker	*Spirits (40% alc)*	*Wine (12% alc)*	*Normal beer (5% alc)*
Men	75 ml (180 kcal)	240 ml (170 kcal)	600 ml (180 kcal)
Women	50 ml (120 kcal)	160 ml (115 kcal)	400 ml (120 kcal)

Of course, to make matters more complicated still, recommended alcohol intakes for everyone else in the United Kingdom are measured in units. Basically, 30 grams of alcohol equates to about 2.2 units, and 20 grams to 1.5 units.

When is a beer not a beer? When it's an extra-strong beer. Some kinds of popular beer and lager, like canned 'super-strength' lager, have almost twice as much alcohol as 'normal-strength' beers and lagers. Even wine can vary between 9 and 13 per cent alcohol, so some versions have 50 per cent more alcohol than others. That means you *must* check the alcohol content of all the alcohol you drink.

In addition to the calories, alcohol plays other roles in diabetes. Taking alcohol without food can cause low blood glucose by increasing the activity of insulin without food to compensate for it. Some alcoholics, even without diabetes, go to bed with several drinks and are unconscious the next morning because of very low blood glucose. They can suffer brain damage unless their body is able to manufacture enough glucose to wake them up.

A hypoglycaemic episode can go unnoticed if you're inebriated. Go to Chapter 4 to remind yourself of the symptoms of hypoglycaemia. You are much more prone to hypoglycaemia if you are using either insulin or sulphonylurea drugs to control your diabetes.

If you're having a couple of glasses of wine or other alcohol, make sure that you eat some food along with it.

Substituting Sweeteners (Caloric and Artificial)

Fear of the 'danger' of sugar in the diet has led to a vast effort to produce a compound that can add the pleasurable sweetness without the liabilities of sugar. Interestingly enough, despite the availability of a number of excellent sweeteners, some containing no calories at all, the incidence of diabetes continues to rise. Still, if you can reduce your caloric intake or your glucose response by using a sweetener, it does have an advantage. Sweeteners are divided into those that contain calories and those that don't.

Among the calorie-containing sweeteners are:

- **Fructose found in fruits and berries:** Fructose is actually sweeter than table sugar *(sucrose)*. It's absorbed more slowly from the intestine than glucose, so it raises the blood glucose more slowly. The liver takes up the fructose and converts it to glucose or triglycerides.

- **Xylitol, found in strawberries and raspberries:** Xylitol is like fructose in terms of sweetness. It is taken up slowly from the intestine so that it causes little change in blood glucose. Xylitol does not cause cavities of the teeth as often as the other nutritive sweeteners, so it's used in sugar-free chewing gum.

- **Sorbitol and mannitol, sugar alcohols occurring in plants:** Sorbitol and mannitol are half as sweet as table sugar and have little effect on blood glucose. They change to fructose in the body. If you've read Chapter 5, you may remember sorbitol. When taken as a food, sorbitol doesn't accumulate and damage tissues.

The non-nutritive or artificial sweeteners are often much more sweet than table sugar. Therefore, much less of them is required to accomplish the same level of sweetness as sugar. The current artificial sweeteners include:

- **Saccharin:** This sweetener is 300 to 400 times sweeter than sucrose. It is rapidly excreted unchanged in the urine.

- **Aspartame:** This sweetener is more expensive than saccharin, but people seem to prefer its taste. It's 150 to 200 times sweeter than sucrose.

- **Cyclamate:** Because it's been associated with cancer when given in huge doses, cyclamate is banned in the United States. It is 30 times as sweet as sucrose.

The use of sugar in the diet of the person with diabetes has been changed so that some sugar is permitted. The point is to count the calories eaten as sugar and subtract that from your permissible intake. If you do this, you're likely to have little use for either the nutritive or the non-nutritive sweeteners.

The possibility of a link between aspartame and cancer has caused a few scares. In fact, aspartame is one of the most thoroughly researched food additives out there. In May 2006, after studying the subject, the European Food Standards Agency confirmed that there is no evidence linking aspartame with cancer at even the highest amount most Britons would use. Of course, in an ideal world, none of us would use sugar or sweeteners at all (and dentists would be out of a job!). But if you struggle to do without sugar, using a sweetener instead can save lots of calories and has no hidden health risks.

Special Nutritional Considerations for People with Type 1 Diabetes

If you have type 1 diabetes, you take insulin (see Chapter 10 for more details on this) to control your blood glucose. At this time, doctors and their patients cannot match the human pancreas in the way that it releases insulin just when the food is entering the bloodstream, so that the glucose remains between 4.4 and 6.6 mmol/l. Therefore, you need to make sure that your food enters as close to the expected activity of the insulin as possible.

When you eat

Most people with type 1 diabetes are taking two different types of insulin:

- ✔ Insulin that acts soon after the injection and has a brief period of activity. This rapid-acting insulin is meant to cover the food eaten at meals.

- ✔ Insulin that acts more slowly and lasts longer. This slower-acting insulin covers the rest of the time, particularly overnight when a lot of circumstances tend to raise the blood glucose.

Fortunately, you can take a new type of insulin when you start to eat or even in the middle or at the end of the meal (see Chapter 10 for more information on this insulin). This insulin overcomes the problem that has always existed – that the injection had to be taken 30 minutes before eating to give it time to be active. A person with diabetes who had a meal delayed for any reason often became hypoglycaemic using the old preparation.

Because a person with type 1 diabetes always has some insulin circulating, whether food is available or not, you should not miss a meal. A mid-morning snack, a mid-afternoon snack, and even a bedtime snack, if necessary, are particularly good ideas.

If you have type 1 diabetes, you need to be willing to test your blood glucose frequently. That way, you can identify problems in advance. If, for example, blood glucose is low before exercise (there are more details on this in Chapter 9), you can take some nutrition to avoid hypoglycaemia.

Other considerations

If you have type 1 diabetes, you need to be more careful in drinking alcohol. Alcohol increases the activity of insulin and can bring the blood glucose way down if food is not taken with it. See the section 'Adding Alcohol', earlier in this chapter, for more information on how alcohol can affect you.

Because hypertension is prevalent in type 1 diabetes (as it is in type 2 diabetes), and because it makes diabetic complications occur earlier, you need to reduce your salt intake, too.

Special Nutritional Considerations for People with Type 2 Diabetes

Because most people with type 2 diabetes are overweight, weight control and reduction should be the major consideration. (See the following section 'Reducing Your Weight' for specific techniques to lose weight.)

You see the benefits of weight loss rapidly, even when you lose relatively little weight:

✔ There is a rapid fall in your blood glucose.

✔ Your blood pressure declines.

✔ Your cholesterol falls.

✔ Your triglycerides drop and your good cholesterol (HDL) rises.

As you can find out earlier in this chapter, even a modest reduction of 10 per cent of body weight has a significant positive effect on coronary heart disease.

If you have type 2 diabetes, you must be very aware of the fats in your diet. The metabolic syndrome (see Chapter 5) is commonly found in this type of diabetes. You must pay attention to foods that increase triglycerides, which lead to the production of small, dense LDL particles that are connected to coronary artery disease.

High blood pressure, which makes diabetic complications occur earlier, is common in people with type 2 diabetes. So reducing your salt intake is an important consideration.

Reducing Your Weight

Losing weight is very easy in theory. If you take in any fewer calories than you use up, you lose weight. You can do this either by eating less or by exercising more. Best of all, you can eat less and exercise more at the same time!

Weight reduction is difficult for many reasons. Many overweight people get frustrated by slow rates of weight loss. Their frustration is mostly due to unrealistic expectation. In our experience, most patients do very well initially but tend to return to old habits. There is evidence that this tendency to regain weight is built into the human brain. When fat tissue decreases or even increases, a central control system in the brain acts to restore the fat to the previous level. If you undergo liposuction, for example, the remaining cells swell up to hold more fat.

Still, losing weight and keeping it off are possible. At one time, estimates claimed that only one out of 20 people who lost weight kept it off. Now the figure is closer to one out of five. But while losing weight is all about achieving goals, keeping weight off is a lifelong commitment.

Mathematics of weight loss

A pound of fat contains 3,500 kilocalories. In order to lose a pound of fat, therefore, you must eat 3,500 kilocalories less than you need. You can do this in a week by a daily reduction of 500 kilocalories or by doing 200 kilocalories extra of exercise daily and reducing your diet by only 300 kilocalories per day. Using the first method, a man eating 1,700 kilocalories per day needs to decrease his diet to 1,200 kilocalories per day. Eating 200–500 kilocalories a day less than you expend allows you to lose 2–4 pounds a month.

In the next chapter, we cover the value of exercise in a weight-loss programme. At this point, you need to realise that successfully maintaining your weight loss requires a willingness to make exercise a part of your daily life. (If, for some reason, you cannot move your legs to exercise, you can get a satisfactory workout using your upper body alone.) A recent study showed that 92 per cent of the people who maintained weight loss were exercising regularly, while only 34 per cent of those who regained their weight continued to exercise.

Types of diet

A seemingly endless array of 'new' weight-loss diets comes out all the time. Each one claims that it's more effective, easier, and more efficient than the last. In fact, you can only lose weight in one way – by taking in fewer calories than you use up in energy.

The reason for this huge number of different diets is simple. The media is well aware that huge proportions of the British population are desperate to lose weight and haven't succeeded in the past. If they give out the same message (exercise more and eat less), they won't get new customers, prepared to pay a fortune for the books, slimming products, and other merchandise that go along with these diets.

Some of these diets are fairly drastic in the degree to which they cut calories, and weight loss is fairly rapid. But these methods are particularly prone to result in the original weight being regained. Worse still, some of these diets are frankly dangerous, especially if you're diabetic. Among the many more drastic diets are the following:

- **Very low-calorie diets:** These diets provide 400 to 800 kilocalories daily of protein and carbohydrate with supplemental vitamins and minerals. They are safe when supervised by a physician and are used when you need rapid weight loss – for example, for a heart condition. However, they aren't a good idea as a rule. First, if you restrict your calorie intake too much, your body may start burning muscle rather than fat. Secondly, unless you're very carefully monitored, you may be more prone to hypoglycaemia on this kind of diet. And thirdly, you are more likely to regain the weight after you 'stop' dieting if you haven't altered your basic eating habits.

- **Animal protein diets like the Atkins diet:** These diets limit food to animal protein sources in an effort to maintain body protein, along with vitamins and minerals. Patients often complain of hair loss. People regain their weight rapidly when they discontinue the diet. Such diets are not balanced and we cannot recommend that you use them for more than a few weeks at most.

- ✔ **The cabbage soup diet:** On this diet, most of your daily intake of calories comes from an unlimited supply of thin, watery cabbage soup. Not only does this have very few calories, it's so boring that most people can't eat too much of it. Again, you're not retraining your body's eating habits, and the moment you stop the diet you're likely to revert to your old ways. You also probably regain the weight you've lost quickly.

- ✔ **Fasts:** A *fast* means giving up all food for a period of time and taking only water and vitamins and minerals. A fast is such a drastic change from normal eating habits that you can't remain on the fast for very long, and you regain weight.

Several diets are associated with large organisations and may require that you purchase only their foods. The support given by these organisations does seem to be extremely helpful in weight-loss maintenance. In addition, the slower loss of weight and the connection to more normal eating seems to result in a greater tendency to stay with the programme and keep the weight off.

In the United Kingdom, by far the biggest provider of this type of diet is Weight Watchers. This organisation emphasises slow weight loss, exercise, and behaviour modification. It charges for weekly attendance at its meetings, which are held all over the world as well as in Britain. It doesn't require that you purchase any products. Foods are available for purchase. Weight Watchers' points programme for increasing fibre in your diet may be especially helpful to people with diabetes.

Surgery for weight loss

Surgery is used in the most severe and resistant cases of obesity. Available on the National Health Service, surgery is only for people who are extremely overweight and who have found it impossible to lose weight by other means. It has impressive effects, such as correction of high glucose and reduction or discontinuation of glucose-lowering drugs. Results are so successful in some patients that some surgeons consider type 2 diabetes to be a surgical disease. You may agree that this seems a little extreme.

Some of the reasons for having bypass surgery include:

- ✔ You have a body mass index that is greater than 40.

- ✔ You have an obesity-related physical problem, such as inability to walk.

- ✔ You have a high-risk obesity-related health problem like heart disease.

Traditionally, the best surgical treatment for obesity has been the *vertical banded gastroplasty,* where doctors staple the upper stomach to create a small pouch above, a narrow opening, and a larger pouch below. Because the upper pouch is small, you have a feeling of early fullness and you tend to eat less. More recently, the laparoscopic gastric banding procedure has been used. A constricting band containing an inflatable balloon is placed around the upper end of the stomach. The balloon can be inflated or deflated to control the size of the upper stomach. The usual loss of weight is two-thirds of the excess in two years. Some of the problems of gastric bypass and banding include:

- The pouch may stretch.
- The staple line can break down, or the band slip.
- Malabsorption of iron and calcium may occur.
- There may be reflux of acid from the stomach into the oesophagus (or gullet), causing heartburn.
- Anaemia may occur from lack of vitamin B12.
- The dumping syndrome may occur. In this condition, stomach contents move too fast into the small intestine, provoking a loss of insulin with resultant hypoglycaemia.

When you have bypass surgery for obesity, you must be willing to be committed to lifelong medical follow-up. You must also be willing to give up large meals and be determined to lose weight. There is no question that severely obese patients with type 2 diabetes do well with surgery. As the patients lose weight, their blood glucose falls, their cholesterol falls, and their blood pressure improves. They sleep better and are less depressed.

As for the possible role of liposuction in the treatment of type 2 diabetes, few studies exist on the subject and both short-term and longer-term studies are needed before we assume that the early promise is maintained. For example, a report in the *Annals of Plastic Surgery* in January 2004 showed a fall in glucose, cholesterol, and insulin secretion after liposuction, but this was only three weeks after surgery.

Behaviour modification

If you 'stop' dieting once you've achieved your target weight, you're likely to regain, over the next year, 60–70 per cent of the weight you've lost. The best way to avoid regaining the weight is to incorporate weight loss into a complete, lifelong rethink of your whole way of eating. Think of a weight-loss diet as an extension of normal healthy eating.

The first behaviour changes you need in order to lose weight are diet and exercise. After that, you can change your eating behaviour to make the diet easier to follow. Some of the best techniques include the following:

- Eat according to a schedule to avoid snacking and unscheduled eating.
- Find a single place to eat all your food.
- Slow down your eating to make the meal last.
- Eat from a smaller plate – the food looks more.
- Put high-calorie foods away. Remove serving dishes and bread from the table.
- Concentrate on cooking tasty, lower-calorie foods that the rest of the family can share. That way, you don't feel too left out at mealtimes.
- Don't dispense food to others to avoid exposure for yourself.
- Don't feel you have to clean your plate. Stop eating when you've had enough.
- Set realistic goals for weight loss.
- Allow yourself the occasional treat to stop yourself getting too frustrated by your diet.
- If you're going to go out for a meal, reduce the rest of your day's eating to take account of the excess calories.
- When eating out, be careful of salad dressing, alcohol, and bread.
- Get a 10-pound weight and carry it around for a while to appreciate the importance of a loss of even that little.
- Make a shopping list before you go to the supermarket, and stick strictly to the list.
- Never go shopping for food when you're hungry.

You can incorporate one technique into your life each week (or even longer) until you feel you have mastered it and have added it to your eating style. Then go on and adopt another technique.

As you go about this difficult task of losing weight and keeping it off, remember to seek the help of those around you. A loving partner can be a great help through the roughest days.

Coping with Eating Disorders and Diabetes

The Duchess of Windsor is supposed to have coined the phrase, 'You can never be too rich or too thin.' How much damage has this statement done to society, especially the thin part? Many young people are preoccupied with their body weight. In a survey of students, 60 per cent had dieted over the previous year, even though only 9 per cent had a BMI over 25 (see Chapter 7 to find out more about BMI).

When this preoccupation becomes too great, it can result in an eating disorder. The young girl (90 per cent of sufferers are female) either starves herself and exercises excessively, or eats a great deal and then induces vomiting and/or takes laxatives and water pills. The one who starves herself has *anorexia nervosa,* while the one who binges and purges has *bulimia nervosa.* By themselves, these conditions can result in severe illness and even death when carried to extremes. When combined with diabetes, there is very great danger to the person's health.

Understanding anorexia

The 'typical' anorexic is a girl in her teens. She often comes from a middle- or upper-class background and excels academically or in sports. She is often seen as the 'perfect child' and may find it difficult to rebel. If she experiences a lot of pressure to perform (either academically or at sports), she may feel that she's not in control. Keeping very tight control of her diet may be her way of being in control of her life, or it may be a form of passive rebellion.

Anorexia often starts with people eating a relatively normal diet, and others may not notice any difference for some time. Anorexics are very good at disguising their symptoms. They often conceal their shape under baggy clothes or hide food at the table to make it look as if they have eaten more than they have. They make a lot of excuses to avoid eating in company, and may exercise excessively.

 Although anorexia is very uncommon before puberty, and ten times more common in girls than in boys, it doesn't only happen to teenage girls. Anorexia can happen to anyone. If you think your child may be anorexic, don't confront her or him with it immediately. Anorexics are very sensitive about their weight, and often get defensive and aggressive when someone confronts them about it directly. Talk to your doctor about the best ways to help.

A diagnosis of anorexia nervosa is made on these criteria:

- ✔ Refusal to maintain body weight over the minimum recommended BMI of 18
- ✔ Intense fear of becoming fat, even when underweight
- ✔ Disturbance in body image (the person feeling he is overweight when he is underweight, or feeling one part of his body is disproportionately fat)
- ✔ In girls, the absence of at least three consecutive periods
- ✔ The absence of other serious mental or physical illness to account for the criteria above

The symptoms

The main symptoms of anorexia can be divided into physical symptoms and psychological symptoms.

Physical symptoms include:

- ✔ Reduced basal metabolic rate (BMR)
- ✔ Tiredness
- ✔ Loss of muscle bulk
- ✔ Reduced heart rate and blood pressure
- ✔ Reduced body temperature
- ✔ Reduced wound healing
- ✔ Absence of periods and shrinkage of the ovaries and uterus
- ✔ Thinning of the bones
- ✔ Lanugo hair (fine, downy hair, mostly on the back and arms)
- ✔ In severe cases, hypoglycaemia, seizures, and cardiac failure, which can lead to death

Mental symptoms include:

- ✔ Preoccupation with food
- ✔ Poor concentration
- ✔ Obsession with others' eating
- ✔ Food rituals
- ✔ Embarrassment at eating in company

> ✔ Depression and social isolation
>
> ✔ Mood swings

Anorexia and diabetes

Anorexics are in a constant state of starvation. When they have diabetes, their condition is just like that of people with type 1 diabetes before the availability of insulin. They have very low blood glucose levels, so they require little or no insulin (see Chapter 10 for more about this). Anorexia nervosa is a serious condition for anyone, but is far more dangerous for a diabetic.

Management of diabetes requires a certain amount of routine from day to day. Achieving such systematisation is impossible when the amount of food coming into the body is so uncertain. The girl with severe anorexia may need intravenous feeding until she has stabilised a little. This sometimes leads to very high blood glucose levels, necessitating the use of insulin. Once the life-threatening starvation is under control, good blood glucose control can be achieved with help from the patient and a therapist who can help her to understand her distorted body image. If the person suffers from clinical depression, antidepressant medication may be necessary.

Understanding bulimia

Bulimia involves eating large quantities of easily digested food and then purging it by vomiting and taking laxatives or water pills. Patients with bulimia are not as severely thin as those with anorexia are. In fact, they may be slightly overweight. Their background is similar to the anorexia patients. They may represent up to 40 per cent of college-age female students. Because their weight is closer to normal, they usually menstruate normally.

Girls with bulimia are more likely to go on to adult obesity and are harder to treat. They actually do not do as well with therapy as those with anorexia. They may end up with more psychiatric problems later in life.

Their food intake is extremely variable, but is less restricted than that of anorexics. Therefore, their diabetes is a little easier to treat. They may get other complications, though, such as rotten teeth from the stomach acid they vomit, or malnutrition and fluid imbalances from laxatives.

Both of these conditions make controlling blood glucose impossible, but one other activity worsens the problem: Some diabetic women and men skip insulin injections in order to lose weight. When they do this, they lose weight as the body turns to fat for fuel because glucose can't be used (see Chapter 2).

Again, people suffering from bulimia experience loss of muscle mass, and the blood glucose rises very high.

For more information

To find out more about anorexia and bulimia, you can contact the Eating Disorders Association:

First Floor
Wensun House
103 Prince of Wales Road
Norwich, NW11 1DW

Phone: 01603-621-414.

Their offices are open 8.30 a.m. to 6.30 p.m., Monday to Friday.

You can also go to these Web sites:

✔ www.mentalhealth.com/icd/p22-et01.html

✔ www.eduak.com (Eating Disorders Association)

✔ www.nami.org/helpline/anorexia.htm (National Alliance for the Mentally Ill)

Chapter 9

Keeping It Moving: Exercise Plan

● ●

In This Chapter

▶ Understanding the importance and benefits of exercise

▶ Exercising for the person with type 1 and type 2 diabetes

▶ Determining duration and proper amount of effort

▶ Choosing your activity

● ●

More than 60 years ago, the great leaders in diabetes care declared that diabetes management had three major aspects:

✔ Proper diet

✔ Appropriate medication

✔ Sufficient exercise

Since then, millions of pounds and man (and woman) hours have been spent to define the proper diet and the right medication, but exercise has rarely received its proper place in the triad of care. This chapter looks at how you can correct this omission.

Getting Off the Sofa: Why Exercise Is Important

When they wrote their recommendations just after the isolation and administration of insulin, the experts were really talking about type 1 diabetes. In fact, many studies have shown that exercise doesn't normalise the blood glucose or reduce the haemoglobin A1c (you can read about this in Chapter 7) in type 1 diabetes. Many other studies have shown that exercise does normalise blood glucose and reduce haemoglobin A1c in type 2 diabetes.

ANECDOTE

Exercise your way to health

John Plant is a 46-year-old male who has had type 1 diabetes for 23 years. He takes insulin injections four times daily and measures his blood glucose many times a day. He follows a careful diet.

Prior to developing diabetes, John was a very active person, participating in vigorous sports and doing major hiking and mountain climbing. At the time of his diagnosis, John's doctor warned him that he would have to give up many of the most strenuous activities because he would never know his blood glucose level and it may drop precipitously during his heavy exercise. John ignored this advice and continued his active way of life. He has found that he can do with much less insulin than his doctor prescribed, and he rarely becomes hypoglycaemic. He has been able to continue these activities without limitation. His blood glucose level is

generally between 4.2 and 7.8. His last haemoglobin A1c was slightly elevated, at 6.7. A recent eye examination showed no diabetic retinopathy. He had no significant microalbuminuria in his urine and no tingling in his feet.

Is John lucky? You bet he is. But like most 'luck', John's is based on a realisation that both mind *and* body make up a human being. Why would humans have all these muscles if they were meant to spend their lives munching sweets and crisps in front of a television set?

When a new diabetic patient enters my surgery, I give him a bottle of 50 pills. I instruct him not to swallow the pills but to drop them on the floor three times daily and pick them up one pill at a time. After all, the condition a person is in can be judged by what she takes two at a time – pills or stairs.

But while exercise cannot replace medication for the type 1 diabetic, its benefits are crucial for patients with both types of diabetes.

The main benefit of exercise for both types of diabetes is that it helps prevent cardiovascular disease (you can read about this disease in Chapter 5). Cardiovascular disease affects the entire population – diabetics and non-diabetics alike – but it's particularly severe in people with diabetes. Exercise does prevent cardiovascular disease in numerous ways:

- Exercise helps with weight loss in type 2 diabetes.
- Exercise lowers bad cholesterol and triglycerides, and raises good cholesterol.
- Exercise lowers blood pressure.
- Exercise lowers stress levels.
- Exercise reduces the need for insulin or drugs.

✔ Exercise helps maintain your muscle mass and reduces fat.

✔ Exercise may have a beneficial effect by reducing your body's plasmino-gen activators, which can influence the 'stickiness' of your blood and increase your risk of cardiovascular disease.

The feeling of fatigue that occurs with exercise is probably due to the loss of stored muscle glucose. (See the sidebar 'How exercise works its magic' for more detail.) Of course, this fatigue is short term, and if you exercise regularly, you find that your overall energy levels increase.

With exercise, insulin levels in non-diabetics and people with type 2 diabetes decline because insulin acts to store and not release glucose and fat. Levels of glucagon, adrenaline, cortisol, and growth hormone increase to provide more glucose. Studies show that glucagon is responsible for 60 per cent of the glucose, and adrenaline and cortisol are responsible for the other 40 per cent. If insulin does not fall, glucagon cannot stimulate the liver to make glucose.

You may wonder how insulin can open the cell to the entry of glucose when insulin levels are falling. In fact, two things are at work here:

✔ Glucose is getting into muscle cells without the need for insulin.

✔ The rapid circulation that comes with exercise delivers the smaller amount of insulin more frequently to the muscle. The muscle seems to be more sensitive to the insulin as well.

This is exactly what the person with type 2 diabetes hopes to accomplish when insulin resistance is the major block to insulin action.

One way to preserve glucose stores is to provide calories from an external source. Any marathon runner knows that additional calories can delay the feeling of exhaustion. Of course, you don't need to eat every time you're about to exercise, but the more stamina you're likely to need, the more helpful food can be. The timing of this food intake is important. If you take the glucose an hour before exercise, it metabolises during the exercise and increases endurance. However, if you take it 30 minutes before exercise, it may decrease stamina by stimulating insulin, which blocks liver production of glucose. (See the sidebar 'How exercise works its magic' for more information.)

Fructose can replenish you when you're doing prolonged exercise. This sweetener can replace glucose because, although it's sweeter, you absorb it more slowly and it doesn't provoke the insulin secretion that glucose provokes. Your body rapidly converts fructose into glucose. (Chapter 8 tells you more about fructose.)

How exercise works its magic

To understand how exercise reduces the blood glucose in type 2 diabetes and helps prevent cardiovascular disease in both types, you need to have some understanding of the dynamics of metabolism during exercise.

As exercise begins, the demand for both glucose and fat for energy increases. Glucose and fat leave the sites where they're stored and enter the bloodstream, heading for muscles. At first, glycogen, the storage form of glucose in the liver, begins to break down and release glucose. With continued exercise, glycogen is used up, and the liver begins to make large amounts of glucose from other substances to continue to provide energy.

With steady, moderate exercise, the body eventually looks to fat as the glucose production begins to diminish. This situation is wonderful, especially because most people with type 2 diabetes have plenty of fat to offer. On the other hand, if the exercise is very vigorous, the liver actually makes more glucose than the muscles can use immediately, and the blood glucose begins to rise. This explains some of the instances where the glucose is higher after exercise than it is before exercise. The reason the liver makes so much glucose is that very vigorous exercise depletes the stores of glucose in the muscle very rapidly. You do not continue vigorous exercise for very long, and the extra glucose is there to replenish the muscle tissue once exercise ends.

That's why, on the whole, you notice that all the recommendations are for aerobic exercise rather than anaerobic exercise. See the sidebar 'What are aerobic and anaerobic exercise?' if you want to know more about the difference between the two.

Glucose is a better source of energy when the exercise is very vigorous because you convert it to energy much faster than you convert fat. For less intense exercise, fat is preferred because it provides more energy than an equal amount of glucose.

Exercising When You Have Diabetes

If you have diabetes and haven't exercised previously, you should check with your doctor before you start an exercise programme, especially if you're over 35 or have had diabetes for more than ten years. You should also check with a doctor if you have any of the following risk factors:

- ✔ The presence of any diabetic complications like retinopathy, nephropathy, or neuropathy (explained in Chapter 5)
- ✔ Obesity
- ✔ A physical limitation
- ✔ A history of coronary artery disease or elevated blood pressure
- ✔ Use of any medications (most are fine, but check with your doctor)
- ✔ A history of recurrent hypoglycaemic episodes

You need to discuss any of these problems with your doctor in order to choose the best forms of exercise for you. You can read more about the types of exercise in the section 'Is Golf a Sport? Choosing Your Activity', later in this chapter.

Once you begin your exercise programme, you can do a lot to maximise the benefits and minimise the risks, whether you have type 1 or type 2 diabetes. Some important steps to take include:

✔ Wearing an ID bracelet

✔ Testing your blood glucose very often

✔ Choosing proper socks and shoes

✔ Drinking plenty of water

✔ Carrying treatment for hypoglycaemia

✔ Exercising with a friend

Lycra is not mandatory! Apart from the right shoes and socks, which are essential to protect your feet (you can find out why in Chapter 5), and possibly padded shorts if you're a cyclist, you don't need to buy special clothing.

Most forms of exercise involve using your feet, and *any* such exercise can put your feet at risk if you have diabetic foot disease (see Chapter 5 for information on that). Even swimming can cause problems, if you bang your feet against the side of the pool or walk barefoot to the changing rooms. If you do any form of exercise that involves training shoes, make sure that your shoes provide good support and don't rub. Also be sure you follow the advice on examining your feet in Chapter 7 *every* time you exercise.

Exercise for a person with type 1 diabetes

If you have type 1 diabetes, you depend on insulin injections to manage your blood glucose. You don't have the luxury of a 'thermostat' that automatically shuts off during exercise and turns back on when exercise is finished. Once you take an insulin injection, the insulin is active until you use it up.

If you have type 1 diabetes, be sure not to overdose on insulin before you exercise. Overdosing can lead to hypoglycaemia; underdosing can lead to hyperglycaemia. If your body doesn't have enough insulin, it turns to fat for energy. Glucose rises because you're not metabolising it, but its production is continuing. If you exercise particularly vigorously and you don't have enough insulin, your blood glucose can rise to extremely high levels. Here are some ways to prevent hypoglycaemia:

✔ **Reduce the insulin dosage prior to exercise.** In one study, an 80 per cent reduction in the dose allowed the person with diabetes to exercise for 3 hours, while a 50 per cent reduction forced the person with diabetes to stop after 90 minutes due to hypoglycaemia. Of course, these figures vary according to your level of fitness and how vigorously you exercise. Each person with diabetes varies, and you must determine for yourself how much to reduce your insulin by measuring your blood glucose before, during, and after you exercise.

✔ **Eat some carbohydrate.** You need to have some carbohydrate (which quickly raises blood glucose) available during exercise.

✔ **Choose the right injection site.** The site of the insulin injection is important because this determines how fast the insulin becomes active. If you are running and inject insulin into your leg, your body takes up the insulin more quickly than if you had the injection in your arm.

✔ **Pick an exercise time you can stick to.** You can exercise whenever you will do so faithfully. If you like to sleep late and schedule your exercise at 5.30 a.m., you're not likely to exercise consistently. Your best time to exercise is probably about 60 to 90 minutes after you eat, because this is when the glucose peaks. Exercising at this time provides the calories you need, avoids the usual post-eating high in your blood glucose, and burns up those food calories.

Exercise for a person with type 2 diabetes

Even though you have type 2 diabetes, many of the suggestions for the type 1, other than the insulin discussion, apply to you, too. If you haven't already, read the section 'Exercising When You Have Diabetes' earlier in this chapter.

With sufficient exercise and diet, some people with type 2 diabetes can revert to a 'non-diabetic' state. This doesn't mean that you no longer have diabetes, but it certainly means that you don't develop the long-term complications that can make things so miserable later in life (which you can read about in Chapter 5).

Determining How Much Exercise You Can and Should Do

Unless you have a physical abnormality, you're not limited on what you can do. You need to select an activity that you enjoy and will continue to perform.

What are aerobic and anaerobic exercise?

Aerobic exercise is exercise that can be sustained for more than a few minutes, uses major groups of muscles, and gets your heart to pump faster during the exercise, thus training the heart. It's the kind of exercise that leaves you mildly out of breath. This chapter has many examples of aerobic exercise.

Anaerobic exercise, on the other hand, is brief (sometimes a few seconds), intense, and usually cannot be sustained. Lifting large weights is an example of an anaerobic exercise. A 100-yard sprint is another example.

Whichever form of exercise you're doing, you need to warm up and cool down for about five minutes before and after you exercise. You can warm up by stretching or just standing in one place and hitting a ball before starting to run around.

Exerting enough effort

In the recent past, exercise physiologists said that you needed to make sure that you monitored your exercise intensity by periodically checking your heart rate during exercise.

The younger you are, the faster your exercise heart rate may be. Like everything in this book, your exercise heart rate is an individual number. If you are a world-class athlete training for your ninth marathon, your exercise heart rate may be higher than most people's. If you have some heart disease, your exercise heart rate may be significantly lower.

Figuring out your exercise heart rate

Your exercise heart rate is based on your age and, for aerobic exercise, is supposed to be between 50 and 70 per cent of the range between your basal (or resting) heart rate and your maximum heart rate, which is taken as 220 (beats per minute) minus your age. So, for example, for a 50-year-old man with a resting heart rate of 70, the range would be taken as 50–70 per cent of 70 (his basal rate) and 170 (220 minus his 50 years of age); 50 to 70 per cent of the range between these two numbers is 120–140.

Now studies have shown that people can sustain aerobic exercise at higher heart rates. Perhaps the best way to know whether you're meeting your exercise goals is to use the 'perceived exertion scale', explained in the following section.

Once you know your maximum exercise heart rate, you can choose your activity and use the perceived exertion scale to be sure that you achieve that level during exercise.

Using the perceived exertion scale

Measuring your pulse during exercise (or even at rest) may be hard for you. Instead, you can use the perceived exertion scale. Exercise is given a descriptive value from 'Very, very light' to 'Very, very hard', with 'Very light', 'Fairly light', 'Somewhat hard', and 'Very hard' in between.

If you exercise at a level of 'Somewhat hard', you're at your target heart rate in most cases. As you get into shape, the amount of exertion that corresponds to 'Somewhat hard' increases.

Regardless of what your exercise heart rate is or where your workout falls on the perceived exertion scale, do not continue exercising if you have tightness in your chest, chest pain, severe shortness of breath, or dizziness.

How long and how often?

The number of kilocalories you use for any exercise is determined by your weight, the strenuousness of the activity, and the time you spend actually doing it. To have a positive effect on your heart, you need to do a moderate level of exercise for 30 to 45 minutes at least four times a week, and ideally every day. (See the earlier section 'Using the perceived exertion scale' for an explanation of what constitutes moderate exercise.)

You can do your daily exercise in one go, or you can divide it into sessions of at least 10–15 minutes. That doesn't mean that taking the stairs rather than the lift is a waste of time – it certainly helps your overall level of fitness, and walking upstairs is a great habit to get into. However, to do the most for your heart, you need to exercise in bursts of at least 10–15 minutes.

To stretch or not to stretch

As you've been reading through, and if you have eagle eyes, you may have noticed that I haven't explained much about stretching. That's because doctors can't agree on the place of stretching for the healthy exerciser. One study showed that a group of runners who didn't stretch did better than a group who did. Most doctors agree that stretching after an injury is appropriate, but whether all the advice about stretching before exercise for an uninjured person is much ado about nothing is yet to be determined. If you do stretch, do not stretch to the point that it hurts. This is where muscle tears occur. See the excellent book *Fitness For Dummies,* 2nd Edition, by Suzanne Schlosberg and Liz Neporent (published by Wiley) for more about stretching.

When you need support

The Diabetes Exercise and Sports Association is an organisation that you can turn to for help, instruction, and friendship as you add exercise to your good diabetes care. See the Web site at `http://www.diabetes-exercise.org/index.html`. Its Web site also has details of events in the United Kingdom and Europe.

An hour (not an apple) a day keeps the doctor away! 30 minutes is a minimum, not a maximum, and you can always build up over time. Moderate aerobic exercise done for an hour every day provides enormous physical, mental, and emotional benefits.

Moderate exercise is a moving definition. If you're out of shape, moderate exercise for you may be slow walking. If you're in good shape, moderate exercise may be jogging or cross-country skiing. Moderate exercise is simply something you can do and not get out of breath. For ideas on the types of exercise you can do, see the next section.

Is Golf a Sport? Choosing Your Activity

The best choice for you is an exercise you enjoy and can stick with. The choices are really limitless. The following factors can help you determine your choice of activity:

- Do you like to exercise alone or with company? Pick a competitive or team sport if you prefer company.

- Do you start the year full of good intentions about getting fit, then find your enthusiasm waning? Consider making a regular date to exercise with a friend, so you're able to inspire each other to keep up the good work.

- Do you like to compete against others or just yourself? Running and walking are sports you can do alone.

- Do you prefer vigorous or less vigorous activity? Less vigorous activity over a longer period is just as effective as more vigorous activity.

- Do you live where you can do activities outside all year round, or do you need to go inside a lot of the year? Find a sports club if weather prevents year-round outside activity.

Fore!

Golf may not be as much of an obsession for the British as it is for the Americans or the Japanese, but we're catching up fast. Unfortunately, we're picking up some of their bad habits, too, like using a motorised golf buggy to get from hole to hole. This virtually eliminates the exercise associated with golf.

If you enjoy golf, by all means continue to play it as often as you like, but leave the golf buggy at the nineteenth hole and get the whole experience. A few hours strolling round the golf course is a marvellous way to enjoy the scenery and relax your mind as well as your body.

✔ Do you get bored easily? Consider doing a variety of sports, or take up circuit training, which involves doing the round of several 'stations' with different exercises.

✔ Do you need special equipment or just a pair of running shoes? Having the right materials can make all the difference in both how effective and how safe your exercise programme is.

✔ What benefits are you looking for in your exercise: Cardiovascular, strength, endurance, flexibility, or body fat control? You should probably look for all these benefits, but you may have to combine activities to get them all in.

✔ Do you have a particularly busy life? That's no excuse for not exercising, but setting aside the time you need certainly takes more planning. Getting off the bus or tube a couple of stops earlier every day and walking briskly the rest of the way to work, for instance, is a great way of incorporating exercise into your daily routine. Cycling to work saves on parking charges and helps the environment at the same time!

Your choice of activity must take into account your physical condition. If you have diabetic neuropathy (you can read about this in Chapter 5) and cannot feel your feet, for example, you should not do pounding exercises that may damage them without your awareness. You can swim, cycle, row, or do arm-chair exercises where you move your upper body vigorously.

The good it does you

As your body becomes trained with regular exercise, the benefits for your diabetes are very significant. Your body starts to turn to fat for energy earlier in the course of your exercise. At the same time, the hormones that tend to raise the blood glucose during exercise are not produced at the same high rate because they aren't needed. Because you don't require as much insulin, your insulin doses can be reduced, and you find it much easier to avoid hypoglycaemia during exercise.

Perhaps a good starting point in your activity selection is to focus on the benefits. Table 9-1 gives you some ideas.

Table 9-1	Match Your Activity to the Results You Want
If You Want to . . .	*Then Consider . . .*
Build up cardiovascular condition	Swimming, vigorous basketball, squash, volleyball, cross-country skiing, football, hockey
Strengthen body	Swimming, low-size, high-repetition weight lifting, gymnastics, mountain climbing, cross-country skiing
Build up muscular endurance	Gymnastics, swimming, gym workouts, rowing, cross-country skiing, vigorous basketball
Increase flexibility	Gym workouts, gymnastics, judo and karate, yoga, football, surfing
Control body fat	Swimming, squash, cross-country skiing, vigorous basketball, singles tennis

You can tell from Table 9-1 that living in the mountains where you have plenty of snow is helpful because cross-country skiing is in practically every list. On the other hand, so is swimming, so there's no excuse for giving up exercise if you live outside the Scottish Highlands!

The special needs of many of these sports may turn you off exercise. The curious thing is that the best exercise that you can sustain for life is right at your feet. A brisk daily walk improves heart function, adds to muscular endurance, and helps control body fat. So many people drive their cars to the gym and try to park as close as possible so that they can get to the building with as little effort as possible. Seems a little strange, doesn't it?

Of course, the social benefits of exercise are very important. You are together with people who are concerned with their health and appearance. These people usually share many of your interests. Someone who likes to jog often likes to hike and climb and camp out. Many lifetime partnerships begin on a tennis court (and some end there as well!).

Walking 10K a Day

The idea of walking 10,000 steps a day may seem like a huge, unattainable goal to you, but you may be surprised. This is certainly a goal worth striving towards because, as we discuss earlier in this chapter, walking is one of the most beneficial exercises you can do.

Buy a *pedometer,* a device that you wear on your waist that counts each step you take. Don't waste money on a fancy one – all you need is to be able to count your steps and, if you want, to convert the steps into miles. To do this, you need to know how far you walk each time you take a step. Walk ten steps, measure the distance, and divide by ten to get your stride length. Input this number in the appropriate place in the pedometer, and it will give you the miles that correspond to the steps you walk.

Begin by doing your usual amount of exercise each day. Remember to record the steps at the end of the day and reset the button on the pedometer to zero. After seven days, add up the steps and divide by seven to get your daily count. You'll probably find you are doing between 3,000 and 5,000 steps a day. Next, you want to build up your daily number. Here are some tips to help:

 ✔ Get a good pair of walking shoes or trainers and replace them as soon as they begin to wear out.

 ✔ Leave your car parked. If you can make a trip in an hour or less by foot, save on petrol and pollution and add substantially to your daily step count.

 ✔ Try to add a few hundred steps a day. Begin by identifying a baseline day in your first week when you did the most steps, and make every day like that one. Each week add a few hundred more to your daily goal.

 ✔ Find an exercise buddy to walk with you. It's much more fun.

 ✔ Keep a record of the number of steps involved in various walks you take, so you can easily get the steps you are missing on any given day.

 ✔ Use stairs instead of the lift, whether you're going up or down.

 ✔ Take a walk at lunchtime daily.

 ✔ Stop if you feel pain, and check with your doctor before continuing.

Combine healthy exercise with some of the most glorious scenery the United Kingdom has to offer. The South Downs Way and the Pennine Way are just two of the dozens of trails you can follow on a walking holiday. Be realistic about the number of miles you can cover in a day (there may be far more hills than you're used to!). As an alternative, check out some of the walking or cycling holidays on offer from specialist travel companies. Many of them can transport your luggage from one location to the next, and offer a variety of packages to suit all levels of fitness.

If you don't have a pedometer, or if you want to count other types of exercise towards your walking goal, use the following conversions:

- ✔ 1 mile = 2,100 average steps
- ✔ 10 minutes walking = 1,200 steps on average
- ✔ Biking or swimming = 150 steps per minute
- ✔ Weight lifting = 100 steps per minute
- ✔ Rollerskating = 200 steps per minute

A study in the *Archives of Internal Medicine* in June 2003 provides the best evidence for the benefits of walking. Diabetics who walked for at least 2 hours a week had a 40 per cent lower death rate than inactive diabetics. What are you waiting for? Take the first steps!

Making the most of your exercise

Cross-training, where you do several different activities throughout the week, is a good idea. Cross-training reduces the boredom that may accompany one thing done day after day. It also permits you to exercise regardless of the weather because you can do some things indoors and some outside.

If you have a tendency to make excuses for not doing your planned exercise, why not team up with a friend? You can do this if you like two-person sports, such as tennis or squash, but you can also team up for jogging or going to a class at the gym. The prospect of letting someone else down is a great incentive to persevere when you don't feel like exercising.

If you worry about the cost of organised exercise, check out your local council's facilities. Most councils now offer special rates to people on low incomes, or for using council sports facilities at off-peak times. You can get the details from your local library. Some general practitioners can also offer exercise 'on prescription' through arrangements with local gyms and swimming pools.

Everything you do burns calories. Even sleeping and watching television use 20 kilocalories in 20 minutes if you weigh 9 stone (126 pounds). Table 9-2 lists a variety of exercises that you can try and tells you how many kilocalories you can burn by doing these activities for 20 minutes.

Table 9-2	Exercise and the Amount of Calories You Burn	
Activity	*Kilocalories Burned (125 pounds)*	*Kilocalories Burned (175 pounds)*
Standing	24	32
Walking, 4 mph	104	144
Running, 7 mph	236	328
Gardening	60	84
Writing	30	42
Typing	38	54
Carpentry	64	88
House painting	58	80
Cricket	78	108
Dancing	70	96
Football (except in goal when your team is winning!)	138	192
Golfing (without a buggy!)	66	96
Swimming	80	112
Skiing, downhill	160	224
Skiing, cross-country	196	276
Tennis	112	160

Find a form of exercise that fits in with your lifestyle. Many examples of the benefits of exercise are listed in this chapter, but these don't last forever if you stop. In fact, evidence suggests that you start to lose the benefits of regular training as little as three to ten days after you cease.

How long can you stop exercise before you start to get out of condition? It takes only about two to three weeks to lose some of the fitness that your exercise has provided. Then it takes up to six weeks to get back to your current level, assuming that your break from exercise doesn't go on for too long.

Particular considerations for people with special conditions

If you have diabetic retinopathy (explained in Chapter 5), you don't want to do exercises that raise your blood pressure (like weight lifting), cause jerky motions in your eyes (like bouncing on a trampoline), or change the pressure in your eye significantly (like scuba diving or high mountain climbing). You also shouldn't do exercises that place your eyes below the level of your heart, such as when you touch your toes.

If you have nephropathy (which is explained in Chapter 5), you should avoid exercises that raise your blood pressure for prolonged periods. These exercises are extremely intense activities that you do for a long time, like marathon running.

Some people have pain in the legs after they walk a certain distance. This may be due to diminished blood supply to the legs so that the needs of the muscles in the legs cannot be met by the inadequate blood supply. It's called peripheral arterial disease, and you can find out more about it in Chapter 5. Although you should discuss this problem with your doctor, you do not have to give up walking. You can determine the distance you can walk up to the point of pain. Then you should walk about three-quarters of that distance and stop to give your circulation a chance to catch up. Once you have rested, you may find that you can go about the same distance again without pain. By stringing several of these walks together, you can get a good, pain-free workout. You may even find that you are able to increase the distance after a while because this kind of training tends to create new blood vessels.

Is there a medical condition that should absolutely prevent you from doing exercise? Short of chest pain at rest, which must be addressed by your doctor, the answer is no. If you cannot figure out an exercise that you can do, get together with an exercise therapist. You may be amazed at how many muscles you can move that you never knew you had.

Weight lifting versus weight training

Weight lifting is a form of anaerobic exercise. (See the sidebar earlier in this chapter if you're not sure what anaerobic exercise is.) When you lift weights, you move heavy weights for brief periods. The results of weight lifting are significant muscle strengthening and increased endurance.

Heavy weight-lifting exercises can increase your blood pressure and the pressure inside your chest. This can be dangerous, especially if you have high blood pressure or retinopathy.

Weight training, on the other hand, which uses lighter weights, can be a form of aerobic exercise. Because the weights are light, you can move them for prolonged periods. The result is improved cardiovascular fitness along with strengthening of muscles, tendons, ligaments, and bones. Weight training is an excellent way to protect and strengthen a joint that is beginning to develop some discomfort.

We recommend that you do seven different exercises with light weights every other day, or daily if possible. Choose weights that allow you to do each exercise ten times in a row for three sets of ten with a rest in between. You should need only 5 to 10 minutes to complete all seven, and the benefits are huge. You can find a description of each in *Weight Lifting For Dummies* (Wiley), among other sources. They are the bicep curl, shoulder press, lateral raise, bent-over rowing, good mornings, flys, and pullovers.

Older people in nursing homes who were given weights of just a few pounds have shown excellent return of strength to what appeared to be atrophied muscles. The benefits for you will be that much greater.

Weight training may be good for the days that you do not do your aerobic exercise. You can also do weight training a few minutes after you finish your aerobic activity. Weight training is also good for working on a particular group of muscles that you feel is weak. Very often, this muscle is the back. Weight-training exercises can isolate and strengthen each muscle.

If you do a lot of aerobic exercise that involves the legs, you may want to use upper-body weight training only. We can tell you from personal experience that you not only feel a stronger upper body, but your ability to do your usual exercise is enhanced as well.

Chapter 10

Medication: What You Should Know

- -

In This Chapter

▶ Considering drugs taken by mouth – oral agents

▶ Combining oral agents

▶ Using insulin

▶ Combining insulin and oral agents in type 2 diabetes

▶ Avoiding drug interactions

- -

*Y*ou don't know how lucky you are. You are the beneficiary of the greatest advances in medication for diabetes in the history of this disease. From 1921, when insulin was isolated and used for the first time, to 1955, when a class of glucose-lowering drugs called *sulphonylureas* became available, insulin was all there was. Now four new classes of drug, each in its own unique way, lower blood glucose. In Chapter 16, you see that even more drugs are coming, and soon.

In this chapter, you find out all you need to know to use these drugs effectively and safely. (You need to take medication if diet and exercise are not keeping your blood glucose under control; see this part for more information.)

This chapter helps you become an educated consumer. Not only can you find out about the medication you're taking and how it works, but you discover when to take it, how it interacts with other medication, what side effects it may cause, and how to use several of these types of medication together, if necessary, to normalise your blood glucose. Right now, today, this year, you have all the tools needed to control your diabetes, and more is yet to come. In the immortal words of the great entertainer Al Jolson, 'You ain't seen nothin' yet.'

Some of the drugs we talk about in this chapter are relatively new, and some are a lot more expensive than the 'traditional' drugs that have been used to control blood sugar for years. Because all general practitioners these days are under close scrutiny from prescribing advisers, who monitor the costs of the drugs that general practitioners prescribe for their patients, many are reluctant to prescribe a more expensive medication. If you think this may be the situation in your case, try blinding your doctor with a little science of your own: Even though diabetics make up only about 3 to 4 per cent of the British population, the National Health Service spends about 6 to 7 per cent of its annual budget on treating them. The huge bulk of that cost comes from inpatient treatment costs. Oral medicines used to control blood glucose in type 2 diabetics (who make up over 90 per cent of the diabetics in the United Kingdom) only account for 2 per cent of the yearly expenditure on diabetes. So if your general practitioner wants to reduce his costs, tell him that improving your blood sugar control by using some of the newer drugs if they're needed is in his interest – as well as yours. That way, you're less likely to get complications that need to be treated at his Primary Care Trust's expense!

Taking Drugs by Mouth: Oral Agents

Most people do not like injections. You may be an exception, but we doubt it. Fortunately, drugs that you can take orally have been available for some time. One thing you should know about these pills: you can take them or leave them, but they work much better if you take them.

Sulphonylureas

Sulphonylureas are drugs that reduce blood glucose by making your pancreas produce more insulin. Scientists discovered sulphonylureas accidentally in the 1940s, when they noticed that soldiers given certain antibiotics called *sulphonamides* developed symptoms of low blood glucose. When scientists began to search for the most potent examples of this effect, they came up with several different versions of this drug. The first sulphonamides – carbutamide and tolbutamide – were produced in the 1950s. In the 1960s, acetohexamide, tolazamide, and chlorpropamide followed. These drugs are known as the *first-generation sulphonylureas.* The 1970s and 1980s produced a succession of similar drugs, called the *second-generation sulphonylureas.* These include glibenclamide, gliclazide, and glipizide. The most recent sulphonylurea to come on the market, glimepiride, was introduced in the mid-1990s.

The following sections explain characteristics of all the sulphonylureas.

How sulphonylureas work

All sulphonylureas work by making the pancreas release more insulin. How well they work depends on whether or not your pancreas is capable of producing enough insulin when stimulated. They are not effective in type 1 diabetes where the pancreas is not capable of releasing any insulin. Here are other things to know about sulphonylureas:

- ✔ They are well absorbed, and most of them reach their peak level in the bloodstream within two to four hours.

- ✔ They are all metabolised by the liver.

- ✔ If they are given on their own, they usually lower your fasting blood glucose by about 2–4 mmol/l. This translates into a reduction in haemoglobin A1c of about 1 to 2 per cent.

- ✔ Your age or body weight doesn't influence their effect.

- ✔ Although they sometimes don't work when first given (primary failure), they almost always stop working later on (secondary failure). Every year, secondary sulphonylurea failure occurs in about 5 to 10 per cent of people taking them.

- ✔ When you use any of a class of antibiotics called *sulphonamides,* the glucose-lowering action of the sulphonylureas is prolonged.

- ✔ They can be given in combination with any oral drug from the other groups discussed later in this chapter. When given in combination with one of the other classes of oral agents, sulphonylureas can be fairly potent.

- ✔ If you have problems with your kidneys or liver, or if you have a condition called porphyria (don't worry too much about this, because if you haven't heard of it, you haven't got it!), you need to use these drugs with caution.

Side effects

All sulphonylureas can cause the following side effects:

- ✔ **Hypoglycaemia.** Severe hypoglycaemia brought on by sulphonylureas is a medical emergency. It can cause coma, convulsions, and even death. If your blood glucose is below about 3 mmol/l, it's quite likely that you have severe hypoglycaemia. If you do, you're unlikely to be conscious. Carry an identity card or bracelet at all times, and make sure that those around you know how to recognise the symptoms of severe hypoglycaemia and call an ambulance immediately.

- ✔ **Sensitivity reactions such as rashes.** These reactions rarely occur.
- ✔ **Weight gain.** This is usually in the order of 1–4 kilograms, and stabilises after about six months.

Other side effects are uncommon, but include wind, diarrhoea, and headache.

Who should not take sulphonylureas?

The following people should not take sulphonylureas:

- ✔ Pregnant women. Women who are expecting should not take sulphonylureas except in exceptional circumstances and certainly not in the third trimester of pregnancy.
- ✔ Women who are breastfeeding. These drugs can theoretically cause hypoglycaemia in your baby if you use them when you are breastfeeding.
- ✔ Anyone who has ketoacidosis (refer to Chapter 4).

Sulphonylureas – when, which, and how?

Diet, weight loss, and other non-drug measures (refer to Chapters 8 and 9) are the first-line treatment in type 2 diabetes. Your doctor prescribes medication only if your blood sugar doesn't come down to acceptable levels using these measures. An important thing to know is that these medications can really help only if you stick with your healthy lifestyle. Even if your doctor starts you on medication, you must still pay just as much attention to your diet, weight, and exercise levels.

Sulphonylureas are one of the most common drugs for type 2 diabetes in the United Kingdom. Only metformin (which you can find out about later in this chapter) is more commonly prescribed as a first-line treatment for type 2 diabetics in Britain. Your doctor is more likely to prescribe a sulphonylurea, rather than metformin, if you are not overweight, because of sulphonylureas' tendency to cause weight gain.

Whichever type of sulphonylurea you take, your doctor will start you on a low dose. You usually have your blood sugar checked every two weeks when you first start taking a sulphonylurea, although you should check it yourself between visits. Your doctor will increase your dose at two- to four-week intervals until your blood sugar is adequately controlled.

Occasionally, you may reach a stage where increasing your dose of sulphonylurea doesn't improve your blood sugars or haemoglobin A1c. This can sometimes happen at a dose much lower than the maximum recommended dose. If it does occur, your doctor should reduce your dose back to the highest dose that actually made a difference.

If you develop symptoms of hypoglycaemia when you start taking a sulphonylurea, you should try to confirm your blood sugar at home when you have one of these episodes. If blood testing confirms that you have had a hypoglycaemic episode, your doctor may reduce your dose or change you to a different type of sulphonylurea.

Which drug your doctor prescribes first may be partly dictated by which one he uses most often and is most familiar with. However, other factors in your history may make one sulphonylurea more suitable than another for you. For instance:

- ✔ Long-acting sulphonylureas, like chlorpropamide and glibenclamide, are associated with a higher risk of hypoglycaemia. They are less suitable for elderly patients.

  If your eating habits are irregular, you may be at higher risk of hypoglycaemic episodes when you are taking sulphonylureas, especially if you are using a longer-acting version like glibenclamide. Drinking alcohol while taking a sulphonylurea can also increase your risk of hypoglycaemia.

- ✔ Gliclazide and tolbutamide, which are relatively short acting, may be more suitable for elderly patients.

- ✔ Chlorpropamide is the longest acting of the sulphonylureas. It has several potential side effects that are not seen with other sulphonylureas. It can cause fluid retention, low sodium in your blood, and facial flushing if you drink alcohol while you are taking it. It also gives rise to more frequent, and more severe, hypoglycaemia than is seen with the shorter-acting sulphonylureas. For all these reasons, chlorpropamide is no longer generally recommended in the United Kingdom.

- ✔ Glibenclamide and tolbutamide have a mild diuretic action, meaning that they tend to make you pass more water. This can be a disadvantage if your lifestyle is very busy.

Metformin

Metformin is an entirely different kind of glucose-lowering medication. One of the earliest traditional remedies for diabetes in Europe was a plant called French lilac. More than 80 years ago, French lilac was found to contain high levels of guanidine. Metformin is derived from this active ingredient. Interestingly, other guanidine derivatives were used for the treatment of diabetes in the 1920s, but were discontinued and forgotten for decades before the introduction of metformin in 1957.

Metformin has been used in Europe for years without much trouble. In the United States, a sister medication called Phenformin was banned more than 20 years ago because of an association with a fatal complication called lactic acidosis. That may be why metformin was only approved in America in 1995. Metformin is rarely, and perhaps never, associated with the fatal complication that caused Phenformin to be banned. Worldwide, metformin is the single most commonly used oral medication for type 2 diabetes, and is licensed as first-line drug treatment in type 2 diabetes, or in conjunction with any of the other oral drugs for type 2 diabetes. In the United Kingdom, metformin is the first-choice drug for most people starting tablets for diabetes for the first time. This medication is particularly popular and useful because most people with type 2 diabetes are overweight, and metformin has no weight gain side effects (although it is equally effective for people who are not overweight). In fact, some people who take metformin eat less because of nausea, which is one of its side effects. This actually makes them more likely to lose weight.

Metformin is available in 500 milligram and 850 milligram tablets, and the maximum dose is 2,500 milligrams, taken in divided doses with each meal. About 10 per cent of patients fail to respond to metformin when first taken, and the secondary failure rate (when the medication has worked at first but stops working later) is 5 to 10 per cent a year. It does not depend on stimulating insulin to work, as the sulphonylureas do.

The following sections explain the characteristics of metformin.

How metformin works

Metformin can be a very useful drug, especially when *fasting hyperglycaemia* (high blood glucose on awakening) is present.

Metformin is passed out of the body in the urine without being broken down. It should only be taken if your kidney function is good enough to stop it building up in the body.

Metformin has some positive effects on the blood fats, causing a decrease in triglycerides and LDL cholesterol and an increase in HDL cholesterol. Other effects of the drug include:

- ✔ Lowering the blood glucose mainly by reducing the production of glucose from the liver (the hepatic glucose output).
- ✔ Possibly increasing the sensitivity of the muscle cells to insulin and slowing the uptake of glucose from the intestine.

Side effects

Metformin has the following side effects:

✔ Gastrointestinal irritation. Because of this problem, you must take metformin with food; however, this side effect declines with time.

✔ Weight loss. The possible cause of the weight loss may be from the gastrointestinal irritation or because of a loss of taste for food.

✔ A decrease in the absorption of vitamin B12. Metformin occasionally causes a decrease in the absorption of vitamin B12, a vitamin that is important for the blood and the nervous system.

Who should not take metformin?

The following people should not take metformin:

✔ Those who have impaired kidney function

Because of the small risk of lactic acidosis, which is increased if you have significant kidney disease, you must not take metformin if your kidney function is even mildly impaired.

✔ Those who have significant liver disease or heart failure

✔ Alcoholics

✔ Pregnant women or nursing mothers

Drug interactions

The following are drug interactions involving metformin:

✔ When metformin is given in combination with the sulphonylureas, hypoglycaemia can occur. If persistent, the dose of sulphonylurea is reduced. By itself, however, metformin does not cause hypoglycaemia.

✔ Using metformin at the same time as the anti-indigestion drug cimetidine can cause levels of metformin in the body to rise.

✔ Because metformin doesn't bind much to proteins in the blood, it doesn't interfere with other drugs that are bound to proteins.

✔ Metformin is usually stopped for a day or two before surgery or an X-ray study using a dye.

Acarbose

Acarbose, the first of a group of drugs called *alpha-glucosidase inhibitors,* was introduced in the early 1990s. The brand name is Glucobay. Recently, two other drugs in this group, miglitol and voglibose, have been introduced in some countries; however, these drugs are not available in the United Kingdom.

The following sections outline the main characteristics of acarbose.

How acarbose works

Acarbose blocks the action of an enzyme in the intestine that breaks down more complex carbohydrates into smaller molecules like glucose and fructose so that they can be absorbed. The result is that the rate of rise of glucose in the bloodstream is slowed after meals. These carbohydrates are eventually broken down by bacteria lower down in the intestine and produce a lot of gas, abdominal pain, and diarrhoea, which are the major drawbacks to this drug. Other things you should know include the following:

- It is licensed as first-line drug therapy in type 2 diabetes, or in combination with any of the other oral drugs used in type 2 diabetes.
- It does not require insulin for its activity.
- The lowering of glucose and haemoglobin A1c is modest at most.
- It's supplied in 50 milligram and 100 milligram strengths.
- The recommended starting dose is 50 milligrams once a day. This dose can be increased to 50 milligrams three times daily, and after 6–8 weeks to 100 milligrams three times daily, depending on the blood glucose. The highest dose is not given unless the patient weighs more than 9½ stone.

Side effects

Acarbose does not cause hypoglycaemia when used alone, but it can when used in combination with sulphonylureas. If hypoglycaemia is persistent, the dose of sulphonylurea is decreased. It can cause wind, loose stools or diarrhoea, bloating, and stomach pain.

Many of our patients are very troubled by the side effects of acarbose. We always advise them to avoid potentially embarrassing social situations just after they start taking the drug. One of our patients was mortified to find the dinner party she was attending brought to a complete standstill by her tummy rumbling and, even worse, uncontrollable wind. These side effects do subside with time in some patients, but in this woman's case we had no hesitation in complying with her request for a change of treatment!

Because its action is to block the breakdown of complex carbohydrates, hypoglycaemia occurring with acarbose and sulphonylurea combinations must be treated with a preparation of glucose, not more complex carbohydrates.

Who should not use acarbose?

The following people should not use acarbose:

✔ Women who are pregnant or breastfeeding

✔ People who suffer from inflammatory bowel disease, such as ulcerative colitis or Crohn's disease

✔ People who have liver disease, severe kidney disease, a hernia, or a history of abdominal surgery.

Thiazolidinediones (the glitazones)

The glitazones are the first group of drugs for diabetes that directly reverse insulin resistance. The antidiabetic effect of the glitazones was first described in the early 1980s.

The first drug in this group to be marketed was troglitazone. Troglitazone was launched in the United States, Japan, and the United Kingdom in 1997. However, because it was found to cause severe, sometimes fatal, liver damage in a few patients, it was withdrawn in the United Kingdom within a few weeks of its launch, and taken off the market worldwide in 2000.

In 2000, two other glitazones, called rosiglitazone and pioglitazone, were launched in Europe. Neither of these drugs has been linked to liver damage.

Both rosiglitazone and pioglitazone are broken down in the liver. The breakdown products of rosiglitazone are passed out of the body more in the urine than the bile produced by the liver. The products of pioglitazone are passed out of the body mostly in bile from the liver. Even though neither rosiglitazone nor pioglitazone has been connected with the liver damage that led to the withdrawal of troglitazone, neither of them is recommended if you have liver disease. You should also have your liver function tests checked while you are taking the drug.

How rosiglitazone and pioglitazone work

The glitazones actually reverse insulin resistance. They do this by causing changes in the muscle and fat cells where the insulin resistance resides. They also enhance the actions of insulin in the liver.

The glitazones share the following characteristics:

✔ Tablets are taken once a day, with or without food.

✔ They should be started at a low dose – 2 milligrams once or twice a day for rosiglitazone and 15 milligrams once a day for pioglitazone.

✔ They may take up to two or three months to have their maximum effect.

✔ They are quickly absorbed, with peak levels in the blood seen within two hours (one hour for rosiglitazone).

✔ Because they improve insulin resistance, the glitazones have their greatest effect on the blood glucose after eating, rather than the first morning glucose.

✔ Glitazones are insulin sparing, meaning that the body does not have to make as much insulin to control the blood glucose when a glitazone is given.

✔ So far, secondary failure (the drug works initially but stops working later) does not seem to be a problem.

Glitazones take 10 to 12 weeks to give you the maximum benefit, so don't expect miraculous results overnight! This long run-in period is one of the reasons that glitazones are preferred in the United Kingdom as an 'add-in' medication, rather than as an alternative to the treatment you're already taking.

The National Institute for Health and Clinical Excellence (NICE) has brought out guidelines on when pioglitazone and rosiglitazone should be used in the United Kingdom. It recommends the following:

✔ If you can tolerate them, you should be offered a combination of metformin and a sulphonylurea before a glitazone is added in. This means that for most people with type 2 diabetes, a glitazone will be a third-line therapy, the third drug you take to bring your glucose levels down.

✔ You should usually be prescribed a glitazone only if your blood sugars aren't well enough controlled on a combination of metformin and a sulphonylurea.

✔ If you're starting a glitazone as your second-line therapy (in other words, you're already taking one drug to help keep your glucose down and a glitazone is the second), you should be offered a glitazone in combination with metformin rather than with a sulphonylurea, if possible.

✔ You should only be given a glitazone in combination with a sulphonylurea if you can't tolerate metformin, or there is some reason why you shouldn't take it.

✔ You should, if possible, be offered a glitazone in addition to metformin and a sulphonylurea if your blood sugars aren't well enough controlled, as an alternative to starting on insulin.

Drug interactions

Following is information regarding drug interactions involving the glitazones:

✔ They are very strongly bound to protein, but because their concentrations are generally low, they don't interact much with other protein-bound drugs.

✔ By themselves, the glitazones do not cause hypoglycaemia. They can cause hypoglycaemia if they are used in combination with insulin or sulphonylurea. If a glitazone is given to a patient who is already taking a sulphonylurea, the dose of sulphonylurea often needs to be reduced after a while because of hypoglycaemia.

✔ If a glitazone is given to a patient on sulphonylurea or metformin, those drugs must not be stopped when the glitazone is started.

Side effects

Following are the side effects of the glitazones:

✔ They can cause weight gain. This is typically 1–4 kilograms, and the weight levels off after 6–12 months.

✔ They can cause fluid retention and anaemia.

✔ Glitazones have been found to have unexpected effects in women of child-bearing age; specifically, an unintended pregnancy due to improved fertility. Many such women have reduced fertility as a result of insulin resistance. When these women take a glitazone, their fertility may improve, and they may become pregnant.

Who shouldn't take glitazones?

The following people should not take glitazones:

✔ Those who have liver problems, congestive heart failure, oedema (swelling of the legs), or anaemia

✔ Women who are pregnant or breastfeeding

Meglitinides (the prandial glucose regulators)

Repaglinide (brand name Prandin) and Nateglinide (brand name Starlix) belong to a group of drugs called *meglitinides*. Meglitinides are the last of the current group of new medications for type 2 diabetes.

How meglitinides work

The *meglitinides* are chemically unrelated to the sulphonylureas, but they work by squeezing more insulin out of the pancreas just like the sulphonylureas do. The meglitinides, however, are taken just before meals (either just before or up to 30 minutes before your meal) to stimulate insulin for only that meal. You need to take the medication before each main meal, usually three times a day. They come in tablet form.

Keep in mind these things about meglitinides:

- Because meglitinides are mostly broken down in the liver and leave the body in the bowel movement, the dosage has to be adjusted downwards if any liver disease is present. If you have severe liver disease, you shouldn't take a meglitinide.

- Despite the lack of excretion through the kidneys, increases in the dose have to be made more carefully when kidney impairment is present.

As a rule, we try to avoid giving patients tablets that have to be taken several times a day. This is because the more times you take tablets, the more often you forget them. One of our patients (whom we rename here) proved recently that exceptions to this rule do exist. Terry Harding was a 42-year-old mature student and had the irregular lifestyle to prove it. One week, he might be up all night partying; the next week, he might be up every day at 5 a.m., revising. Terry's blood sugars were all over the place, and he admitted that he often forgot his tablets. When we talked about adding repaglinide to his drugs, we looked at ways he could remember to take them before every meal. His meal-times may have been irregular, but at least he couldn't afford to eat out much! Keeping notes on the inside of his fridge and plate cupboard worked for him. No matter how irregular his meals, he was reminded about his tablet when he was cooking. His haemoglobin A1c came down by over 1 per cent as a result.

Drug interactions

Following is information regarding drug interactions involving meglitinides:

- They're not used with the sulphonylureas but can be combined with metformin. Use in combination with a glitazone has not been studied.

- They lower the blood glucose and the haemoglobin A1c effectively when used in combination with metformin.

Side effects

Following are the side effects associated with meglitinides:

- Because they act through insulin, they can cause hypoglycaemia.

- They can cause a variety of tummy upsets, including pain, diarrhoea, constipation, nausea, and vomiting.

- It's possible to be allergic to them, in which case you may develop a rash.

Who shouldn't take meglitinides?

Meglitinides are not recommended for use in the following people:

- ✔ Women who are pregnant or breastfeeding
- ✔ Patients who are over 75 or under 18
- ✔ People who have severe liver disease

Insulin

If you're a person with type 1 diabetes, insulin is your saviour. If you have type 2 diabetes, you may need insulin late in the course of your disease. Insulin is a great drug, but you have to take it through a needle at present, and that is the rub (or the pain). Inventors have come up with many different ways to administer insulin, and in the United Kingdom, insulin pens have proved more popular as a way of giving insulin than any other. Most people in Britain who switch from using a needle and syringe to using an insulin pen prefer the pen. We tell you about the newer methods, including insulin pens, in this section. If you're still using a needle and syringe, you may want to consider switching to one of these methods because they are easier and possibly more accurate than the old way.

Forms of insulin

In the human body, insulin is constantly responding to ups and downs in the blood glucose. No simple device is currently available to measure the blood glucose and give insulin as the pancreas does. In order to avoid having to take many injections a day, forms of insulin were invented to work at different times. These forms of insulin include the following:

- ✔ **Rapid-acting lispro and aspart insulin:** The newest preparations and the shortest acting, lispro and aspart insulin (called, respectively, NovoRapid and Humalog), begin to lower the glucose within five minutes after their administration, peak at about one hour, and are no longer active by about three hours. These extra-fast-acting insulins are a great advance because they free the person with diabetes to take an injection just when he eats. With the previous short-acting insulin (regular insulin), the person had to take an injection and eat within 30 minutes or hypoglycaemia might occur. Because their activity begins and ends so quickly, lispro and aspart insulin do not cause hypoglycaemia as often as the older preparations.

Animal insulin versus human insulin

Until a few years ago, insulin could only be obtained by extracting it from the pancreas of cows, pigs, salmon, and some other animals. This was not entirely satisfactory because those insulins are slightly different from human insulin. Using them resulted in an immune reaction in the blood and certain skin reactions. The preparation was purified, but tiny amounts of impurities always remained. In 1978, researchers were able to trick bacteria called *E. coli* into making human insulin. Almost all insulin is now perfectly pure human insulin. In a short while, no insulin besides human insulin will be available.

✔ **Short-acting regular insulin:** Regular insulin takes 30 minutes to start to lower the glucose, peaks at three hours, and is gone by six to eight hours. This insulin is the preparation that was used before meals to keep the glucose low until the next meal.

✔ **Intermediate-acting NPH or lente insulins:** Both begin to lower the glucose within 2 hours of administration and continue their activity for 10 to 12 hours. They can be active for up to 24 hours. The purpose of this kind of insulin is to provide a smooth level of control over half the day so that a low level of active insulin is always in the body. This attempts to parallel the situation that exists in the human body.

✔ **Long-acting ultralente insulin:** This insulin begins to act within 6 hours and provides a low level of insulin activity for up to 26 hours. It was invented to provide a smooth, basal level of control requiring only one injection a day. It can act differently in different people, looking more like intermediate insulin in some patients.

✔ **Long-acting insulin glargine:** Aventis is selling a new insulin called *insulin glargine* or Lantus. Studies have shown that insulin glargine has its onset 1 to 2 hours after injection, and its activity lasts for 24 hours without a specific peak time of activity, which is exactly what is needed to control the blood glucose over an entire day. Insulin glargine is released in a smooth fashion from the site of injection, and it doesn't matter what part of the body is injected. Because of its smooth and predictable activity, insulin glargine does not often cause low blood glucose at night, which often happens with NPH insulin. We have used this insulin in a number of patients with type 1 diabetes and have been extremely pleased with the results. We are now using it with most new type 1 diabetes patients.

If you do not have good diabetic control (haemoglobin A1c of 7 per cent or less is good control) with NPH insulin, ask your doctor to consider using insulin glargine.

> ✓ **Premixed insulins:** These contain 70 per cent NPH insulin and 30 per cent regular insulin. Some contain a 50–50 mixture. These insulins are helpful for people who have trouble mixing insulins in one syringe, have poor eyesight, or are stable on a preparation that doesn't change.

You need to know a few things that are common to all insulins:

✓ Insulin may be kept at room temperature for four weeks or in the refrigerator until the expiration date printed on the label. After four weeks at room temperature, you should discard the insulin.

✓ Insulin does not take too well to excessive heat, such as direct sunlight, or excessive cold. Protect your insulin against these conditions.

✓ You can safely give an insulin injection through clothing.

✓ If you take less than 50 units in an injection, there are ½ cc syringes that make it easy to measure up to 50 units. The same is true if you take less than 30 units, which would use ³⁄₁₀ cc syringes.

✓ Shorter needles may be more comfortable, especially for children, but the depth of the injection helps to determine how fast the insulin works.

✓ You can reuse disposable syringes (on yourself) a couple of times.

✓ You must dispose of used syringes and needles in a puncture-proof container that is sealed shut before being placed in your rubbish bin.

Combining insulin and oral agents in type 2 diabetes

Sometimes the characteristics of the currently available oral agents do not provide the tight control needed to avoid complications. This is particularly true after many years of type 2 diabetes. Then, insulin may be required. Insulin may be added in a number of ways, but often an injection of NPH insulin at bedtime is all that is needed for the patient to start the day under control and continue with oral agents.

As type 2 diabetes progresses, the oral agents may be less effective, and insulin is taken more often. Two injections a day of intermediate and short-acting insulin may do the trick. Usually the patient takes two-thirds of the dose in the morning and one-third before supper, because they need short-acting insulin to control the supper carbohydrates. This is a situation where premixed insulin may be useful, allowing the patient to measure from only one bottle, or to use a premixed combination in a pen. This combination is especially valuable in older people with diabetes, where the tightest level of control is not being sought because the expected lifespan of the patient is shorter than the time necessary to develop complications. In this kind of patient, doctors want to prevent problems like frequent urination leading to loss of sleep or vaginal infections, so they give enough to treat these symptoms, but not so much that a frail, elderly patient is having hypoglycaemia on a frequent basis.

Delivering insulin with a syringe

In the United Kingdom, more and more people are choosing to give their insulin with a pen, rather than with the old-fashioned needle and syringe. However, a needle and syringe work very well for some diabetics using insulin. Fortunately, the new syringes and needles are just about painless.

Previously, insulin came in two different strengths, U40 and U80, which meant 40 units per millilitre or 80 units per millilitre. This measurement was confusing, especially if the wrong syringe was used – you had to use a U40 syringe for U40 insulin. This double standard was eliminated in the United Kingdom, and now all insulin is U100 or 100 units per millilitre, and all syringes are U100 syringes. This standardisation is not necessarily used in all parts of Europe or elsewhere, so check the strength of the insulin and the markings on the syringe.

How to shoot yourself

Whatever the type, drawing up insulin is done in the same way. If you look at the syringe in Figure 10-1, you see that it's lined. Starting at the needle end of the syringe, you can see nine small lines above the needle, followed by a tenth, longer line where the number 10 may be found. Each line is one unit of insulin up to ten units. Above the 10 unit line, you see a succession of four small lines followed by a larger line representing 15, 20, 25, and so on.

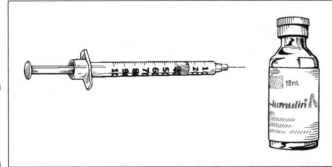

Figure 10-1:
The insulin syringe and bottle.

Keep these tips in mind when you inject insulin:

✔ **Where you inject the insulin helps determine how fast it will work.** Insulin injected into the abdomen is most rapidly absorbed, followed by the arms and legs, and then the buttocks. You can use these differing rates of uptake of the insulin to get faster action when your blood glucose is high. If you exercise the body part that gets the insulin, the insulin enters more quickly. If you use the same site repeatedly, the absorption rate slows down, so rotate the sites.

✔ **When you inject the insulin helps to determine the smoothness of your glucose control.** The more regular you are in your injections, your eating, and your exercise, the smoother your glucose level.

If the insulin is lispro, aspart, or regular, it should be clear and you do not have to shake the bottle. The other kinds of insulin are cloudy, and you need to shake the bottle a few times to suspend the tiny particles in the liquid. A new bottle has a cap on the top, which you break off and discard. When you're ready to take insulin, follow these steps:

1. **Wipe the rubber stopper in the top of the bottle with alcohol.**

2. **Pull up the number of units of air that corresponds to the number of units of insulin you need to take.**

3. **Turn the insulin bottle upside down and penetrate the rubber stopper with the needle of the syringe.**

4. **Push all the air inside and pull out the insulin dose you need. Because air replaces the insulin, the pressure inside the bottle is unchanged, and no vacuum is created.**

5. **Check and make sure that you have the right amount of the right insulin and no air bubbles in the syringe.**

6. **To give the injection, use alcohol to wipe off an area of skin on the arm, the chest, the stomach, or wherever you're injecting.**

7. **Insert the needle at a right angle to the skin and push it in. When the needle has penetrated the skin, push the plunger of the syringe down to zero to administer the insulin.**

Mixing insulins

If you're taking two kinds of insulin at the same time, you can mix them in one syringe, thus avoiding two injections. Here's how you do that:

1. **Wipe both bottles with alcohol.**

2. **Draw up the total units of air corresponding to the total insulin you need.**

3. **Push the units of air into the longer-acting insulin bottle that corresponds to the number of units of longer-acting insulin that you need and withdraw the needle.**

4. **Push the rest of the units of air into the shorter-acting insulin bottle and withdraw the correct units of insulin.**

5. **Go back to the longer-acting bottle and withdraw the correct units of insulin from there.**

By doing this, you do not contaminate the shorter-acting insulin with the additive in the longer-acting insulin.

Aids to insulin delivery

For those of you still using the old needle and syringe method, we want you to be aware of the numerous aids that can make taking your insulin easier:

- **Spring-loaded syringe holders:** You place your syringe in the holder, hold it against the skin, and press a button. The needle enters, and you've administered the insulin.

- **Syringe magnifiers:** These help the visually impaired administer insulin.

- **Syringe-filling devices:** You can feel and hear a click as you take up insulin.

- **Needle guides:** You can use these guides when you can't see the rubber part of the insulin bottle to insert the needle to take up the insulin.

Delivering insulin with a pen

Several drug manufacturers have sought ways to make delivering insulin easier. The insulin pen, shown in Figure 10-2, is one useful tool. The pen comes with the cartridge already inserted, or the cartridge is placed inside the pen just like the old ink cartridges used to be put in pens. Each cartridge contains 3.0 millilitres of either NPH, regular, lispro, or a premixed combination of NPH and regular insulin. You can dial the amount of insulin that you need to take. Each unit (sometimes two units) is accompanied by a clicking sound so that the visually impaired can hear the number of units. The units also appear in a window on the pen. If you dial up too many units, one of the pens forces you to waste the insulin by pushing it out of the needle while the other allows you to reset the pen and start again. Depending on the pen, you can deliver from 30 to 70 units of insulin. You screw on a new needle as needed.

Patients tell us that whichever kind of pen they use, the Novo Fine Pen Needles are less painful to use.

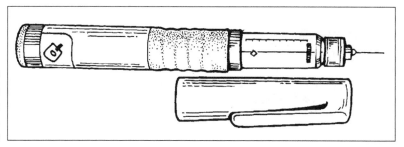

Figure 10-2:
The insulin
pen.

Should you shift from your syringe and needle to a pen? Well, ask most of the people with diabetes in the United Kingdom who use insulin – more of them use pens than anything else. If you're comfortable with the syringe and needle and feel your technique is accurate, you probably have no reason to change. If you're new to insulin, have some visual impairment, or feel that you're not getting an accurate measurement of the insulin, then a pen may be the solution for you.

Delivering insulin with a jet injection device

Jet injection devices (see Figure 10-3) are for the person who just can't stick a needle into his or her skin. At around £600 or more, they're expensive, but they last a long time and replace the syringe and needle. They're made by at least three different manufacturers:

- **Antares Pharma (formerly Medi-Ject Corporation).** Antares Pharma is the leading manufacturer of jet injection devices. Its device, the Medijector Vision, is easy to dose, has a safety lock on it so that the insulin isn't delivered until it's fully measured, and uses the newer technology of so-called needle-free syringes. This advance allows the patient to see the insulin and doesn't require washing a stainless-steel nozzle. (The stainless-steel nozzle was a feature of the older jet injection devices. The nozzle had to be cleaned regularly, or the correct dose of insulin may not be delivered.)

- **Activa Corporation.** Activa makes the Advanta Jet injection device. It also makes the Gentle Jet for children and the Advanta Jet ES for especially tough skin. However, Activa continues to use the old stainless-steel technology, which puts its device at a disadvantage.

- **Bioject.** Bioject devices are similar to the Medijector. Bioject's current device is the VitaJet 3, which uses the newer technology but may not be as easy to dose as the Medijector.

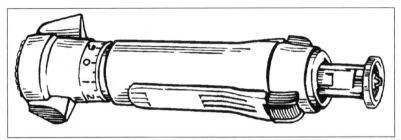

Figure 10-3:
A jet
injection
device.

A large quantity of insulin is taken into the injection device, enough for multiple treatments. The amount of insulin to be delivered is measured, usually by rotating one part of the device while the number of units to be delivered appears in a window. You hold the device against the skin, and when you press a button, a powerful jet of air forces the insulin through the skin into the subcutaneous tissue, usually with no pain perceived by the patient. The devices come in a lower power form for smaller children. These devices can deliver up to 50 units at one time.

Should you try an insulin jet injector? If you have no trouble with the syringe and needle or find the pen to be an easy substitute, you don't need a jet injector. If you hate needles or need to give frequent injections to a small child who is very resistant to them, then a jet injector may solve your problems.

Delivering insulin with an external pump

For some people – and you may be one of them – the external insulin pump (see Figure 10-4) is the answer to their prayers. These devices are as close as you currently can come to the gradual administration of rapid-acting insulin that is normally taking place in the body. They're expensive, costing more than £2,500, but the insulin pump may be the answer for patients who simply cannot achieve good glucose control with syringes, pens, or jet injectors.

Currently, three companies – Animas, MiniMed, and Disetronic Medical Systems – sell these pumps, which are the size of a pager. Inside the pump is a motor. A syringe filled with short-acting insulin is placed within the pump, with the plunger against a screw that slowly pushes the plunger down to push insulin out of the syringe. The end of the syringe is attached to a short tube, which ends in a needle pushed into the skin of the abdomen. Insulin is slowly pushed under the skin.

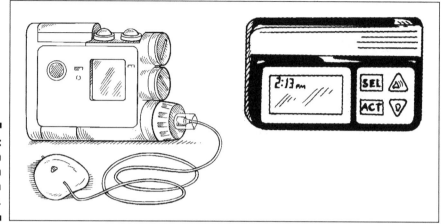

Figure 10-4:
The insulin pump with its infusion set.

The rate at which insulin slowly enters the abdomen is called the *basal rate*. It can be set, by way of a computer chip, to vary as often as every half hour to an hour. For example, from 8 a.m. to 9 a.m. the pump may deliver 0.8 units, while from 9 a.m. to 10 a.m. the pump may deliver 1.0 unit, depending on the needs of the patient. This amount is determined, of course, by measuring the blood glucose with a meter (see Chapter 7).

When a meal is about to be eaten, the patient can push a button to deliver extra insulin, called a *bolus* of insulin. (You determine the amount by carbohydrate counting.) You can get extra insulin if your blood glucose is too high at any time.

Pump usage has its advantages:

- ✔ It's flexible because the bolus (see the previous paragraph) is taken just before the meal.
- ✔ It often smoothes out the swings of glucose during the day because the insulin is administered slowly and in small doses.
- ✔ It can be rapidly disconnected and reconnected for you to take a shower or swim, but can take a little getting used to when worn to bed.
- ✔ It's safe from overdosage because it has built-in protective devices to prevent this occurrence.

On the other hand, pump usage has definite disadvantages, besides the high cost:

✔ Infections of the skin are frequent because the infusion set is left in place for several days. These infections are usually mild, however.

✔ Overall diabetic control is not necessarily better with the pump than with other ways of delivering insulin, especially with the new insulin glargine.

✔ Because short-acting insulin is the only form the patient receives, if insulin stops entering, ketoacidosis may come on rapidly (see Chapter 4).

✔ Some patients are allergic to the tape that holds the infusion set onto the abdomen.

✔ You must measure blood glucose often to adjust the pump for optimal control.

Pump usage is definitely not treatment to be done on your own at the beginning. You need a diabetes consultant to help with dosages, a dietician to help with amounts of boluses based on carbohydrate intake, and someone from the manufacturer to teach you how to set the pump and to be there for any malfunctions.

Is an insulin pump for you? If you're willing to invest the time and effort at first, if your schedule is very uncertain, particularly with respect to meals, and if your control has not been good with other means, it may be worth looking into this option.

Our experience with patients has generally been positive. None of those who have the pump are willing to give it up. Occasionally, they disconnect the pump to allow their skin to heal. They have generally shown improved control and a better haemoglobin A1c.

Do we recommend using an insulin pump? With the new form of insulin called insulin glargine, you can accomplish a continuous basal control of your blood glucose much like the pump does. The pump proponents say that you need to be able to alter the basal dose for different conditions throughout the day, and you can't do that with a single injection of insulin. Although this is true, we're not sure that it makes a great difference in the course of controlling the blood glucose.

Is one pump better than another? All seem to have excellent mechanical features, and all provide you with the ability to adjust your insulin in numerous ways. They all have alarms for any eventuality like blockage of the tube, an electrical failure, and so forth. They try to differentiate themselves by offering different options for how the insulin is delivered, but you may find that you need the help of a rocket scientist to figure them out.

Inhaling insulin

Sounds great, doesn't it? An end to injections is the dream of most patients with diabetes. Unfortunately, while the development of the first inhaled insulin is a step on the way to this goal, we aren't there yet.

Inhaled insulin comes in the form of a fast-acting, dry-powder preparation of human insulin. You inhale it into your lungs using a specially designed inhalation device, and take it before meals. If you use long-acting insulin as well, you need to continue to take this by injection. The only form of inhaled insulin that has been licensed for use in the United Kingdom is called Exubera.

Blood sugar control using inhaled insulin seems to be about the same, overall, as with injected insulin regimens. The rate of hypoglycaemia (low blood sugar) also seems to be about the same with inhaled insulin as with injected versions.

As well as needing to continue with your longer-acting 'background' insulin injections, you also need to monitor your blood glucose using finger-prick testing. In fact, as with any change in treatment, you have to monitor your blood glucose levels more frequently when you first start using inhaled insulin.

Some other drawbacks of inhaled insulin include:

- It is not licensed for use in children.
- You can't use it if you're a smoker.
- You need to have good enough lung function to use it, so you need to have a test of your lung function before you start it.
- It can cause coughing, and about 1 in 100 people taking it have to discontinue it for this reason. It can also cause dry throat, shortness of breath, and irritation of the throat.
- It is extremely expensive compared to other versions of insulin, costing about £1,100 a year. In the United Kingdom, where funding for medication depends largely on the approval of the National Institute for Health and Clinical Excellence (NICE), which looks at cost effectiveness as well as medical effectiveness, the cost is proving a major barrier to the widespread introduction of inhaled insulin.

NICE has issued draft guidance on who should be eligible for inhaled insulin. We still await the final guidance, which will effectively determine who will get funding for this treatment on the National Health Service. At the moment,

NICE has recommended that inhaled insulin should be available only for people with diabetes who:

✔ Are unable to inject insulin because of an injection phobia

✔ Have severe persistent problems with injection sites

Conducting intensive insulin treatment

Intensive insulin treatment is essential in type 1 diabetes if you hope to prevent the complications of the disease. This means measuring your blood glucose at least before each meal and at bedtime, and using both short-acting and longer-acting insulin to keep the blood glucose between 4.5 and 5.5 mmol/l before meals and less than 8 mmol/l after eating. How you do this is the subject of this section.

In the human body (except in type 1 diabetes), a small amount of circulating insulin is always present in the bloodstream and, after eating, insulin increases temporarily to control the glucose in the meal. Intensive insulin treatment attempts to mirror the normal human pancreas as much as possible.

In intensive insulin treatment, you usually take a certain amount of longer-acting insulin at bedtime (you may prefer insulin glargine, because it produces a smooth basal level of glucose control over 24 hours). In addition, you take a dose of rapid-acting insulin before each meal. You may prefer lispro or aspart because it is more convenient and less hypoglycaemia occurs. The dose of lispro or aspart is determined by the expected grams of carbohydrates in the meal about to be taken plus the blood glucose at that moment. Your doctor should provide you with a list of how much insulin to take for a given situation. Each patient is different, and the instructions must be individualised.

When you use the carbohydrates in the meal to determine the insulin dose, it is called *carbohydrate counting*. You can quickly figure out how much carbohydrate is in each meal if you know how large your portion is and how much carbohydrate is in it. This calculation is especially easy for breakfast, because most people eat the same things at breakfast time. Figuring out the carbohydrate content at lunch and supper gets harder, because meals tend to be different. But with a little practice, carbohydrate counting isn't too difficult then either.

You also need to know how many grams of carbohydrate are controlled by each unit of insulin. For example, one person may need 1 unit to control 20 grams of carbohydrate, while another person needs 1 unit to control 15 grams of carbohydrate. If both of them eat a breakfast of 75 grams of carbohydrate, the first person might take 4 units of lispro, while the second person takes 5 units of lispro. Then you add more units for the amount that the blood glucose needs to be lowered. A typical schedule is to take 1 unit for every 3 mmol/l that the blood glucose is above 6 mmol/l. Insulin can also be subtracted if the blood glucose is too low. For every 3 mmol/l that the glucose is below 6 mmol/l, subtract 1 unit. (To see how carbohydrate counting works in practice, see the sidebar 'Carbohydrate counting to maximum health'.)

The key to this system is to know the carbohydrates in your food. Here is where you make use of your friendly dietician, who can go over your food preferences and show you how many carbohydrates are in them. The dietician can also show you where to find carbohydrate counts for any other foods that you might eat.

By measuring your blood glucose frequently, you can find out how different carbohydrates affect your blood glucose. By using the carbohydrate sources that have a low glycaemic index, you need to use less insulin to control them. (See Chapter 8 for more on carbohydrates.)

In an attempt to mirror normal insulin and glucose dynamics, you often have to deal with a greater frequency of hypoglycaemia with intensive insulin treatment. The best way to handle hypoglycaemia is by eating slightly smaller meals and using the unused calories as between-meal snacks. This technique smoothes out the ups and downs.

At what point do you adjust your long-acting insulin? If you find that several mornings in a row your fasting blood glucose is too high, you may add a unit or two to your bedtime long-acting insulin. If the fasting blood glucose is too low, you may reduce your long-acting insulin by a unit or two or try eating a small bedtime snack. A high blood glucose level throughout the day is an indication to raise the long-acting insulin. Getting a lot of hypoglycaemia at different times of day is a reason to lower this insulin. These adjustments are best done in consultation with your doctor, but sometimes your doctor is not available or you are away. As a knowledgeable person, you can make these adjustments on your own.

Adjusting insulin when you travel

As you travel through time zones, you lose or gain hours in the day, depending on the direction. Time changes of under three hours require no modifications, but changes above three hours require progressively more changes, and you should probably discuss these with your doctor before you go.

ANECDOTE

Carbohydrate counting to maximum health

To find out how you can accomplish carbohydrate counting in everyday life, take a typical type 1 patient. A 41-year-old patient of ours has had type 1 diabetes for 31 years. He has been well controlled because he follows a good diet, does lots of exercise, and takes his insulin appropriately. He takes 30 units of insulin glargine at bedtime. He has a list of dosages of lispro insulin that tells him to take one unit of insulin for each 20 grams of carbohydrate. He is about to have breakfast and knows that it will contain 80 grams of carbohydrate. Therefore, he needs four units of lispro insulin. He measures his blood glucose before breakfast and finds that it is 11 mmol/l. His doctor has told him to take an extra unit of lispro insulin for each 3 mmol/l above 6 mmol/l. He adds two more units for a total of six units of insulin taken just before breakfast.

At lunch, his blood glucose measures 3 mmol/l. He is about to have a lunch of 120 grams of carbohydrate, so he needs 6 units for that, but he reduces it by 1 unit for the low measurement that is approximately 3 mmol/l lower than 6 mmol/l for a final dose of five units.

Before supper, his blood glucose measures 6 mmol/l. His supper contains only 60 grams of carbohydrate, so he needs three units for that. He does not have to adjust the dose because the glucose is close to 6 mmol/l, so he takes only three units. When he measures his blood glucose at bedtime, it's 6 mmol/l, so he is doing very well. Unless the blood glucose is 11 mmol/l or greater, he does not need to take any bedtime lispro because he is taking insulin glargine to control his glucose overnight.

Avoiding Drug Interactions

In some studies, patients are taking as many as four to five drugs, including their diabetes medication. These drugs often interact and end up costing millions of pounds in drug toxicity. Sometimes (believe it or not) even your doctor is not aware of the interactions of common drugs. You need to know the names of all the drugs you take and whether they affect one another.

Many common medications used for the treatment of high blood pressure also raise the blood glucose, sometimes bringing out a diabetic tendency that doctors may otherwise not have recognised:

- **Thiazide diuretics** may raise the glucose by causing a loss of potassium.
- **Beta blockers** reduce the release of insulin and include such drugs as atenolol and bisoprolol.

- ✔ **Calcium channel blockers** also reduce insulin secretion and include nifedipine and amlodipine.

- ✔ **Minoxidil** can raise blood glucose.

Drugs used for other purposes can also raise blood glucose:

- ✔ **Corticosteroids,** even topical use, can raise blood glucose (see Chapter 2 for more on corticosteroids).

- ✔ **Cyclosporine,** used to prevent organ rejection, can raise the blood glucose by poisoning the insulin-producing beta cell.

- ✔ **Oral contraceptives** were accused of causing hyperglycaemia when the dose of oestrogen was very high, but current preparations are not a problem.

- ✔ **Nicotinic acid and niacin,** used to lower cholesterol, can bring out a hyperglycaemic tendency.

- ✔ **Phenothiazines,** such as chlorpromazine, promazine, thioridazine (which isn't often used any more in the United Kingdom), fluphenazine, and tripfluoperzaine, can block insulin secretion and cause hyperglycaemia.

- ✔ **Thyroid hormone,** in elevated levels, raises the blood glucose by reducing insulin from the pancreas.

Many common medications, either on their own or by doing something to make the oral hypoglycaemic agents more potent, also lower the blood glucose. The most important of these include the following:

- ✔ **Salicylates** commonly known as aspirin, can lower the blood glucose, especially when given in large doses.

- ✔ **Ethanol,** in any form of alcohol, can lower the blood glucose, particularly when taken without food.

- ✔ **Alpha-blockers,** another group of antihypertensives that includes doxazosin, lower the glucose as well.

- ✔ **Fibric acid derivatives** like fenofibrate or bezafibrate, used to treat disorders of fat, cause a lowering of blood glucose.

If you start a new medication and suddenly find that your blood glucose is significantly higher or lower than usual, ask your doctor to check for the possibility that the new medication has a definite glucose-lowering or glucose-raising effect.

Chapter 11

Diabetes Is Your Show

● ●

In This Chapter

▶ Understanding your role as the person in charge of your diabetes

▶ Figuring out who's who on your medical team

▶ Tapping into the support of your family and friends

● ●

*A*s the old song goes, 'There's no business like show business . . . let's go on with the show!' And diabetes is certainly your show. As the person with diabetes, you're the author, director, and star, all rolled into one.

Of course, being the star, director, and author of any show is a major responsibility, even for shows that have finite life spans. But unlike programmes that run for a few seasons and then go away, diabetes *doesn't* go away. It's not like a cold, or even a nasty case of flu, which knocks you for six at the time but is all over in a matter of days. Diabetes is a condition that lasts for life.

Fortunately, diabetes isn't a one-man (or one-woman) show. It includes a cast of characters: doctors, nurses, dieticians, and more. When it comes down to it, you're responsible for pulling all these cast members together.

This chapter takes a look at some of the medical personnel in your cast and explains what you can do to help these people help you manage your diabetes.

You're Author, Director, and Star

Diabetes is a condition that lasts for life. If you don't direct yourself and the members of your production team properly, your long-term health suffers. The key to treating your diabetes is working closely with the other people on your team. Building up a good working relationship with your healthcare professionals can really make a difference. These people can help you understand your disease and encourage you to do what you need to (like take your medication and follow your diet and exercise regime) to control your diabetes and stay healthy.

Even though diabetes lasts for life, it doesn't have to control you. You can control it and reduce the impact it has on your life. Head to Chapters 4 and 5 for advice on how to reduce short-term and long-term complications. You can find plenty of invaluable information on keeping the effects of diabetes to a minimum.

Here are some things you have going for you:

- **The most important member in your cast is fully committed.** Yes, that's you we're talking about, and reading this book shows that you realise that the most important person, in terms of your diabetes management, is you! A survey in 2006 suggested that only a minority of patients with diabetes consider themselves to be well informed about their own condition. Considering that 95 per cent of diabetes care is self-care, that's a huge amount of self-help these patients are missing out on. By buying – and using – this book, you're already going a long way to ensuring that you get the very best of care.

- **You're in charge.** Because you're always going to have diabetes, you get to live with your condition day by day. As such, you come to understand your diabetes better than anyone else. Your general practitioner or diabetic specialist nurse may know more about interpreting your blood results than you – but no one knows how you feel as well as you do. That knowledge gives you the chance to be where you should be as far as your diabetes is concerned: In control.

- **You have a team of professionals ready to help you.** These days, health professionals have moved a long way from the attitude of 'doctor knows best'. Apart from anything else, there aren't enough trained staff in the National Health Service to keep the show running without your help. But that doesn't mean they aren't worth listening to. As with all successful productions, teamwork is the key. So think of your healthcare team as your production assistants. All of them have different skills, and the show wouldn't run as smoothly without them. They're there to help you understand more about the different aspects of your diabetes.

All general practice surgeries and hospitals have slightly different ways of working and different facilities available to them. Get to know how your local system works so that you can get the best out of it. If you move to a new area, you can find out all about the local practices from your Primary Care Trust (look it up in the phone book). Alternatively, your local library has details of all the qualifications and interests of the general practitioners in your area. You may find that one of the local doctors lists diabetes among her special interests. You can then contact the surgery to get more details on the way its diabetes services are managed before you register with that practice.

- **Your family and friends are part of your team.** They're your audience, your prompt, and, in case of emergency, your understudy. Never forget that they can't perform their roles unless they, too, know their lines.

Being the star of the show is both an honour and a responsibility – even if you never auditioned for the role. Times are always going to occur when you resent having landed the part. But by taking control and working with your family, friends, and healthcare professionals you have on board, you should have enough help to make the job much less demanding.

The Surgery Diabetic Clinic – Your Stage

About 50 per cent of people with type 2 diabetes in the United Kingdom are never referred to hospital. If you're one of them, the general practice surgery is your stage. Over 70 per cent of surgeries in the United Kingdom now run dedicated diabetic clinics. The staff members making up the team vary from surgery to surgery, but you should be able to access most of them. You don't need to see all of them at each appointment, but you should have an annual check-up where every aspect of your diabetes is monitored. If you can't, think seriously about asking for a hospital referral – none of these cast members is entirely dispensable.

The Receptionist – Your Box Office Staff

Over 98 per cent of general practices in the United Kingdom now have a diabetic register, which can be used to remind you when you need a check-up. A receptionist, practice administrator, or practice nurse is the one who usually runs this register.

Getting a good reception

Receptionists at general practice surgeries have an unjustified reputation for being obstructive. In fact, they can be your most useful allies. For example, if you ring during surgery hours and ask to speak to your doctor or practice nurse, the receptionist will probably refuse. This isn't because they're bolshy or power crazed (well, not always!) – if your doctor is in surgery and seeing another patient, the receptionist is also protecting that patient from having her consultation interrupted.

Almost all general practitioners, though, do have a set time every day when they take phone calls from patients. Your surgery should also have a system for dealing with emergencies – the sort of medical problems that can't wait until you can get an appointment. To find out, go into the surgery at a relatively quiet time (say, late morning or early afternoon) and have a chat with the receptionist about how the system in your surgery works. She can explain all the quirks of your surgery, answering any questions you have about phone calls, getting results, ordering repeat prescriptions, and so on.

Check with your surgery to find out what its recall system is and who runs it. That way, you know who to call if you think you've been overlooked.

Even the most efficient of surgeries makes mistakes sometimes, and you can't expect the surgery to keep track of exactly when you're due for what checks. That responsibility falls to you. Make sure you never leave one appointment without making the next one, or at least make a note in your diary to chase your appointment at a later date.

The General Practitioner – Your Assistant Director

Everyone in the United Kingdom has the right to be registered with a general practitioner, and over 95 per cent of people are. Your general practitioner may work in a partnership, in which case 'your' doctor may not run the diabetic clinic in your practice. You may want to be registered from the outset with a general practitioner who has a special interest in diabetes, or at least one with a partner who runs the regular clinic.

There are four main reasons for the rise of the general practitioner to the heady heights of assistant director of your diabetes:

✔ Although general practitioners in the past suffered from the description of 'jack of all trades, master of none', these days the training for general practice is as tough as that for any other specialism, and most general practitioners are highly qualified and highly skilled.

✔ The number of patients with diabetes is rising so rapidly (the figures in the United Kingdom for people diagnosed with diabetes look set to rise from 1.8 million in 2004 to 3 million by 2010) that hospitals simply cannot cope with the work. As such, your general practitioner is your primary resource for your diabetes.

✔ With more and more doctors working as part of a primary healthcare team, general practitioners have far more support to help them provide a comprehensive service.

✔ Most importantly, your general practitioner knows all about you. He is the one doctor who provides real continuity of care in every area of your health. That puts him in a good position to look at your diabetes in the context of your other illnesses, as well as focusing on the multi-system nature of diabetes.

If you've already read about long-term complications in Chapter 5, you know that diabetes can affect almost all parts of your body. More and more, diabetes is being considered as a multi-system disease. Major studies like the United Kingdom Prospective Diabetes Study (UKPDS) have shown that looking after your heart is just as important to a diabetic as looking after your blood sugar. Your general practitioner can help you to pull all the different strands together – but only with your help.

If things aren't working out with your general practitioner, you're free to change to another doctor in your area, without giving a reason. You can just take your National Health Service medical card to the new surgery you want to join. (If you've lost your card, you can fill in a form when you get there.) Be sure to check, though, that other doctors in your area have room to take you on to their list.

The Practice Nurse – Your Technical Assistant

Virtually all general practice surgeries in the United Kingdom now have at least one practice nurse. The role of the nurse varies between surgeries, but you can often look to the practice nurse for the following:

- To take most of the measurements (blood pressure, weight, blood tests, and so on) that you need to get done regularly.
- To be a very useful source of advice about lifestyle measures like diet and exercise (you can read more about these in Chapters 8 and 9).

Practice nurses usually have more time than your general practitioner, which means that they can offer much more detailed practical advice.

Some practices now also employ a *nurse practitioner,* a kind of 'super-nurse' who can make limited clinical decisions and prescribe some medicines. If you're not sure whether you need to see your general practitioner about a problem, your nurse practitioner will be able to pass you on to them if she can't sort it out herself.

The Diabetic Consultant or Endocrinologist – Your Technical Consultant

Diabetic consultants or endocrinologists are consultant physicians based in hospitals, but they've had years of extra training. As such, they should have the most in-depth knowledge of the management of diabetes. If they're endocrinologists, they have specialised in disease of the glands, such as diabetes, thyroid problems, and so on. Even if they deal with other medical problems as well as diabetes, they spend more of their time on 'your' disease than any other. This makes them great sources of information about the latest advances and new treatments.

Your diabetic consultant works as part of a team with more junior doctors and nurses running the clinic alongside her. You're unlikely to see your consultant every time you go to the hospital. For most of your appointments, you see another member of the team. Because the less senior doctors in the team move from job to job as part of their training, you're unlikely to meet them at more than one appointment. In reality, you may be met by an ever-changing stream of doctors, each of whom may have moved on to another post by your next appointment. Your consultant and diabetic specialist nurse (explained in the next section) are likely to be more constant. If you want to see them, ask as soon as you arrive for your appointment.

Depending on the type of diabetes you have, you're helped in different ways:

- ✔ If you have type 1 diabetes, you're referred to a consultant. Your consultant works mainly from a hospital, but some areas may run an outreach clinic nearer to you. This is a clinic in a local surgery, where the consultant attends every so often with other medical staff to run an outpatient clinic.

- ✔ If you have type 2 diabetes, you may not be referred to a hospital at all. If you aren't satisfied with the management you're getting from your primary care team, you have the right to ask your general practitioner for a referral to a hospital consultant. Your general practitioner may try to put you off because all referrals affect her practice budget – but don't let the general practitioner tell you that you're not allowed to be referred.

Getting the best from your general practitioner

In a recent survey, one of the three most unpopular phrases among general practitioners was 'I'm just here to get a referral to hospital'. General practitioners in the United Kingdom are very highly trained, and it's not entirely surprising that treating them as barriers to 'proper' care is a pretty good way to get their backs up! You do have the right to be referred to hospital, but remember that you have to carry on seeing your general practitioner for all sorts of other problems, so you want to try avoiding an argument.

Before you see your general practitioner to complain, write out a list of queries and concerns and try presenting them to yourself in the mirror or to a long-suffering family member. Try to avoid launching straight in with your grievances. If you explain your concerns, you may find that your general practitioner can answer them – or may agree with them! That way, you're more likely to get what you want without wrecking your relationship with your doctor.

The Diabetic Specialist Nurse – Your Props Provider

Most hospitals now have at least one diabetic specialist nurse. She is highly trained in all aspects of diabetes management, especially the practicalities. She is, perhaps, the person most likely to know the answer to questions like 'How do I change my treatment if I join a gym?' or 'Can I have champagne at Christmas?' She should also have samples of most of the devices you're likely to consider using for giving insulin or checking your blood sugars.

If you have type 1 diabetes, you're very likely to meet a diabetic specialist nurse. She'll probably come and visit you on the ward during your first admission and keep in close contact as you get to grips with your diabetes. She has the skills necessary to advise on changes in your medication and to prescribe and order devices to help in your management.

Unfortunately, as with so many other services in the National Health Service, diabetic specialist nurses are a rare breed. They're often expected to divide themselves between primary care (where they may teach practice nurses about running diabetic clinics or managing diabetes), community clinics, hospital clinics, and managerial tasks.

If you attend a hospital, ask at your next clinic appointment about talking to the diabetic specialist nurse or phone her directly. If your care is dealt with entirely in primary care, you may still be able to get the specialist nurse's help by talking to your general practitioner or practice nurse.

The Chiropodist – Your Dance Instructor

One of the first rules of diabetes is never to forget your feet. This is especially true if you have neuropathy (you can read about this in Chapter 5), which can affect your ability to feel problems with your feet.

You should have your feet checked at least once a year, at your annual check-up. At other times, you may be referred to a chiropodist if you have a problem or for regular checks. Some areas have open-access clinics, where you can refer yourself – ask your general practitioner or diabetic specialist nurse about services in your area.

You may think you've got more important things to worry about than your feet, but remember, as a diabetic you're 15 to 70 times more likely than a non-diabetic to need part of your leg amputated if you don't look after your feet!

The Eye Doctor – Your Lighting Designer

An eye doctor is called an *ophthalmologist*. She's the one who ensures that your diabetes doesn't damage your vision. You should have a detailed examination of your eyes at least once a year, at your annual check-up. The doctor looks for conditions like diabetic retinopathy (damage to the back of the eye) and cataracts, and you can read more about these in Chapter 5. In some areas, your general practitioner (or the doctor at another community-based clinic) is the one who examines your eyes – but if you have any problems, you should certainly be referred to an ophthalmologist.

You need drops put into your eyes to dilate your pupils when you have a proper eye examination. These sting and make you sensitive to bright lights for a while. Make arrangements for someone to drive you home after your eye examination.

You may think of restoring or protecting eyesight as a good thing, but matters are not always that simple. One ophthalmologist in America tells of restoring the vision of a diabetic patient with laser treatment. The patient promptly bought a gun and nearly shot someone he had a long-standing grievance against!

The Dietician – Your Food Services Provider

The expression 'you are what you eat' is never more true than when you're a diabetic. Your dietician doesn't just give you information about keeping your blood sugar down. She can also provide very detailed eating plans that help you lose weight (type 2 diabetes is much more common if you're obese) and look after your heart. Of course, it's really important that your dietician gives you flexible advice that fits in with your lifestyle – if you think her suggestions are too rigid, tell her.

To make the most out of your visits to the dietician, fill in a food diary for a few days beforehand – and don't bother to cheat! The diary gives your dietician a good idea of where you need to concentrate most of your dietary work. Some dieticians can provide recipe sheets with diabetes-friendly versions of your favourite meals.

If you're a type 1 diabetic, you must know how your food interacts with your insulin injections. The dietician can teach you how to count carbohydrates so that you know how much insulin to take for your meals (see Chapter 10 for more on carbohydrate counting).

Dietician or nutritionist?

In the United Kingdom, all dieticians are legally obliged to undertake professional training at a hospital, pass a professional exam, and then register with the Council for Professions Supplementary to Medicine (CPSM). They keep their knowledge up to date with continuing education and abide by the CPSM's code of conduct. That sets them apart from nutritionists, who don't need any professional training at all – and don't need to have their standards checked by any reputable body.

Of course, many nutritionists have undergone training in nutrition. Without the guaranteed qualifications that a dietician holds, though, you can't guarantee the nutritionist is of high quality. So if a friend tells you that she's got the most wonderful nutritionist who discovered all sorts of problems that her doctor missed – beware!

You're much more likely to stick to a healthy diet if everyone you live and eat with is on your side. If you don't do most of the cooking in your household, take the cook along to your appointment. The dietician will be delighted to see them. And do tell the dietician if you eat food corresponding to a particular ethnic background – they're able to tailor their advice to suit you.

The Pharmacist – Your Usher

The role of usher may not sound important, but how are you going to enjoy the play if you can't find your way to your seat? The pharmacist is your guide to all the medicines and tools you need to manage your diabetes, including any complications you may develop. She ushers you through the use of all these strange and new products – and unlike a general practitioner, you don't need an appointment to see a pharmacist!

Following are some services your pharmacist may provide:

- Many pharmacists collect your repeat prescription from your general practitioner and even deliver the medication to you at home. This service is great if you're housebound, but you may find they have more time to chat and give advice if you go to the pharmacy to collect your prescription.

- Some pharmacists are now able to issue repeat prescriptions without you seeing your general practitioner at all. Ask your local pharmacist what services she provides.

- Most pharmacists prepare a repeat prescription list of all the medicines you take regularly. This list tells you the strength and dosage frequency of each medication. You can carry it around in case any doctor ever needs to know what you take, and it's especially useful if you travel away from home.

✔ Every time you're issued with a new medicine, good pharmacists check to make sure that the new medication doesn't conflict with other medicines you're taking. They may also be able to tell you whether side effects you're experiencing are related to one of your medicines.

✔ These days, most pharmacists are highly trained and can give preliminary advice about minor ailments. If you're having problems getting to see your general practitioner or aren't sure if you need a doctor's appointment, ask your pharmacist to help.

If you have diabetes, you're exempt from the National Health Service prescription charge. That means that some medicines you can buy over the counter, such as thrush treatment and simple painkillers, are free if you get your general practitioner to prescribe them. Your pharmacist may have an arrangement with your surgery that lets the pharmacist give you these medications on prescription and get the prescription from your general practitioner later.

Your Family and Friends – Your Captivated and Caring Audience

Your audience consists of the people you live with, eat with, and play with. Your family and friends can be a tremendous source of help, but you must clue them in to the fact that you have diabetes. If you have type 1 diabetes, you can teach your family and friends how to recognise when your glucose is too low, in case you're ever too ill to take care of yourself. If you have type 2, ask your family to moderate their diet so that you can follow yours. Complying with your diet is difficult enough, and you don't need your family exposing you to high-calorie foods. Besides, a diabetic diet is good for anyone.

Your family and friends can also become your exercise partners. Sticking to a programme is a lot easier when someone is counting on you to show up to work out. They can also accompany you when you visit the doctor and remind you to ask the doctor a question or to follow the instructions you receive.

Let your family and friends know about your diabetes and buy them a copy of this book (or let them borrow yours) so that they understand something about what you're going through and how they can best help you.

Chapter 12

Putting Your Knowledge to Work

· ·

In This Chapter

▶ Improving your frame of mind

▶ Optimising your use of tests and monitoring

▶ Taking medication properly

▶ Following a diet

▶ Benefiting from exercise

▶ Getting help from others

· ·

*I*f you read this entire part, you can get a good idea about what the experts know. But knowing is often quite a distance from doing. The key thing is to start acting on your knowledge now. Don't wait another day to begin to do the things that can prolong your life and increase its quality. You don't want to regret your life the way poor George Burns did. When a beautiful girl walked into his hotel room and said, 'I'm sorry, I must be in the wrong room,' he told her, 'No, you're not in the wrong room. You are just 40 years too late.'

Developing Positive Thinking

Studies have shown fairly conclusively that if you start with a positive frame of mind, your body can work with you and not against you. Even when things go wrong, if you're optimistic, you can pick yourself up and move forward. If you're pessimistic, you can become depressed and believe that nothing can help you. A pessimistic attitude, therefore, doesn't help you control your blood glucose and avoid complications.

We have a patient who came to us to improve his glucose control just after having a toe amputated. This patient is one who sees manure and knows there is a beautiful horse in the area. He refuses to believe that a temporary setback is a permanent defeat. We got him on a programme of tight diabetic control with the newer oral medications. His eyes have got better, and his neuropathy (diabetic nerve disease, see Chapter 5) has improved. He believes in his ability to control his blood glucose, and all his actions are directed towards doing just that. The result has been an amazing turnaround in his haemoglobin A1c. With his attitude, he is willing to make the changes necessary because he knows these changes pay big dividends for his health.

Achieving a positive attitude has a lot to do with how you interpret problems. If you see problems as permanent and unchangeable, you have trouble being positive. If you see them as temporary and something you can change given enough time, you're much more optimistic and able to solve most of your troubles.

Monitoring and Testing

Many of my patients ask me about a cure for diabetes. A cure doesn't exist yet, but the future looks very promising. So far, doctors don't have a portable machine that can measure blood glucose and respond with the right amount of insulin. Such a gadget wouldn't be of much use for the people who take pills anyway. Therefore, you have to use your brain to make the calculation that your pancreas would make automatically if it could. The calculation is, of course, how much medicine to take for a given glucose level. To make the calculation, you need to know the glucose. This is where monitoring comes in.

If you use insulin, you should have one of the monitors that I describe in Chapter 7. If you have type 1 diabetes, you should probably monitor before meals and at bedtime at least. If you have type 2 diabetes, you should discuss with your health professionals whether or not you need to monitor your own glucose levels. Even if you don't monitor the levels regularly, you should be monitoring your glucose levels when you're unwell. Chapter 10 is where you can find information about what to do in response to your test results.

Remember, however, that blood glucose tests are only a moment in time. What you need to know is whether you are in control 24 hours a day. That is where the haemoglobin A1c comes in. Your doctor should order this test at least every six months if you're stable, and every three months if you're not. If you have close to normal results in this test, you don't have to worry about long-term complications (see Chapter 5) and probably don't suffer from short-term complications (see Chapter 4) either.

Even with near-normal haemoglobin A1c results, you still want to be checked for any sign of complications. That means regular eye examinations, regular blood and urine tests for kidney damage, and regular tests for sensation in your feet. Your doctor should perform these checks on schedule; if he doesn't, remind him.

Great treatment exists for every diabetic complication, and the earlier treatment starts, the less likely it is that the complication leads to serious damage. Routine monitoring and testing allow you to discover the problem as early as possible.

Using Medication

Medication can be tricky. Even the most potent medication doesn't work if you don't take it. Doctors use the word 'noncompliance' when they talk about the tendency of patients not to take their medication. Consider the compliance rate of patients with high blood pressure, for example: Only about half take their medication regularly in the long term. Not a good idea. Some of the things you need to know when you take your medication include the following:

- ✔ Are you taking the right dose at the right time?
- ✔ Are you taking it with or without food, as recommended by the medication?
- ✔ Does it mix with your other medication?
- ✔ Are you aware of side effects, and are they being monitored?
- ✔ Can the desired effect sometimes be too strong?
- ✔ Do you have an antidote to the effect available if necessary?
- ✔ Do you need to adjust the dose when you're not feeling well?

Your doctor, your pharmacist, your practice nurse, or your diabetic specialist nurse can all help you with your medication, but you're on your own when it comes to taking it. If you have trouble remembering, get yourself a plastic case containing seven sections for the seven days of the week, then fill each section with each day's pills. These cases are called *dossette boxes*, and are available for under £5 from most pharmacists. This trick lets you see easily whether you took all your medication or not. Alternatively, talk to your pharmacist about getting your tablets packaged in *blister packs.* These packs can be dispensed once a month and contain all the medication you need to take at different times, packed and labelled clearly.

For more on medication, see Chapter 10.

Following a Diet

If you look at Appendix A and its recipes, it should be clear to you that you're not sacrificing very much by following an appropriate diabetic diet, unless you consider avoiding being overweight to be a sacrifice. You can enjoy delicious food that provides plenty of energy for your needs.

Although the emphasis in the last few years has been on reducing fat in your diet, especially cholesterol and saturated fat (see Chapter 8), when it comes to diabetes you have to be aware of your carbohydrate intake as well. And it doesn't hurt to know something about the quality of the carbohydrate as well as the quantity. Try to choose low glycaemic index carbohydrates, like basmati rice instead of white rice. Any carbohydrate with lots of fibre is a low glycaemic source. You have a lower blood glucose as a result of eating it and require less insulin to control it. Not only does that mean better diabetic control, but your fats, particularly triglyceride, are also lower, and this decreases the severity of the insulin resistance syndrome if you have type 2 diabetes.

Most people can make changes in their diet over the short term, but maintaining these changes over the long term is difficult. The best way to accomplish a long-term change is to have a plan and try to carry it out. Unplanned situations are probably the most damaging to your diabetic control. When you enter a restaurant, for example, you're presented with a menu. The job of the menu's author is to entice you with the description of the foods. If you have in mind what foods are good for your diabetic diet, you're more likely to order what helps you, not what messes up your control.

A few restaurants are just starting to include menu selections that offer dishes geared towards people with diabetes. It will take a long time before more restaurants offer these selections, and some will never do it (especially in Paris!). Until then, you must go out to eat prepared to order appropriately.

The same thing holds when you eat at someone else's home. If your hosts know you have diabetes, hopefully they will prepare something you can eat. If they don't, you must select with great care. Don't be afraid to say no. Your friendly dietician can give you a lot of help on what to select and what to reject.

Having a fair amount of order in your life helps a lot when you have diabetes. If your life is disorganised, controlling your diabetes is much more difficult. You must take your medication at about the same time and eat at about the same time each day. You must test at about the same time and exercise at about the same time. But you don't have to eat the same thing all the time. An endless variety of delicious foods is available to you. For more on your diet, see Chapter 8.

Exercising

The more you exercise regularly, the better you can control your blood glucose (and your weight as well). If you have type 2 diabetes and exercise regularly, you need less or no medication. If you have type 1 diabetes, you need less insulin. Your exercise choices are unlimited (see Chapter 9). Yes, even a game of golf is exercise, though most people (who are not professional golfers) do not play the sport more than once or twice a week.

If you're having trouble exercising, follow these tips:

- ✔ **You need to do something daily if possible, but no less than three or four times a week.** If you can't exercise regularly on your own, get an exercise partner. You don't need a sports club to find step aerobics. Just walk up a few flights of stairs where you work. Go for a 30-minute walk outside if the weather permits.

- ✔ **Set up a programme with goals so that you do not stay stuck at a low level of exercise.** If you do not know how to create exercise goals yourself, check with an exercise physiologist. If you're older than 40, have not exercised, and are overweight, check with your doctor before beginning a strenuous programme.

- ✔ **Don't limit yourself to aerobics.** A little weight lifting a few days a week can make an amazing difference to your strength, your stamina, and your physique. If your sport is tennis, you may find that you can play that third set with much greater ease once you start on a weights programme. All other sports benefit from weight lifting in a similar fashion.

Exercise is definitely a way to get high without drugs. It's good for depression or any unhappy state of mind. Don't take my word for it – get out and find out for yourself. See Chapter 9 for more on exercise.

Using Other Expertise

People are usually eager to help you with your diabetic condition. (See Chapter 11 to find out more about your supporting cast.) So much knowledge is out there just waiting to be tapped. The National Health Service recognises the value of resources like the dietician and the diabetic specialist nurse. Most general practices and all hospital diabetic clinics have access to one.

You can get lots of free sources of information from your friendly pharmacist, the Internet, and other people with diabetes. You may want to be careful of these last two groups, however. A great deal of misinformation is shared on the Internet and among diabetic patients. Before you make a major alteration in your treatment on the basis of uncertain information, check with your doctor. (You can find out about some of the most common bits of misinformation in Chapters 17 and 19.)

Every time you have a question about your diabetes, write it down and save it for your next surgery visit to your doctor, unless the question is urgent. If you don't know whether something is urgent, call your doctor and let him determine the urgency of your problem.

Don't neglect your family and friends as a helpful source. These are the people who love you and know that you would help them if the tables were turned. The problem is that they cannot help you if they don't know what you're dealing with. Tell them that you have diabetes and explain the risks, such as hypoglycaemia, that you face. Tell them how to help you if the need arises. You'll find that the result is a much closer relationship.

Part IV

Special Considerations for Living with Diabetes

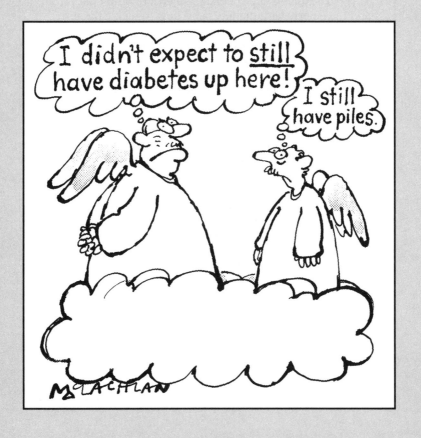

In this part . . .

Diabetes in growing children and the elderly often produces problems that the average adult with diabetes does not have to deal with. Children have to grow normally and develop sexually, while the elderly often have other illnesses and, in any case, are more frail. Both groups have emotional problems that are unique. Children are learning to fit in with their peers while separating from their parents. The elderly are losing friends and relatives at the same time as their mental processes are declining. This part explains the special problems of both children and the elderly with diabetes and how to tackle them.

Even the middle-aged adult has unusual problems, in this case often relating to driving and employment. Fortunately, the barriers are rapidly coming down, but you still need to know about certain areas. Discrimination cannot be tolerated, and you can find out what to do about it here.

Finally, we tell you about the huge number of new developments in diabetes treatment, putting them into perspective as to their usefulness and appropriateness. After that, we expose the false promises that some people make. So many things have been proposed for diabetes care without the benefit of careful evaluation. We present the scientific evidence for and against each development so that you can make up your own mind.

Chapter 13

Your Child Has Diabetes

. . . .

In This Chapter

▶ Managing your child's diabetes, from infancy to young adulthood

▶ Dealing with obesity and type 2 diabetes in children

▶ Finding sick-day solutions

▶ Appreciating the extra value of team care

. . . .

C hildren with diabetes present special problems that adults with diabetes do not have. Not only are they growing and developing from babies to adults, but they have problems of psychological and social adjustment. Diabetes can add complications to a period of life that is not exactly smooth, even without diabetes.

Many doctors believe that if a child has diabetes, the whole family really has the disease because everyone must adjust to it. Because diabetes is the second most common chronic disease in children after asthma, it is no small problem. In this chapter, you find out how to manage diabetes in your child at each stage of growth and development.

As recently as 20 years ago, type 1 diabetes was often referred to as 'juvenile onset diabetes' and type 2 diabetes as 'maturity onset diabetes'. With the explosion in obesity in the last few years, people in their teens are now developing type 2 diabetes. That's why we no longer use the terms 'juvenile' and 'maturity' onset diabetes. You can find out more about how the two types of diabetes affect young people later in this chapter.

Dealing with Your Child's Diabetes through the Years

Every stage of childhood diabetes presents its own challenges. The following sections tell you what you need to know to manage your child's diabetes.

When your child has diabetes, keep these things in mind:

✔ You have a great responsibility, but it's one that you can handle. Just don't try to cope alone. Follow the advice in this section and use the medical experts available to you, as well as your family and friends, to make the challenges manageable.

✔ Your child is first a child and *then* a child with diabetes. You're not to blame for your child's diabetes (and neither is your child). Diabetes is not a form of retribution for your sins.

When your baby has diabetes

Although type 1 diabetes does not usually show up in babies, it can, and you should know what to expect when it does. Obviously, your baby is not verbal and cannot tell you what is bothering her. For this reason, you may miss the fact that she is urinating excessively in her nappy. If your baby loses weight and vomits or has diarrhoea, you may ascribe this to a stomach disorder rather than diabetes. When the diagnosis is finally made, the baby may be very sick and require a stay in a paediatric intensive care unit. If this happens to you, don't blame yourself for not realising that your baby was sick.

Once the diagnosis is made, the hard work begins. You must learn to give insulin injections and to test the blood glucose in a child who is reluctant to have either one done. You have to learn when and what to feed the baby, both to encourage growth and development and to prevent low blood glucose.

At this stage, you're not as worried about tight control as you will be later on. There are several reasons for this. First, the baby's neurological system is still developing. Frequent, severely low blood glucose damages this development, so the glucose is permitted to be higher now than later on. Second, studies show that changes associated with high blood glucose leading to diabetic complications don't begin to add up until the pre-pubertal years, so you have a grace period during which you can allow less tight control.

On the other hand, a small baby is very fragile. There is less of everything, so small losses of water, sodium, potassium, and other substances can more rapidly lead to a very sick baby. If you keep your baby's blood glucose around 8.3 to 11.1 mmol/l, you are doing very well.

For a time of variable duration, called the *honeymoon period*, your child seemingly regains the ability to control the blood glucose with little or no insulin. This period always ends, and it isn't your fault that it finishes. When the honeymoon period is over, you have to work with the doctor, the dietician, and the diabetic specialist nurse to find out how to control diabetes with insulin. You'll need to be able to do the following:

✔ Identify the signs and symptoms of hyperglycaemia, hypoglycaemia, and diabetic ketoacidosis (see Chapters 4 and 5). Each child has a particular way of expressing low or high blood glucose, for example by becoming quiet or loud. Discover the signs for your child and let anyone else who cares for the child know them.

✔ Administer insulin (see Chapter 10). Thanks to rapid-acting insulin, you can wait to see how much the baby is eating before you decide on the amount of insulin.

✔ Measure the blood glucose and urine ketones (see Chapter 7). Toddlers who are toilet-trained may have an 'accident' when their glucose is high, which causes a large quantity of urine. Very frequent blood glucose measurements are essential. The more information you have, the better the control and the less frequent the hypoglycaemia. However, most children should need no more than 4–7 blood glucose measurements a day to achieve excellent control.

✔ Treat hypoglycaemia with food or a medicine called glucagon (see Chapter 4). Toddlers require half of the adult dose of glucagon. Glucagon may cause the toddler to vomit but it still raises the blood glucose.

✔ Feed your diabetic child (see Chapter 8).

✔ Set an example for lifelong exercise for your child by exercising with her.

✔ Know what to do when your child is sick with another childhood illness. If it is necessary to go to the hospital, this should be approached as a positive experience, a chance to get a tune-up.

The honeymoon period

Given that name because it represents a period of improvement in type 1 diabetes that does not last, the honeymoon period occurs in most patients. Once diabetes has been diagnosed and treated so that the blood glucose levels are close to normal, the child may require little or no insulin for a time. This is a period of remission in the disease and means that there is still some function in the beta cells of the pancreas (see Chapter 3 to understand how the pancreas functions). The honeymoon period lasts longer in the following situations:

✔ When the age at onset of diabetes is older

✔ When the disease is milder at initial diagnosis

✔ When the amount of islet cell antibody (explained in Chapter 2) is lower

This is a temporary remission and ends with a sudden or slowly increasing requirement for insulin. By three years after the diagnosis, there is complete loss of insulin production in young children. Older children may have some preservation of function.

Your responsibilities as the parent of a diabetic baby or pre-school child (discussed in the following section) are extensive and time-consuming. Training your usual helpers to take over, even for a short time, is especially difficult. Unless you hire a professional to take over for a while, you may not get very much time away from your diabetic infant.

Your other children may resent the attention that you pay to the child who has diabetes. If your other children start to misbehave, this jealousy may be the reason.

When your pre-school child has diabetes

Diagnosing diabetes in your pre-school child may be just as difficult as diagnosing an infant's diabetes (see the preceding section for details). The child may have very limited language skills and still be running around in nappies. Administering the necessary medication and performing the required test may be even harder.

A pre-school child is beginning the process of separating from her parent and starting to learn to control the environment (by becoming toilet-trained, for example). This separation process makes it more difficult for you, the parent, to give the injections and test the glucose. You must be firm in insisting that these things be done, and you need to do them yourself. A small child neither knows how to perform the tests, nor does she understand what to do with the information that the glucose meter generates.

Here are other things to keep in mind when your pre-school child has diabetes:

- ✔ If a honeymoon period occurs after the diagnosis, this period is usually briefer than if a diagnosis is made in a teenager. See the sidebar 'The honeymoon period' for an explanation of this temporary remission period.

- ✔ Because a child's eating habits may not be very regular, the use of very short-acting insulin like lispro is especially helpful (see Chapter 10).

- ✔ Very soon, people with diabetes should have a way of measuring the blood glucose in a painless fashion, which will be of great assistance in monitoring young children with diabetes.

When your primary school child has diabetes

For the rest of this section, we assume that your primary school child has type 1 diabetes rather than type 2, because the vast majority of primary school children with diabetes have type 1. Sadly, as you can find out later in the chapter in the section on obesity and type 2 diabetes in children, that may not be the norm for long.

In some ways, diabetes care gets a little easier with a primary school child, but in other ways it gets more difficult. Your child can finally tell you when she has symptoms of hypoglycaemia, so this condition is easier to recognise and treat. But you must begin to control the blood glucose more carefully because your child is reaching the stage where control really counts. The challenges you face include the following:

- ✔ You still have a child who is growing and developing, so nutrition remains very important. You need to make sure that your child gets enough of the right kinds of calories. A snack such as 4 ounces of apple juice and a cracker between breakfast and lunch, between lunch and supper, and at bedtime helps to smooth out control and avoid the lows.

- ✔ As the child goes to school, she is interacting with other children, is looking for their approval, and wants to fit in. The child may consider diabetes as a stigma. She may be very reluctant to share the fact that she has diabetes with other children. A plan of treatment that interferes with school and friendships may be very unwelcome. Diet may also suffer at school as the child tries to fit in and not stand out by eating the things that diabetes requires.

- ✔ Your child is going to do more to separate from you. She may insist on giving insulin injections and doing blood tests herself. Studies again indicate that you should not relinquish these tasks to your child, certainly not completely. Your child may not be physically capable of performing them and, in an attempt to hide the disease from peers, may not carry them out at all during school.

Because you are beginning to tighten the level of control, hypoglycaemia is more of a risk, especially at night. You can avoid hypoglycaemia by taking any or all of the following steps at this stage and from now on:

- ✔ Give a bedtime snack regularly.

- ✔ Measure and treat a low blood glucose before bedtime.

- ✔ Occasionally check the blood glucose at 3 a.m.

- ✔ Ask about symptoms of night-time low blood glucose, such as nightmares and headaches.

- ✔ Be sure that your child does not skip meals.

- ✔ Have your child eat carbohydrates before exercising.

Make sure that some member of your family can administer glucagon by injection to treat hypoglycaemia if you are unable to get your child to eat or drink.

> ## Diabetes and the Disability Discrimination Act of 1995
>
> The Disability Discrimination Act of 1995 protects anyone with a disability, defined as a physical or mental impairment that has a substantial and long-term effect on your ability to carry out normal day-to-day activities. This includes diabetes. Local Education Authorities, schools (both private and state), and higher education establishments are all covered by the Act. The Scottish Parliament has introduced a similar Act, and the Act now applies to Northern Ireland.
>
> The Act requires that schools make reasonable adjustments to ensure that a child with diabetes is not treated less favourably than anyone else, without a justifiable reason. Under the Act, a child with diabetes should be able to participate fully in all school and after-school activities, including school trips, even those abroad. This means that the school must make provisions for blood glucose testing, for treatment with insulin, and for taking snacks or going to the toilet as needed.

Once your child is off to school or a daycare setting, you need to address new problems. For the first time, your child is under the care of someone other than you for much of the time. That person, or persons, may not know as much as you about your child's diabetes. They may have different priorities. Fortunately, there are lots of steps you as a parent can take to minimise any problems that may arise.

Try to think of every possible problem in advance and share this information with your child's teacher and other staff so that they know what to do on every occasion. If, for example, your child can recognise the signs of hypoglycaemia and knows that she needs to eat something quickly, your child's teacher should be aware of that possibility so that, if it occurs, the teacher can respond appropriately. Being proactive in this way can stop any embarrassing misunderstandings. You also may want to bring the subject out into the open with your child's classmates. Schedule a time to go in to the classroom and talk about the condition and how it can affect your child and those around her. Alternatively, ask your child's teacher or diabetic specialist nurse to talk about the disease.

To ensure that the people in your child's school understand diabetes and know what to do in various situations, you, your doctor, and the school nurse can develop a written treatment plan. In this plan, relevant people in the school have assigned roles. In most cases, the diabetic specialist nurse visits your child's school to talk to your child's teacher and other staff about diabetes. The plan should include information about the following:

- ✔ Blood glucose monitoring
- ✔ Insulin administration
- ✔ Meals and snacks
- ✔ Recognition and treatment of hypoglycaemia
- ✔ Recognition and treatment of hyperglycaemia
- ✔ Who to contact in an emergency

As the parent, you are responsible for providing all supplies for testing and treatment. It is the responsibility of the relevant person from the school to understand and treat hypoglycaemia, to test the blood glucose and provide treatment when the level is outside certain parameters, to coordinate meals and snacks, and to allow time for appointments to the doctor as well as toilet use. There is no reason that your child should not participate fully in school.

Talk to your general practitioner or diabetic specialist nurse about getting spare supplies of testing equipment and sticks to keep at your child's school.

Your child has a right not to be discriminated against because of her diabetes. If you think your child may be suffering discrimination, you can contact the Disability Rights Commission Helpline, which is open from Monday to Friday, 8 a.m. to 8 p.m. The helpline staff can advise you about whether your child's school is in breach of the Disability Discrimination Act (see the sidebar 'Diabetes and the Disability Discrimination Act of 1995' for information on this Act), and what you can do about it. You can reach the helpline at:

DRC Helpline
Freepost MID 02614
Stratford-Upon-Avon
CV37 9BR

Phone: 08457-622-633 (all calls charged at local rate)

Web site: www.drc-gb.org
e-mail enquiries: ddahelp@stra.sitel.co.uk

When your adolescent or teen has diabetes

The comments in this and the next section refer to type 1 diabetes in children. The goal in type 2 diabetes remains normalisation of weight and increased exercise to achieve normal blood glucose levels, and management of the disease is very similar to that of adults with type 2 diabetes. This can be accomplished in type 2 diabetes in children, but is much more difficult in type 1 diabetes.

Your adolescent or teenager with diabetes provides some of your biggest challenges. This is the time that most childhood diabetes begins. On the plus side, the Diabetes Control and Complications Trial showed that tight control can be accomplished beginning at age 13, and that this control can prevent complications. Another plus is that the higher frequency of severe hypoglycaemia that accompanies tighter control wasn't found to be damaging to the brain of the child at this age. On the negative side, children at this age don't think in terms of long-term blood glucose control and prevention of complications, so they're not willing to do many of the tasks required to control their diabetes on a regular basis.

During the adolescent and teen years, your child is most eager to become independent. Yet you don't want to give up all control at this time for several reasons:

- ✔ Your child actually does better if she has limits that are clearly stated and enforced.
- ✔ The 'shame' of diabetes may cause the child to skip injections and food, especially around friends.
- ✔ The problem of eating disorders (see Chapter 8) may pop up at this time, especially among the girls trying to maintain a slim body image. Girls with diabetes know that, if they skip their injections, they lose weight. They ignore the high blood glucose that results.
- ✔ Teenagers with diabetes may still be unable to translate levels of blood glucose into appropriate action.

The hormonal changes that occur in puberty are often associated with insulin resistance. These changes may be the source of loss of control rather than any failure of your child to follow the diabetic treatment plan. Upward adjustment of the insulin may overcome this problem.

Strenuous exercise may play an even greater role in the life of your child at this age. The result is a significant reduction in the amount of insulin required after the exercise. Type 1 diabetes is no reason to prohibit strenuous exercise. Your child's blood glucose measurements help you and your child to define her need for insulin.

When your child plays a team sport, the team coach, as well as teammates, have to be aware of her diabetes and allow your child to eat, go to the loo, and take insulin as required. It may be worth talking to your child to check that she's comfortable discussing these issues with her team coach, or offering to bring the subject up tactfully for her.

Make sure that snacking continues throughout the adolescent and teenage years and that snacks are readily available no matter where the child may be.

When your young adult child has diabetes

When your child becomes a young adult, you definitely want to give up the control that has helped her thrive up to this point. At this age, your child should be doing her own testing. She is ready to leave the paediatric level and begin to work with doctors who care for adults. This means that you are probably out of the loop. Your child should now have the skill to choose appropriate insulin treatment based on blood glucose levels and calories of carbohydrate consumed (see Chapter 10 for treatment options and medications).

Your child now has new challenges, including finding work, going to college, finding a future mate, and finding a place to live independently. At the same time, the reluctance to admit to diabetes and the desire for a thin body continue to complicate care.

Diabetes care must be intensive at the point of young adulthood (see Chapter 10 for information about what intensive diabetic care entails). Multiple injections of intermediate and short-acting insulin are taken. Your child must follow a diabetic diet (explained in Chapter 8). An exercise programme is also essential (see Chapter 9). The rest of this book really has to do with the tasks that your young adult child with diabetes faces.

Special considerations for the college student

Once your child leaves for college, she has to take all the responsibility for her diabetes. It is important that she has access to all the equipment for testing her blood glucose and administering insulin. The college must be aware of her medical condition. It is valuable to find one or several people at the college who are prepared to help her (a roommate is ideal if she has one).

Two issues are particularly important to discuss before the student leaves – alcohol use and sexual activity. Alcohol use may significantly increase in college, which leads to many empty calories as well as the risk of severe hypoglycaemia if your child does not eat food with the alcohol. If your budding scholar is male, you need to make sure that concerns about erection problems have been addressed. If you're waving off your daughter, she needs to be fully aware of the increased risk of pregnancy if her diabetes is not in control.

College, like the rest of your child's life with diabetes, can be experienced just as it would be if diabetes were not present. The key is planning.

Obesity and Type 2 Diabetes in Children

In the United Kingdom, the majority of children with diabetes have type 1 diabetes. However, the incidence of type 2 diabetes increases as the country's rate of obesity goes up – and boy, do we have an increase in the rate of obesity! Sadly, the United Kingdom has the fastest increase in obesity rates in the world, and the incidence of obesity is rising fastest among the young. Among British adults, for instance, the rate of obesity has increased by 70 per cent in the last 10 years (up from 14 per cent to 24 per cent of adults). Among children, rates have doubled (that's a 100 per cent increase) over the same period. So among British children today:

- 25 per cent are overweight or obese (up from 15 per cent over the last 10 years)

- 9.2 per cent of pre-school children are obese (up from 5.4 per cent over the last 10 years)

- 18 per cent of 16 year olds are obese (up from 10 per cent over the last 10 years)

That means that a real risk exists that in future years, as many, if not more, schoolchildren will have type 2 diabetes as have type 1. In the United States, for example, where about 39 per cent of the adult population are obese, the proportion of children with diabetes who had type 2, rather than type 1, increased from under 4 per cent in 1990 to 30 per cent in 2003.

Even without diabetes, obesity is a burden for children. The obese child has severe psychological and social consequences:

- Lower respect from peers than other disabled children

- Less comfortable family interactions

- Poor body image

- Low confidence and self-esteem

Adding type 2 diabetes into this mix can be devastating. The consequences of the preceding problems may lead to failure to manage the diabetes because the child wants to avoid any activity that makes her even more different from her peers.

Children at risk of type 2 diabetes

Overweight or obesity is present in as many as 25 per cent of all children. Only a fraction of these children go on to develop diabetes, but it is important to separate type 1 diabetes from type 2 because some of the short-term complications, like ketoacidosis (see Chapter 4), don't occur in children with type 2 diabetes. That is no reason to treat type 2 diabetes in your child less seriously than type 1; far from it. Young people with type 2 diabetes can run into just as many problems in the longer term as those with type 1 diabetes, if they don't manage their condition vigorously.

The child with type 2 diabetes can be treated with pills or diet and exercise alone. However, because children don't appreciate the long-term consequences of their actions, you often have the problem of getting them to comply.

Helping your child lose weight

You must help your obese child lose weight because obese children are nine times more likely than normal-weight children to become obese adults. With the assistance of a dietician, you can figure out the food that your child can eat to maintain growth and development without further weight gain. Following are some tips for helping your child manage her weight:

- ✔ Take your child into the supermarket and point out the difference between empty calories and nourishing calories.
- ✔ Never make high-calorie food, like cake and sweets, a reward.
- ✔ Keep problem foods out of the house. If they aren't there, your child is less likely to eat them.

All kids need to eat! Special considerations for your diabetic child's diet

All of us who are parents are only too well aware of the 'rules' for children's diets. No, we're not talking about the standard rules, about avoiding too much sugar and fat, encouraging five portions of fruit and vegetables a day, and so on. We're talking about the unwritten rules that state that the moment your child finds a food they really love and you stock up on it, they go off it. Or that just because your child loves baked potatoes, they're bound to choose chips at school because that's what all their friends are having.

Children go through a terrifying number of changes in the space of a few short years. We're certainly glad, for this reason alone, that we never have to go through childhood and adolescence again. Children learn many of their life lessons from their peers, and they feel an awful lot of pressure to fit in. By definition, having diabetes in the first place means they're going to be 'different'.

That's why it's especially important for them to understand when they can afford to eat the same as their friends, when a few minor changes can make all the difference, and when they really need to stick to the diabetes rulebook.

Here, then, are a few pointers on your child's diet:

- Don't forget that your child's energy and nutritional needs are changing all the time as she grows. When your child goes through a growth spurt, make an extra appointment with the dietician or have a chat with her on the phone.

- Your child's level of physical activity is likely to vary a lot more than yours does. Remind your child of the effect of exercise on blood sugars, even if it's not planned exercise like physical education lessons. A game of football in the playground can use up a lot of energy!

- Compromise is better than all-out warfare. Your child, and certainly your adolescent, is probably completely convinced that your own adolescence is far too long ago for you to remember what that time of life was like. If you don't have diabetes, that's just another reason why you don't understand. We don't have a magic wand, but letting your child make some of her own decisions on minor matters does increase the likelihood of her cooperating on the major decisions. Keeping the heavy guns for the major conflicts saves on door slamming and shouting in the house!

- Considering the amount of fat in the diet is important to prevent obesity and heart disease later on. However, small children need some fats to help them build a healthy body. If you exclude too much fat from your small child's diet, your child may find getting enough nutrients difficult. For children under 2, or faddy eaters under 5, avoid skimmed milk and very low-fat dairy products.

- Likewise, small children may not get enough energy for their needs if their diet contains too many bulky, fibre-rich cereal foods. Baked beans, unsweetened breakfast cereals, pasta, potatoes, rice, chapattis, and fresh fruit can offer a good compromise.

- Your child can easily cut down on the fat content of some foods without having to have a different meal than the ones her friends eat. At school, for example, she can cut the visible fat off meat and bacon, or take the skin off chicken and turkey. At home, choosing leaner cuts of meat (or choosing fish or poultry instead of beef, pork, or lamb) can help her eat 'normal' foods, without the dangers to her heart. Likewise, low-fat alternatives like turkey sausages and 'turkey ham' let your child enjoy convenience foods without the risks. The vegetarian product Quorn is now available in all supermarkets in lots of different forms. Quorn mince makes fantastic meaty-tasting bolognese sauce or lasagne, and you can use Quorn chunks for casseroles and stir-fries. Your child may probably never know the difference, but you do!

✔ Many schools offer a variety of 'healthy' alternatives in the cafeteria. Some of them, like baked beans, fish fingers, and baked potatoes, are much healthier than the chips and chicken nuggets that parents dread, without being seen as 'health foods'. Schools are required to provide meals that satisfy minimum standards for healthy eating. Get the dietician to have a chat with your child about how to eat more healthily without feeling different at the school lunch table.

✔ There's very little benefit in getting 'diabetic' chocolate, Easter eggs, and similar products. Likewise, your child doesn't need to avoid normal cakes or desserts. She does, though, need to regulate her intake of such foods. Using sweets as a carbohydrate top-up before or during exercise, for example, lets her enjoy her favourite treats without going mad.

✔ Don't be scared to admit that you have anxieties, too. All parents want the best for their children. For most of us, that's only a problem when we're biting our nails over their exam revision. Parents of children with diabetes are faced with anxiety about their welfare every time they have a meal. Do discuss your concerns with the dietician. You may be reassured to discover how many other anxious parents she deals with. You can also raise your anxieties with your child's clinical psychologist and talk about how best to deal with them.

Your child is unlikely to have more than one or two (if any) other diabetics in her school. Getting to know others of the same age who are also suffering from diabetes can be an enormous support. They can share problems, experiences, and, best of all, useful tips. Ask your paediatrician about a diabetic children's support group in your local area. Alternatively, contact Diabetes UK on 0207-424-1000 and ask about local groups.

Sick-Day Solutions

Your child is susceptible to all the usual childhood illnesses, but type 1 diabetes complicates her care (children with type 2 diabetes don't have nearly the same problem with their diabetic control when they're ill). An illness can affect diabetes in opposite ways. An infection may increase the level of insulin resistance so that the usual dose of insulin is not adequate. Or the illness may cause nausea and vomiting so that no food or drink can stay down, and the insulin may cause hypoglycaemia. For this reason, you need to measure the blood glucose in your sick child every two to four hours. If the glucose is over 13.9 mmol/l, you need to give extra short-acting insulin. If the glucose is under 13.9 mmol/l, you give more carbohydrate-containing nutrients.

When your sick child urinates, you can also test for ketones in the urine (explained in Chapter 7). If these become elevated, you need to discuss the situation with your doctor.

Feed your child with clear liquids like tea and squash during sick days. Although milk used to be excluded (people thought it upset the stomach), these days large medical bodies like the World Health Organisation suggest that the benefits of continuing with milky drinks, if your child has them as a major part of her diet, probably outweigh any problems. While the blood glucose remains over 13.9 mmol/l, use tea, water, and diet drinks to avoid adding the calories of carbohydrate. When the blood glucose is less than 13.9 mmol/l, you can use sugar-containing fizzy drinks, squash, or glucose drinks.

As long as your child can hold down clear liquids, you can continue to care for her on your own. If she cannot keep down clear liquids, you must contact your doctor and take your child to the hospital.

Thyroid Disease in Type 1 Children

As type 1 diabetes is an autoimmune disease (see Chapter 2), it's not surprising that children with type 1 have other autoimmune diseases more commonly than unaffected children. The disease found most commonly in association with type 1 diabetes is autoimmune thyroiditis, discovered by obtaining a blood test showing an abnormal increase in proteins in the blood called *thyroid autoantibodies*.

Autoimmune thyroiditis usually results in no symptoms, but occasionally it causes low thyroid function (*hypothyroidism*) and, even more rarely, high thyroid function (*hyperthyroidism*). Autoimmune thyroiditis is found mostly in girls between 10 and 20 years of age, but is easily treated (see *Thyroid For Dummies,* Wiley). In a study of 58 patients (*Diabetes Care,* April 2003), 19 were found to have autoimmune thyroiditis.

Autoimmune thyroiditis is so common in type 1 diabetes that it's recommended that type 1 patients be screened regularly for thyroid disease with a simple blood test called a TSH.

The Extra Value of Team Care

The stress of having a child with diabetes can be overwhelming, especially when your child is first diagnosed. The guilt that comes with this diagnosis may leave you initially unable to be of much help to your child, and it certainly makes it more difficult to discover all that you need to know to master the areas of importance to your child's health. Fortunately, you can depend upon the help of the diabetes care team, more at the beginning, but also throughout the duration of childhood.

In the United Kingdom, all children with diabetes are referred to a hospital specialist team. Your child has most of the changes to her diabetic care made by this team and has most of her outpatient checks in the hospital rather than at the general practice surgery. Your child is also referred to a diabetic specialist nurse, who is based in the hospital. You should be able to contact your child's nurse directly if you have any problems. This specialist nurse often liaises with general practice; check with her about what you can take your child to the surgery for.

Your child's diabetes care team should include the following people:

✔ A consultant paediatrician with a special interest in diabetes

✔ A general practitioner

✔ A paediatric diabetic specialist nurse, who can advise you about issues both in hospital and at home or school

✔ A paediatric dietician, who can give advice about the whole family's diet and how to help your child stick to a healthy diet; the dietician can also advise about the number of calories of which kinds of food your child needs for growth and development

✔ A children's clinical psychologist, who can help with any anxieties or emotional stresses your child might have, either at the time of diagnosis or as the problems arise

All these people work together to provide your child with satisfactory care. Your child's general practitioner, for example, probably prescribes most of the medicines, but which medicines she prescribes are likely to be decided by the hospital team. The hospital then gives you a prescription form, which can either be made up at the hospital pharmacy or taken to the surgery for a general practitioner's prescription to be written out.

Your child's general practitioner still looks after your child for any medical problems that aren't related to diabetes. Of course, make sure, every time you attend your surgery, that the doctor is aware that your child has diabetes. Check with your general practitioner to make sure that the management she's suggested doesn't need to be modified or changed because your child is diabetic. Taking this action is especially important if you call a doctor out of normal hours, or see a doctor who isn't your child's own general practitioner.

SIGN, the Scottish Intercollegiate Guidelines Network, has published a set of guidelines on good practice in the care of children and young people with diabetes. It recommends how the health professionals involved in caring for children with diabetes should work together. If you have any doubts about the quality of your child's care, get hold of these guidelines. You can then show them to your child's paediatrician or diabetic specialist nurse and discuss how the recommendations for your child can be met. You can find these guidelines at www.SIGN.ac.uk.

Chapter 14

Diabetes and the Elderly

· ·

In This Chapter

▶ Diagnosing diabetes in the elderly

▶ Coping with intellectual functioning in the elderly

▶ Dealing with dietary considerations

▶ Focusing on unique eye problems of the elderly

▶ Solving urinary and sexual problems

▶ Individualising treatment considerations

· ·

*E*veryone wants to live a long time, but no one wants to get old. Nevertheless, getting old is better than the alternative. Woody Allen says that the one advantage of dying is that you don't have to do jury duty. We'd rather do jury duty.

Defining 'elderly' is the first problem. Every year our definition seems to change, but it's fair to talk about the age of 70 as the beginning of being elderly. In the United Kingdom, the number of people over the age of 65 has doubled in the last 70 years. The figures for the very elderly are even more dramatic. Predictions are that the number of those over 80 in the United Kingdom will increase by 50 per cent in the 30 years to 2025, and the number of people over 90 will double.

Elderly people with diabetes have special problems. They're hospitalised at a rate that is 70 per cent higher than the general elderly population. Even without hospitalisation, elderly people with diabetes have special problems. In this chapter, you find out about those problems and the way to handle them.

Diagnosing Diabetes in the Elderly

The incidence of diabetes in the elderly is higher for many reasons, but the main culprit seems to be increasing insulin resistance that comes with ageing, even if the elderly person with diabetes is not particularly obese or sedentary.

Doctors don't yet understand why insulin resistance increases. When they look at the pancreas, it seems to be able to make insulin at the usual rate. The fasting blood glucose actually rises very slowly as you get older. The glucose after meals is what rises much quicker and leads to the diagnosis.

Elderly people with diabetes often do not complain of any symptoms. When they do, the symptoms may not be the ones usually associated with type 2 diabetes. Elderly people with diabetes may complain of loss of appetite or weakness, and they may lose weight rather than become obese. They may have incontinence of urine, which is usually thought of as a prostate problem in elderly men or a urinary tract infection in older women. Elderly people with diabetes may not complain of thirst because their ability to feel thirst is altered. Nevertheless, if you have any of these symptoms, see your doctor for a professional diagnosis.

Evaluating Intellectual Functioning

Doctors evaluate the intellectual function of an elderly person with diabetes because management of the disease requires a fairly high level of mental functioning. The patient has to follow a diabetic diet, administer medications properly, and test the blood glucose. Studies have shown that elderly people with diabetes have a higher incidence of *dementia* (loss of mental functioning) and Alzheimer's disease than people who don't have diabetes, making it much harder for them to perform those tasks.

The patient can take *cognitive screening tests* to determine his level of function. Testing makes telling whether the patient can be self-sufficient or needs help much easier. Many older people with diabetes who live alone with no assistance really require sheltered housing or even a nursing home.

Medication and the Elderly

All British citizens aged over 60, like all patients with diabetes, are entitled to free prescriptions. This means that the cost of drugs is not an issue as far as drug compliance is concerned, but complicated drug regimes, medication side effects, and loss of intellectual function all are. Elderly people usually have more medical conditions than younger people, whether or not they have diabetes. That means more tablets, and elderly people are more at risk of side effects from medication, such as dizziness and falls. However, these medications are usually given for a good reason, and the consequences of forgetting regular medication can be serious.

Under the New General Practice Contract of 2004, all patients taking four or more medications should have a regular review of their medication at least once a year. This is usually done by the general practitioner, but can be done by the pharmacist or the district nurse. An elderly person with memory problems can make this review much more effective by making notes on his concerns and possible medication side effects to take with him for review. Dossette boxes and blister packs (you can find out more about these in Chapter 11) can be an invaluable way of ensuring that elderly people take their tablets regularly. Alternatively, an elderly housebound person who's having problems taking his medication can get regular visits from the district nursing service to dispense the medication. The general practitioner can advise about this service.

Considering Heart Disease

Heart attacks are the major cause of death in the elderly diabetic. Strokes and loss of blood flow in the feet are also much more common. These people not only suffer from diabetes but also have high blood pressure, high cholesterol, are overweight or obese, and do little exercise. High blood pressure is a particularly important risk factor for stroke, and the incidence of high blood pressure increases significantly with age. For instance, while 35 per cent of British adults have high blood pressure, 66 per cent of people aged 65–74 and 76 per cent of those over 75 have the same problem.

Although many elderly patients have had a diagnosis of diabetes for a relatively short time, they have suffered from the metabolic syndrome (refer to Chapter 5) for many years before the diabetes. This accounts for their high frequency of cardiovascular disease.

At this point, it is too late to prevent heart disease, but a major effort should be made to control the other risk factors – the glucose, the blood pressure and the cholesterol – in order to postpone the vascular disease.

People with diabetes are at the same high risk of a first heart attack as non-diabetics are of having a second heart attack. The blood pressure drugs called beta blockers have been shown to reduce second heart attacks in non-diabetics, but the same evidence doesn't exist for a heart-protective effect in patients who have not had a heart attack. In June 2006, the National Institute for Health and Clinical Excellence (NICE) issued new guidance recommending that beta blockers should no longer be used as first-line treatment for high blood pressure. However, they do have other benefits, such as preventing second heart attacks and treating heart failure (a condition in which the heart does not pump out efficiently enough). If you're not sure whether you should be taking these drugs, talk to your general practitioner.

Avoiding Hypoglycaemia

Elderly people with diabetes, already somewhat frail, are especially hard hit by the consequences of hypoglycaemia and they are especially susceptible because their intake is uncertain, they are on multiple medications, they skip medications, and they often live alone. Their mental state may not permit them to recognise when they are becoming hypoglycaemic.

Intensive treatment may not be possible when the hypoglycaemia is a frequent problem. Using medication properly and taking a proper diet (as discussed in the sections 'Medication and the Elderly' and 'Preparing a Proper Diet' elsewhere in this chapter) may avoid this problem.

Preparing a Proper Diet

In addition to the intellectual function required to understand and prepare a proper diabetic diet (see the preceding section), the elderly have other problems when it comes to proper nutrition:

✔ They may have poor vision and be unable to see to read or cook.

✔ They may be on a low income and be unable to purchase the foods that they require.

✔ Their taste and smell may be decreased, so they lose interest in food.

✔ They often have a loss of appetite.

✔ They may have arthritis or a tremor that prevents them from cooking.

✔ They may have poor teeth or a dry mouth.

✔ They may be depressed. Depression in all ages commonly affects appetite, but this may be even more marked in the elderly.

✔ They may feel that they are 'too old to worry' about their diet.

Any one of these problems may be enough to prevent proper eating by the elderly person. As a result, the diabetes is poorly controlled.

All areas of the United Kingdom now have access to Meals on Wheels. This service, coordinated by social services, ensures that elderly people can have at least one meal a day delivered to them at home. All Meals on Wheels services now offer a diabetic alternative meal. Some areas also offer variations for people of different ethnic backgrounds, such as Caribbean or South Asian food. Unfortunately, some elderly people aren't mad about these meals. Private alternatives are available, which deliver either every day or in weekly packs that can be heated up individually. You can ask your local social services department about these services.

Dealing with Eye Problems

Elderly people with diabetes are particularly at risk of getting the eye problems that diabetes brings on. These problems can affect all aspects of proper diabetes care. The elderly are susceptible to cataracts, macular degeneration, and open-angle glaucoma in addition to diabetic retinopathy. (See Chapter 5 for more information on these eye problems.) Fortunately, the risk of developing eye diseases associated with diabetes has been found to be lower at any level of haemoglobin A1c as people get older. For example, a 70 year old with a haemoglobin A1c of 11 is at much lower risk than a 60 year old with the same haemoglobin A1c. It's not necessary to control the 70 year old as strictly in order to prevent eye complications. This is fortunate, because elderly people may find it more difficult to cope with the hypoglycaemic episodes that can be linked with very tight glucose control (see 'Avoiding Hypoglycaemia' elsewhere in this chapter).

One of the biggest failures in diabetes care is that as many as one third of the elderly never have an eye examination at all. How can disease be found when it is early enough to treat if no examination is done?

Once these problems are detected, they can be treated and the person's vision can be saved.

Coping with Urinary and Sexual Problems

Urinary and sexual problems are very common in elderly people with diabetes, and they greatly affect quality of life. It is not uncommon for an older person with diabetes to have paralysis of the bladder muscle, with retention of urine followed by overflow incontinence when the bladder fills up. An older person may be unable to get to the toilet fast enough. Sometimes spasms in the bladder muscle lead to incontinence. The result may be frequent urinary tract infections.

Almost 60 per cent of men over the age of 70 are impotent, and 50 per cent have no *libido,* a desire to have sex. These problems can have many causes (see Chapter 6), but older men are especially likely to have blockage of blood vessels with poor flow into the penis. The elderly take an average of seven medications daily, many of which affect sexual function.

To have sex at any age, you need sexual desire and the physical ability to perform, you need a willing partner, and you need a safe, private place. Any or all of these may be missing for the elderly.

It is not always necessary to treat sexual dysfunction if the male and his partner are okay with the situation as it is. If not, Chapter 6 points out a number of treatments for potency problems.

As a medical student, I used to sit in regularly on a hospital diabetic clinic. On one occasion, a male patient of 74 attended with his wife. They had been married for 48 years. When asked if he had anything he wanted to discuss, he raised the question of impotence. The consultant assured him that this was a common complication of diabetes and offered him referral for treatment. As he and his wife left, the wife carefully kicked her handbag beneath her chair before leaving without it. I made to take it to her, but the consultant suggested that she had left it for a reason. Sure enough, she returned without her husband within minutes to 'collect her handbag'. The consultant asked her if there was anything she wanted to discuss without her husband being present. Sure enough, she asked about the causes of impotence. When the consultant confirmed that her husband's impotence was, indeed, due to his diabetes, she looked enormously relieved. 'You see, doctor,' she confided, 'if it was just because he'd gone off me, I was seriously thinking of divorcing him.' Since that early lesson, I have never forgotten that the physical side of a relationship does not always become less important with the passing of the years.

Considering Treatment

When deciding on treatment for an elderly person with diabetes, you first have to consider your goals. Do you have a very elderly person with diabetes with a low life expectancy, or do you have a person with diabetes who is elderly but physiologically young and could live for 15 or 20 more years? A person who has lived to age 65 has a life expectancy of at least 18 more years, plenty of time to develop the complications of diabetes, especially macrovascular disease, eye disease, kidney disease, and nervous system disease (see Chapter 5). Most people who are discharged from a nursing home die within one year after discharge, so treatment decisions may be different for them.

Levels of care

The level of care may be basic or intensive.

✔ **Basic care** is meant to prevent the acute problems of diabetes like excessive urination and thirst. You can accomplish this goal by keeping the blood glucose under 11.1 mmol/l. Basic care is used for an elderly person with diabetes who is not expected to live very long because of the diabetes or other illnesses.

✔ **Intensive care** is meant to prevent diabetic complications in an elderly person expected to live long enough to have them. The goal here is to keep the blood glucose under 7.7 mmol/l and the haemoglobin A1c as close to normal as possible while avoiding frequent hypoglycaemia.

The benefits in terms of prevention of the complications of diabetes are much greater when the haemoglobin A1c is lowered from 11 to 9 than when lowered from 9 to 7. The goal of treatment for many elderly people can be set higher in order to avoid hypoglycaemia in these more fragile patients.

Treatment options and challenges

Treatment always starts with diet and exercise, but exercise may be limited in the elderly person with diabetes. You need to remember that exercise is helpful, even in the very old, as recent studies have shown. Exercise reduces the blood glucose and the haemoglobin A1c. Because elderly patients have more coronary heart disease, arthritis, eye disease, neuropathy, and peripheral arterial disease, exercise just may not be possible. (See Chapter 9 for more on exercise.)

The diet for the elderly person with diabetes is basically the same as that for the younger person with diabetes. (See the section 'Preparing a Proper Diet', earlier in this chapter, and Chapter 8.)

Many elderly patients can't walk at all, but they can still perform resistance exercises sitting in a chair. These exercises make those patients become stronger and their blood glucose falls. Most of the exercises shown in Chapter 9 using weights can be done when seated. Education for the patient who can benefit from exercise can be of great value, especially if the spouse is also involved.

Once diet and exercise have been found to be inadequate, medication must be added. This is complicated by a number of considerations special to the elderly:

✔ The patient may not be able to see the correct dosage.

✔ He may be mentally unable to take the medicine properly.

✔ Physical limitations may prevent taking medication, especially insulin.

✔ Multiple other drugs may interact with the diabetes medicine.

✔ Elderly patients have decreased kidney and liver function, making some diabetic drugs last longer.

✔ Poor nutrition may make the elderly patient more prone to hypoglycaemia.

We explain medication usage in Chapter 10, but, again, drugs in the elderly must be handled more carefully. Here's a very quick rundown of the drugs available:

- **Chlorpropamide** (one of the sulphonylurea drugs) is the longest acting and can cause very prolonged hypoglycaemia, so doctors do not often use it in patients over the age of 65. Glibenclamide is also relatively long acting, and so should be avoided, too. Other sulphonylurea drugs, such as gliclazide or tolbutamide, can be used safely. The newer sulfonylurea-like drugs called the meglitinides (repaglinide and nateglinide) may have an advantage in the elderly because they do not last as long. They cost a lot more than the other sulphonylureas, however. Start with half the usual dose and raise it slowly over weeks.

- **Metformin** can lower the blood glucose without the fear of hypoglycaemia and can be very useful in an older population for this reason. It often causes weight loss, which may be helpful for many patients, but we have seen it cause very excessive weight loss in certain elderly patients. Because the elderly have diminished kidney function, metformin must be used with care in them and not used at all when alcoholism, liver disease, or acute infection exists.

- **Rosiglitazone and pioglitazone** belong to a group of drugs that actually reverse the problem that makes diabetes so prevalent in older people – the insulin resistance. These drugs may play a huge role in the future in preventing diabetic complications as well as the transformation from impaired glucose tolerance to diabetes in the elderly. Recent studies also suggest that for people with diabetes who have had a stroke, pioglitazone can dramatically reduce the risk of a further stroke.

- Drugs such as **acarbose** have a very limited effect on the blood glucose and a lot of intestinal side effects. We do not recommend their use in the elderly.

- If pills fail to provide reasonable control of the blood glucose, so that the haemoglobin A1c is lower than 9, insulin needs to be used. An injection of insulin glargine at bedtime with a pill during the day often accomplishes this level of control. In the worst cases, night-time glargine and daytime short-acting insulin before meals may be necessary, but these circumstances are extremely rare. The infirmities of the elderly make insulin usage much more difficult. They may not see the dose or have the hand–eye coordination to draw up the medication. Help from friends or family becomes essential if the elderly diabetic is not to be forced to live in a nursing facility. Premixed insulins and prefilled insulin pens may make taking insulin a lot easier for these patients.

A patient who is transferred from self-care to institutional care may require a significant reduction in medication because he may not have been taking the medication properly.

Chapter 15

Driving and Occupational Problems

- -

In This Chapter

▶ Getting behind the wheel

▶ Driving safely with diabetes

▶ Driving goods vehicles and people carriers

▶ Knowing how diabetes may affect your choice of job

▶ Recognising and dealing with discrimination in the workplace

- -

*C*an I drive if I have diabetes? In most cases, the answer to this question is yes. If your diabetes is treated with diet or tablets, you are normally allowed to hold a passenger-carrying vehicle (PCV) or a larger goods vehicle (LGV) licence. The situation is more complicated if you are treated with insulin, but this chapter explains what you need to know about driving with diabetes. You can also find out if diabetes affects your chosen career path, and what to do if you find that people are discriminating against you and your diabetes in the workplace.

Getting behind the Wheel

If you're diagnosed with diabetes and want to drive, you need to meet several legal requirements. These requirements may seem harsh, but they protect you, your passengers, other drivers, and anyone else on the roads. The most important things to remember as a driver with diabetes are:

✔ By law, you need to inform your insurance company that you have diabetes, no matter how it is treated.

✔ You don't have to inform the Driver and Vehicle Licensing Agency (DVLA) when you are diagnosed with diabetes, as long as you're being treated with diet alone (in other words, you're not taking tablets or insulin to lower your blood sugar). But if your diabetes is treated with tablets or insulin, the law requires you to inform the DVLA as soon as possible after diagnosis or starting on medication.

✔ If you're applying for a driving licence for the first time, you're legally required to inform the DVLA (or the DVLNI in Northern Ireland) if you have diabetes treated with tablets or insulin. When you apply for a driving licence for the first time, the application form asks you whether you have ever suffered from one of a long list of medical problems. Answer yes to the question about diabetes and give details about your treatment.

✔ You must let the DVLA know if your medical condition changes, for example if you develop any complications that may interfere with your safe driving.

Not informing the DVLA and your insurance company if any of the preceding applies to you invalidates your insurance. You may also be liable to criminal prosecution if you're involved in an accident that is your fault.

As soon as you inform the DVLA that you have diabetes and explain how your diabetes is being treated, they'll tell you what steps to take next:

✔ **If your diabetes is treated with diet or tablets alone,** the DVLA wants to know whether any other medical reasons exist that may impair your ability to drive safely. If none does exist, the DVLA usually issues you a full licence until the age of 70. After that, as with people who don't have diabetes, you have to pay a charge for renewing your licence. All British drivers over the age of 70 have to renew their licences every one to three years. Of course, if your medication or condition changes before your licence expires, you have to let the DVLA know.

✔ **If you have stated that you are being treated with insulin,** the DVLA sends you another form called Diabetic 1. This form asks for more information, the name of your general practitioner and/or hospital doctor, and your consent to approach that person for further information if necessary. Don't worry, receiving this form doesn't necessarily mean you're being refused a licence, but it *does* mean that special limitations apply. For instance, you need to be able to recognise the symptoms of hypoglycaemia, and to meet the required visual standards. The precise visual standards can be found on the Internet at www.dvla.gov.uk/at_a_glance/ch6_visual.htm. Once the DVLA is satisfied that you're safe to drive, it decides how long you can drive for before your situation needs to be reviewed. Here is the process:

1. The DVLA issues you a licence for one, two, or three years. This is the same for full (up to 3.5 tonne vehicle) or provisional driving licences.

2. Before your licence expires, you're sent a reminder and a Diabetic 1 form to complete. You aren't charged for renewing a restricted licence.

3. When you send your application for renewal back to the DVLA, you have to send your old driving licence with it.

4. If you have not received your new licence by the time the old licence expires, for whatever reason, you *must* get advice from your doctor about your fitness to drive. A delay is most likely if the DVLA has to contact your doctor about your condition.

If the DVLA revokes your licence for medical reasons, you're not legally entitled to drive until you get a new one. If you have sent your licence for routine renewal and your doctor has advised you that you don't need to stop driving, you have a legal right to drive under Section 88 of the Road Traffic Act, even if your new licence has not arrived when your old one expires. You don't need to get this advice from your doctor confirmed in writing. However, you should check that your doctor has documented the fact that she hasn't advised you to stop driving.

The DVLA is at pains to point out that it would rather issue licences than take them away, but it has to follow guidelines that prevent even the most unlikely disasters. That means that if you do have to stop driving because of the complications of diabetes, you have to undergo very detailed examinations to prove that you are fit to start again.

Driving for work

The restrictions surrounding *larger goods vehicle* (LGV) and *passenger-carrying vehicle* (PCV) licences are complicated. To drive these types of vehicle, you need to hold a Group II licence. On the whole, there is a blanket ban on anyone treated with insulin holding this kind of licence. If your diabetes is treated with diet or diet and tablets, you are usually allowed to hold an LGV and PCV licence, provided you have no other medical reasons why you shouldn't. Even then, though, you have to fill out lots of forms and have regular examinations. The following sections tell you what you need to know.

Not sure what kind of vehicle you're driving? Maybe this can help: Since 1991, the term *heavy goods vehicle* (HGV) has been replaced by the term *larger goods vehicle* (LGV), and the term *public service vehicle* (PSV) has been replaced by *passenger-carrying vehicle* (PCV).

The Group II licence and types of vehicle

You need a Group II licence to drive any vehicle classed as a Group II vehicle. Group II vehicles are:

✔ Vehicles weighing 3.5–7.5 tonnes are classified as category C1 vehicles.

✔ Vehicles with a trailer, up to a combined weight of 8.25 tonnes, are classified as category C1+E vehicles.

✔ Minibuses are classified as D1 vehicles.

Apart from the exceptions explained in the following section, you aren't allowed to drive any Group II vehicle if you are treated with insulin. If you hold an LGV or PCV licence and you start on insulin, you must inform the DVLA and stop driving any of these vehicles, immediately.

Exceptions to the ban for people on insulin

Under certain conditions and by fulfilling certain requirements, you may be able to get (or keep, as the case may be) a Group II licence, even if your diabetes is treated with insulin:

✔ If you were already treated with insulin before April 1991 and held an LGV or PSV licence before this time, you may be allowed to keep your LGV or PSV licence.

✔ You may be able to get a licence to drive a taxi with fewer than nine seats. Local councils issue these licences, and restrictions vary between councils. Check with your local council for details.

✔ You may be able to get a C1/C1+E licence if you meet the following conditions:

• You've had no episodes of hypoglycaemia requiring assistance in the last 12 months.

• You monitor your glucose levels at least twice a day (before and after you get your licence).

• You monitor your glucose regularly at times relevant to your driving (before and after you get your licence). Examples of relevant times are immediately before, and frequently during, a long drive.

• You've been stabilised on insulin for at least one month.

• You don't have any other medical condition that excludes you from driving a C1/C1+E vehicle.

• You apply for an application pack, which includes forms D1, D750, DIABC1, and D4. You can complete the first three of these yourself. Your general practitioner must fill out form D4 (and can charge you up to £94 for doing so).

You need form D4 filled out when you first apply for your C1/C1+E licence; then you need to fill it out again every five years from ages 45 to 64 years. After that, you fill it out every year.

If the DVLA is happy with your condition based on these forms, it sends you a form C1EXAM. This requires a medical examination at least every 12 months by a hospital diabetic specialist, including blood glucose records for the last three months. The doctor then completes your form C1EXAM, for which she charges you about £100.

• You have to sign an undertaking to report any changes in your condition immediately to the DVLA and to comply with your doctor's recommendations about your fitness to drive.

If you are unsure about whether you can apply for a Group II licence, you can contact the DVLA directly on 0870-240-0010.

You can find out all the latest details on driving with diabetes by visiting the DVLA Web site at www.dvla.gov.uk/at_a_glance/ch3_diabetes.htm.

Driving safely

We all like to think of ourselves as safe drivers. Just because you have diabetes, you don't undergo a Jeckyll and Hyde transformation into a bad driver. However, accidents do happen to people with diabetes, just like everyone else.

If you are on medication that can cause episodes of hypoglycaemia (hypos), you need to take extra precautions. If you have an accident, you may need to prove that you weren't hypoglycaemic at the time. If you are hypoglycaemic when you have an accident, you can be charged with driving under the influence of a drug (insulin), driving without due care and attention, or dangerous driving.

Of course, your incentive for keeping your blood sugar satisfactory while you are driving isn't just to avoid prosecution. Keeping yourself and others safe is an excellent reason in itself. If you follow a few simple precautions, you can make sure that your risks do not increase. You can reduce your risks of hypoglycaemia when you are driving by following these guidelines:

✔ Never drive when you have drunk any alcohol. Alcohol can lower your blood sugar, making you more likely to get a hypo if you are taking insulin or certain tablets. And a hypo can also look like drunkenness, so your low blood sugar may be missed if your breath smells of alcohol.

High glucose levels don't affect a breathalyser result, even if you are ketotic (see Chapter 4).

✔ Check your blood sugar levels before and during your car journey.

- Don't miss or delay a snack or meal when you're driving.

- Don't drive for more than two hours without a snack.

- Avoid long or stressful drives when you're tired.

- Always carry glucose tablets and other carbohydrate food in your car.

- Always carry identification and information about your condition.

- Recognise the early warning signs of hypoglycaemia (which can include hunger, sweating, shakiness, dizziness, nausea, or palpitations) and stop driving as soon as you can do so safely.

If you do experience a hypoglycaemic episode while you're driving, do the following:

- As soon as you feel the first symptoms of hypoglycaemia coming on, take glucose tablets or a glucose drink first followed by another carbohydrate.

- Pull off the road and stop your car as soon as you can.

- Leave the driving seat and remove the ignition keys as soon as you have stopped. Doing so makes it clear that you are not in charge of a vehicle while under the influence of any drugs, including insulin.

- Don't drive again until the episode has passed completely.

- Inform the DVLA immediately if you have a hypo while you are driving.

Diabetes UK publishes books and leaflets, including *Diabetes and Insurance* and *Hypoglycaemia*. You can get more details from Diabetes UK Distribution on 0800-585-088.

Driving with gestational diabetes

If you develop gestational diabetes, or diabetes in pregnancy (see Chapter 6 for more details), and receive insulin treatment, you must inform the DVLA immediately. If your diabetes is unstable, you may need to stop driving. If your diabetes is stable, you are usually allowed to continue to drive a vehicle under 3.5 tonnes. If you're still taking insulin more than six weeks after you have your baby, you must let the DVLA know. You're covered by the same conditions as everyone else with diabetes then.

If you develop gestational diabetes but your condition is controlled by diet alone, you don't have to inform the DVLA.

Diabetes and Your Choice of Job

The good news is that most of us have more sense than to hold Colonel Blimp up as our role model. The bad news is that as a person with insulin-treated diabetes, you can't follow in his footsteps even if you want to. Nor can you make your living as a real-life Inspector Morse.

Yes, having diabetes can have an impact on your choice of job, depending on the type of job and the duties you'd have and how your diabetes is treated. Some jobs don't accept applicants who are treated with insulin, full stop; for other jobs, your status as a person with diabetes is irrelevant. Examples of both are shown in the following sections.

Careers that are not insulin friendly

The armed forces and the police are two of the professions that have a blanket ban on people with diabetes who use insulin. The only exception may be if you develop insulin-treated diabetes while you are already working in one of these jobs. If this happens, you can sometimes make a special appeal.

Here's a full list of jobs that people with insulin-treated diabetes are barred from:

Police service

Armed forces

Merchant navy

Fire service

Prison service

Ambulance service

LGV driver

PSV driver (with a few exceptions; see the earlier section 'Driving for work' for details)

Minicab driver in some areas (see the earlier section 'Exceptions to the ban for people on insulin' for more on this)

Post office worker, if it involves driving

Train driver

Airline pilot or air traffic control

Air cabin crew (on some airlines)

Offshore work (including ferries and oil rigs)

Coal miner

Other jobs: The world is your oyster

For most people with diabetes, your choice of job depends far more on the results of your exams than on the results of your blood sugars. Apart from the conditions above, no reasons exist why having diabetes should restrict your choice of career. Indeed, if you have diabetes, you may pay far more attention to your health and fitness than someone who doesn't have diabetes. That may well make you more, rather than less, reliable and responsible.

Of course, when you're choosing a job, you want to consider how you can fit monitoring and controlling your diabetes into your lifestyle. But then, you've probably been juggling control of your diabetes with the other roles in your life for years. Think of it as another part of life's rich pattern!

Avoiding Discrimination at Work

Over the course of many years in medicine, we've discovered that, unfortunately, a lot of discrimination exists in the world. We've also discovered that most of those who discriminate often give in, if you stand up for yourself or for others weaker than you. So if you think you're being discriminated against, share your concerns with people who can help you and take action. You may just discover, as we have, that for all the litigation, human beings can be a top bunch.

The following sections explain the Disability Discrimination Act and help you figure out whether what you're experiencing is discrimination and what you can do about it.

The Disability Discrimination Act (DDA)

If you're applying for a job that you can do just as well as a person who doesn't have diabetes, in which your diabetes would never put you or others at risk, and the only reason you're not chosen is your diabetes, you are being discriminated against. The Disability Discrimination Act (DDA) of 1995 gives disabled people, including people with diabetes, new rights in employment, access to goods, facilities and services, and buying or renting land or property.

The jobs covered by the blanket ban, as well as work completely or largely outside the United Kingdom, aren't covered by the DDA, however. That means that if you apply for the fire service and it turns you down because you're on insulin, you can't take action against the service. If you're already working when you become diabetic and your job involves working for an organisation that is subject to the rules of the DDA, though, it's a different matter. You can take action.

Every job in the armed services has a blanket ban on people with insulin-dependent diabetes. If you started insulin treatment while you were in the Navy, for example, you'd be given an honourable discharge. As a post office driver, on the other hand, the post office would have to offer you a reasonable alternative job that didn't involve driving. Of course, it can be difficult to prove that you have been turned down for a job purely on the grounds of your diabetes. If you have a job, and lose it when you develop diabetes, the case is much clearer.

You can make a complaint against your employer, or potential employer, by making an application to an employment tribunal. You only have three months from the time of the incident to do this, though.

Knowing discrimination when you see it

Recognising discrimination is terribly simple, really. You can tell it may be discrimination when a situation is just not fair. Of course, we're all grown-ups now, and we don't indulge in childish temper tantrums and patently untrue squawks of 'It's not fair!' Admittedly, most of us feel like doing this sometimes, but we're logical enough to be able to weigh up both sides of the argument. For something that's not fair to constitute discrimination, you must be being treated differently purely on the grounds of your diabetes.

But the odd occasion does occur when you see something happen and you say to yourself, 'That's just not fair.' Maybe you're asked to move in a restaurant so that other customers can't see you inject your insulin; maybe you have to take a day's holiday to have your annual medical examination; maybe your place of employment doesn't allowed flexible work breaks to accommodate your insulin injections.

If you think that something is unfair, it may well be. That's no reason to make straight for the nearest lawyer – here in the United Kingdom we leave that to the Americans. But you can follow a few simple steps to help ensure that you are treated fairly:

> ✔ If your employers treat you less favourably because of your disability or if they fail to make reasonable adjustments for your disability, talk to someone about it. Why not try talking to your diabetic team, a colleague,

a union representative, or a member of the occupational health staff? Formal advice is also available from the following:

- **Disability Rights Commission Helpline**
  Freepost MID 02164
  Stratford-Upon-Avon, CV37 9BR
  Phone: 0845-622-633 (Monday to Friday, 8 a.m. to 8 p.m.)

- **Diabetes UK Careline**
  Phone: 0845-120-2960 (Monday to Friday, 9 a.m. to 5 p.m.)
  e-mail: careline@diabetes.org.uk

✔ When you apply for a job, you may be asked to fill in a health questionnaire. If you feel at all self-conscious about your diabetes, you may be tempted to give a less-than-honest answer. Don't. If you give false information, you basically lose any rights you have regarding your employment. You can, however, explain that your condition is 'well controlled', that you have no hypoglycaemic episodes, and so on. At your interview, answer any questions about your diabetes honestly, as long as the questions are directly relevant to your work or your ability to carry out your job.

✔ Even if you think that the treatment you're receiving is unfair and unjust, try to avoid confrontation. If you have a problem, think of a couple of solutions you're willing to accept before you present your employers with a complaint. Doing so may allow you to be treated fairly and enable your employer to remain on good terms with employees, without any bad feeling.

✔ Be aware of sensitivities over any question of possible discrimination. You may only be asking for equal treatment, but your employer may have had a past experience in which it felt that a disabled employee took advantage of the organisation under the guise of discrimination.

✔ Another thing you can do to ease some possible tension at work is to make sure that your colleagues know about any problems that may arise as a result of your diabetes and how to deal with them (for example, instructing someone what to feed you or how to give you glucagon if you have a hypo at work). The chances are that they take this information completely in their stride, and being forewarned lets them help if they need to without worrying.

Chapter 16

What's New in Diabetes Care

· ·

In This Chapter

▶ Discovering new oral agents

▶ Finding drugs to encourage weight loss

▶ Working with new drugs for neuropathy

▶ Delivering insulin painlessly

▶ Understanding a new form of insulin

▶ Utilising transplantation of the pancreas or insulin-producing cells

▶ Finding unexpected treatments

· ·

*B*etween 1921, when insulin was isolated and used for the first time, and 1980, when blood glucose meters began to be available, relatively little was discovered to improve diabetes care. Between the advances that came in 1980 and about 1995, the same thing could be said. But since 1995, the pace of discovery of new tests, new treatments, and other products for diabetes has been astonishing. Discoveries like metformin (a glucose-lowering medication) and pioglitazone (a drug that acts on insulin resistance), for example, have become established in diabetes care. In addition, doctors and other scientists are aware of the huge need for new therapies to address the growing problem of diabetes, and their response has been truly remarkable.

We used to think of diabetes as a progressive disease. Right now, you and your doctors have all the tools necessary to turn diabetes into a close-to-non-progressive disease. Occasionally, however, these tools – insulin injections, oral medications, and so on – aren't the easiest to use. Fortunately, new medications and treatment options have been developed and others are being tested. The goal of the on-going research and the new products that come as a result is to make managing your diabetes easier; so easy in fact that anyone with diabetes can stop the disease from growing steadily worse. This chapter describes what's new in diabetic care and what you have to look forward to in the future.

New Oral Agents

Pharmaceutical companies are looking for both newer versions of older agents (which may be more effective and have fewer side effects) as well as entirely new agents with different mechanisms of actions. This area is literally exploding, and you are one of the beneficiaries.

✔ **Pramlintide:** This is a synthetic version of another hormone that is secreted with insulin called amylin. The hormone is missing completely in type 1 diabetes. It suppresses glucagon and slows the delivery of food from the stomach to the small intestine, so glucose entry into the blood stream is slowed. Pramlintide, given by injection, has lowered the haemoglobin A1c while not causing weight gain or hypoglycaemia in type 1 diabetes. Patients don't have severe highs and lows when they receive pramlintide. Amylin Pharmaceuticals, the drug's developer, is hoping that this is a great breakthrough in the management of type 1 diabetes. Problems have arisen in that the highest dose did not always lower glucose the most, but few side effects have occurred other than nausea, which does not last. One potential benefit of pramlintide is its tendency to cause weight loss. The drug does not worsen hypoglycaemia, but it must be given by injection, although it can be mixed with the insulin injection.

✔ **Adiponectin:** This is found in fat tissue and is released into the blood stream by fat cells. Interestingly, as fat cell tissue increases, the amount of adiponectin found in the blood decreases. Low levels of adiponectin are associated with increased insulin resistance and when it is given to animals, insulin resistance declines. Humans with insulin resistance have reduced adiponectin and drugs like rosiglitazone increase its level, which reduces insulin resistance. In diabetics with coronary heart disease, levels of adiponectin are further reduced, as they are in high blood pressure. Adiponectin has had healing effects on blood vessel walls in animals. Adiponectin may have a number of clinical uses: It may restore insulin sensitivity, it may reduce obesity, and it may prevent or reduce coronary heart disease.

✔ **Leptin:** Another drug that has shown the promise of weight loss in studies is leptin, which is under trial in the United States. Leptin was discovered to be present in fat cells. As fat cells increase, more leptin is made, and it tells the brain to reduce food intake. In a small study of about 120 people, leptin was given (by injection) to one group; the other group received no leptin. Both groups were put on a weight-loss diet. Those on leptin lost much more weight (4 pounds compared to less than 1 pound on average) than those who did not take the drug. None of the people in this study had diabetes. Much more work needs to be done on leptin, and the problem of the need for injections, the only way it can be administered, is considerable.

✔ **Glucagon-like Peptide-1 (GLP-1)**: This substance, made in the body by pancreatic and intestinal cells, is released into the bloodstream along with insulin. It has the property of increasing insulin secretion along with glucose secretion so that hypoglycaemia is prevented. At the same time it blocks production of glucagon, which tends to raise the blood glucose. It also slows the intestine so that glucose is taken up more slowly from food, and decreases appetite and food intake. These are all very helpful in diabetes, except for the fact that GLP-1 is rapidly broken down by an enzyme called DPP-IV. Novartis, a Swiss drug company, is working on two innovative ways to use GLP-1. The first is a compound like GLP-1 that resists being broken down rapidly but must be given by injection. The other is a pill that blocks DPP-IV so that natural GLP-1 lasts a lot longer. Both of them have been shown to improve glucose control in diabetic patients, especially those with mild type 2 diabetes.

✔ **Working on the PPARs:** In Chapter 10, you can read about the group of drugs called the glitazones, or thiazolidinediones (yes, a scientist out there somewhere really did think this was a reasonable name for a drug!). Glitazones bind to receptors called PPAR-gamma. Some research is going on into drugs to improve the effectiveness of a closely related receptor called PPAR-alpha. These drugs may be able to build on the success of the glitazones.

Drugs to encourage weight loss

Because most people with type 2 diabetes are obese and their glucose control improves with weight loss, the search for weight-lowering drugs has been enthusiastic, to say the least. Such drugs can have an enormous impact, not only on people who have diabetes but on the huge, non-diabetic obese population.

Orlistat

An enormous amount of media coverage in Britain has been given to the 'diet drug' orlistat, which is also known as Xenical. *Orlistat* works by reducing dietary fat absorption. The fat remains in the intestine and the stool. Some patients complain of gas, oily bowel movements, and even bowel incontinence. Usually these side effects disappear after a few weeks, but a few people stopped taking the drug because of this effect.

In a two-year study funded by the drug company that developed orlistat, the people on the drug lost considerably more weight than those who did not take the drug. Once they had lost weight, the patients showed a drop in blood pressure, bad cholesterol, and the need for insulin to control the blood glucose.

In another study also funded by the company, this time specifically of people with diabetes, the orlistat group lost much more weight than the non-orlistat group. The orlistat users were able to reduce their blood glucose, their haemoglobin A1c, their need for oral sulfonylurea medication (which lowers blood glucose), as well as their bad cholesterol levels. Very few of the orlistat takers stopped the drug and left the study because of intestinal or bowel problems.

Orlistat has been assessed by NICE (National Institute for Health and Clinical Excellence), which offers guidance on who can use a drug and for how long. You should be eligible to get orlistat on the National Health Service if:

- Your BMI is over 30, or your BMI is over 28 and you have type 2 diabetes (see Chapter 7 for how to calculate your BMI).

- You are between 18 and 75 years old.

- You have lost at least 5 pounds with diet and exercise alone in the month before you start the medication.

- You are monitored regularly and given advice and support to improve your lifestyle in other ways, while you take the medication.

You can only carry on getting orlistat if you lose at least 5 per cent of your body weight in the first three months of treatment and 10 per cent of your body weight in the first six months of treatment. You are unlikely to be prescribed orlistat for more than a year and never for more than two years.

Sibutramine

Sibutramine, which is also known by its brand name Reductil, works in a slightly different way to orlistat. Sibutramine acts on the brain to reduce the re-uptake of hormones called *serotonin* and *noradrenaline,* making patients feel full sooner and thus helping them feel satisfied with smaller quantities of food.

Sibutramine can increase heart rate and blood pressure, though, which means that patients can only start this drug if their blood pressure is under 145/90 mmHg. If blood pressure goes above this level, or rises by more than 10 mm Hg, the medication has to be stopped.

Sibutramine has also been assessed by NICE. You should be able to get sibutramine on the National Health Service if:

- Your BMI is over 30, or over 28 if you have type 2 diabetes (see Chapter 7 for how to calculate your BMI).

- You've made serious attempts to lose weight in other ways before.

- Your blood pressure is below 145/90 mmHg.

✔ You are monitored regularly and given advice and support to improve your lifestyle in other ways, while you take the medication.

✔ Your blood pressure doesn't rise by more than 10 mmHg or above 145/90 mmHg while you take the medication.

To carry on getting prescriptions, you have to lose at least 4 pounds in the first four weeks of treatment, and at least 5 per cent of your body mass in the first three months of treatment. You will only be prescribed sibutramine for up to a year.

Rimonabant

Rimonabant is a tablet that blocks the cannabinoid-1 receptor (CB-1). If the term 'cannabinoid' sounds a lot like cannabis, that's because the two are closely related! We have long known that cannabis (marijuana, grass, dope – call it what you will) can stimulate the appetite. This led to research to find out if blocking the cannabis chemical receptors in the body reduces appetite.

Unlike the weight-loss drugs above, however, rimonabant has additional benefits for the cardiovascular system over and above those that come from losing weight. Any weight loss reduces total and LDL (bad) cholesterol and increases HDL (good) cholesterol, as well as reducing haemoglobin A1c. In patients taking rimonabant, the improvements in lipid results, and haemoglobin A1c, are calculated to be about twice as great as those that can be expected from weight loss alone. Overall, patients with diabetes using rimonabant for a year can reduce their haemoglobin A1c by up to 0.7 per cent.

On the whole, rimonabant is well tolerated, although it can cause mild (and usually short-lived) nausea, dizziness, diarrhoea, anxiety, and insomnia. Doctors don't recommend rimonabant if you have severe depression or are taking antidepressant medicine.

Of course, none of these drugs is a permanent solution, and they don't teach you to live more healthily. That has to be a lifelong commitment. Hopefully, though, they can 'kick start' your attempts to lose weight, and give you the boost you need to keep up the good work once you've stopped taking them.

New drugs for neuropathy

Two drugs may improve the symptoms of neuropathy (diabetic nerve disease; see Chapter 5 for more on this condition). Both have been on the market for some time for the treatment of other conditions, but a new use may exist for them.

✔ **Gabapentin:** First licensed for the treatment of epilepsy, gabapentin has been shown to significantly reduce the pain of diabetic neuropathy. Also known by its brand name Neurontin, this drug improves not only diabetic neuropathy but the pain of other forms of neuropathy as well. Patients who took gabapentin were able to sleep better (diabetic neuropathy is often worse at night). The drug may work as soon as two weeks after starting treatment.

Gabapentin does have some side effects, namely dizziness, loss of balance, and fatigue.

✔ **Memantine:** This drug is licensed in the United Kingdom for use in moderate to severe Alzheimer's dementia. However, it also seems to reduce the pain of neuropathy, especially at night. Memantine doesn't appear to have any serious side effects, but more study is needed.

Improving Insulin Delivery

The biggest barrier that arises when we tell a patient that he needs to be on insulin is the fear of taking multiple injections. Drug companies are working on ways to deliver insulin without needles. You can find out more about inhaled insulin in Chapter 10. This section provides the latest information about other new ways to deliver insulin, many of which are on the verge of coming to the market.

Oral insulin

The difficulty with taking insulin by mouth is that insulin is a large protein, and digestive enzymes break proteins down into individual amino acids. In order to take insulin by mouth, you need a device to protect the insulin from those digestive enzymes. Scientists have been able to coat insulin with a polymer that prevents the breakdown of the insulin before it is absorbed into the bloodstream from the intestine. The material is one-hundredth the width of the human hair. The coated particles can tether themselves to the upper small intestine, where they are not so exposed to digestive juices and where the insulin can be released. The coating then leaves the intestine over time. So far this coating has worked in animals, but the big problem is getting the right dose into the patient because the dose is so variable from meal to meal. In addition, the timing of the release of the insulin is important to balance the food intake.

An implantable insulin pump

Another way to deliver insulin without the use of needles is an implantable artificial pancreas. The goal of this research is to produce a closed-loop system where a glucose sensor detects the level of the glucose in the blood and transmits the information to the implanted insulin pump, which then releases just the right amount of insulin to cover that glucose through a tube in the peritoneal cavity. Right now we have an open-loop system. The external insulin pump (see Chapter 10) delivers insulin, but only when it is programmed to do so, so that the dosages are fixed. There is even a system with a glucose meter that reads the blood glucose with a finger stick and sends the result to the pump, but the pump only releases insulin based on the instructions of the wearer. The problems that investigators are running into have to do with creating a fool-proof glucose sensor and keeping the pump open and delivering insulin. The pump has to be refilled regularly and this must be done by an injection into the pump reservoir.

Developing a New Form of Insulin

When it comes to rapid-acting insulin, which is needed for the glucose in a meal, lispro insulin (brand name Humalog) is an excellent form (see Chapter 10). Today, however, lispro insulin isn't the only option you have. A new rapid-acting insulin, insulin aspart, has recently been licensed under the brand name Novorapid. Insulin aspart is active almost instantly after the injection is taken, just as lispro insulin is. It acts rapidly and is gone by about the time the absorption of food from the meal is ending. There is less hypoglycaemia with insulin aspart than with regular insulin. Exactly how insulin aspart differs from lispro insulin is not yet clear.

Transplanting Cells for a Cure

One treatment for kidney failure is transplantation of a new kidney (see Chapter 5). If a person with diabetes needs to have a kidney transplant, that may be the best time to do a pancreas transplant as well because the kidney is going to require immunosuppression anyway. Pancreas transplantations have many benefits:

- The new kidney is exposed to normal blood glucose levels.

- Progression of complications already present may be slowed or stopped.

- Patients suffering from hypoglycaemia, hyperglycaemia, or autonomic problems (see Chapter 5) have an improved quality of life.

The choice of the recipient of the transplant is important because certain factors lead to lower success:

- Older age (greater than 45) confers a worse prognosis.
- Hardening of the arteries already present is a negative factor.
- Congestive heart failure results in a poor prognosis.
- Obesity increases the risk of transplant loss.
- Hepatitis C infection also increases the risk of transplant loss.

Simultaneous kidney and pancreas transplantation is, therefore, a definite choice for a younger person without the preceding risk factors, or a person with life-threatening lack of awareness of hypoglycaemia or a poor quality of life due to uncontrolled diabetes.

Another approach is the use of *microencapsulated pancreatic islets,* which are injected into a person who requires insulin. The idea is to surround the insulin-producing cells with a protective capsule so that the cells in the body that want to destroy these injected foreign cells cannot get to them. So far, this approach has not been very successful. Although the cells continue to work and make insulin, they become covered with a layer of other cells. The process is called *fibrosis.* The result is that the blood glucose cannot get in to trigger insulin production and release, and the insulin cannot get out.

Some studies of microencapsulation have been successful in animals. No immunosuppression is needed, and the blood glucose remains normal. The microencapsulated cells rarely function for more than a year, however.

Potentially promising results have come from the University of Alberta in Edmonton, Canada. They are using new drugs to block the autoimmune destruction of islet cells taken from the pancreas of someone who has recently died. As researchers have used the technique on more patients, the results have not been quite as good, with some patients requiring insulin – but still not as much as before the transplantation. These results are promising enough that the National Institute of Health in the United States is funding a multi-centre study to see if the University of Alberta results can be duplicated in other diabetes programmes.

The original researchers in Edmonton have now done more than 91 islet cell transplants in 48 patients with type 1 diabetes. They find that injecting into the liver causes a loss of the protective secretion of glucagon, which helps to prevent hypoglycaemia, so other sites like the abdominal cavity are being considered. Of the 48 patients, 84 per cent are completely free of the need for insulin, but they still have to take immunosuppressive drugs. No patient has died, but there have been some complications including bleeding in the liver requiring transfusion in 11 per cent, clotting in the veins of the liver in 2 per cent, and a temporary rise in liver function test abnormalities in 49 per cent.

Whether other centres can duplicate these good results remains to be determined, but the transplants have required more than one administration of cells that have come from more than one pancreas. Since a pancreas can be divided into several pieces when an organ transplant rather than islet cells is done, it is a better use of an available pancreas. Once the islet cells are functioning properly, they can help to reverse diabetic complications like eye disease and coronary artery disease. At the same time, they reduce the variability in blood glucose levels from very high to very low. Some experts believe that even when the haemoglobin A1c is under 7, the great variability in blood glucose can still cause complications.

Another approach to obtaining cells for transplantation besides using the pancreas is the use of stem cells. These are cells that have not yet changed into a particular kind of cell that has specific functions such as a liver cell, a heart cell, or a brain cell. It may be possible to train these cells to make insulin, grow them, and use them in place of pancreatic islet cells.

Using Other Agents to Fight Insulin Resistance

A study in *Nature* in January 2001 reported the discovery of a hormone called *resistin*. This hormone is made by fat cells and causes insulin resistance, which explains why insulin resistance increases with obesity. Resistin is suppressed by the drug that improves insulin resistance, rosiglitazone. Scientists have also begun to manufacture resistin. When resistin is injected into mice, it causes increased insulin resistance. When antibodies that oppose resistin are given to the mice, insulin resistance improves. This shows that other agents, besides the glitazone class of drugs, may help to improve type 2 diabetes by blocking resistin.

The association is not completely clear, however, since some obese rodents have very low resistin levels. In addition, resistin is not detected in human fat and muscle cells. Although the first report proposed that resistin would be increased in obese humans, recent research has not verified this. The final place of resistin in human metabolism has yet to be determined.

Another possible explanation comes from the discovery published in the *Journal of Endocrinology* in December 2003 that a brain hormone, melanocyte-stimulating hormone (MSH), must be present in obese mice for diabetes to occur. Giving more of this MSH to obese mice made insulin resistance worse. When humans were evaluated, those with higher levels of MSH were more likely to have diabetes. In the future doctors may try to administer drugs that lower levels of MSH in order to improve insulin sensitivity.

Getting Intestinal Cells to Make Insulin

A new technique to get intestinal cells to produce insulin has been described by Dr Ira Goldfine and his colleagues at the University of California in the United States. Dr Goldfine and his associates took the gene that is responsible for producing insulin in mice, broke it into small fragments, and fed it to the mice. The cells of the mice's intestines were able to incorporate the fragments into their DNA and begin to make insulin.

The result is not a cure for diabetes, because the intestinal cells live only a few days, so a pill would have to be taken regularly. Testing of this new treatment will take at least three to five years, but the immediate results, as we can see above, are very promising.

Finding Unexpected Treatments

An article published in *Diabetes Care* in December 2003 provided the very unexpected report from Pakistan that a teaspoon of cinnamon every day improves blood glucose and fats in people with type 2 diabetes. The researchers studied 60 people divided into groups who received 1, 3 or 6 grams of cinnamon daily, or placebo capsules that contained no cinnamon. The trial continued for 40 days.

The results showed that there was a significant reduction in blood glucose, triglyceride, total cholesterol, and LDL cholesterol even at the 1 gram level, while the placebo group showed no change. No one had any problem consuming the cinnamon. The authors thought that even less cinnamon may be successful in lowering these levels.

Cinnamon seems like a pretty benign treatment and is surely worth a try.

Another article, also from *Diabetes Care* published in June 2003, suggested that the use of oolong tea, a type of tea that is partially fermented during processing (compared to green tea, which is not fermented at all and black tea, which is fully fermented), leads to a very significant lowering of plasma glucose. In the study, 20 people were given 1,500 millilitres of oolong tea daily and their glucose fell from 229 to 162 on average. A group who did not drink the oolong tea showed no change. The tea that was used came from China.

Do we recommend this treatment? Again, it seems benign and the possible benefits are great. Your biggest problem may be obtaining the tea. Make sure that it comes from China.

Chapter 17

What Doesn't Work When You're Treating Diabetes

In This Chapter

▶ Critically evaluating information about treatments and 'cures'

▶ Recognising false claims about certain drugs

▶ Discovering why certain diets don't work in the long run

*E*veryone wants a quick and easy solution to problems. For every problem, five people offer a quick and easy answer. Just send in the money. These cheats have got what it takes to take what you've got.

Being fooled by these claims may be a lot more serious for you than for the person who walked up to the man dressed as a polar bear who was promoting soft drinks in a shopping centre. The first man said: 'Don't you feel foolish, dressed like a bear?' The 'bear' replied: 'Me, foolish? You're the one talking to a bear.'

The purpose of this chapter is to tell you about the tests and treatments that don't work. Don't expect to find here everything you have heard or read about that is the 'new wonder cure' for diabetes. As soon as this book is published, new, more seductive claims will be made. When you hear such claims, remain sceptical; use the information in this chapter, especially from the first section, 'Evaluating What You Hear and See', to test the claims out; and check with your doctor before you stop what works and try something that may do more harm than good.

Evaluating What You Hear and See

You're going to see and hear a great deal of information about diabetes from a number of different sources, some reputable, some not. The following sections give you the tools you need to evaluate critically what you hear and see.

Recognising a false claim or promise

Many clues can alert you that a treatment may not work. Here are some of them:

- ✔ **If a pop star or minor film actor endorses a treatment be highly sceptical.** Always consider the source, and make sure that it's reputable. In this case, the company is using the fame of the star to convince you, not any special knowledge that she possesses. The obvious exception is the group of luminaries who have agreed to publicise Diabetes UK. Perhaps the best known of these is the multi-Olympic gold medallist Steve Redgrave, who himself has diabetes.

- ✔ **If the treatment has been around for a long time but is not generally used, don't trust it.** Treatments that really work have been tried in an experimental study, in which some people take or use the treatment and some don't. Doctors and medical texts recommend drugs that pass that test.

- ✔ **If a treatment sounds too good to be true, it usually is.** An example is the claim about chromium improving blood glucose levels (see the section 'Drugs That Don't Work', later in this chapter). The study that 'proved' this claim was done on chromium-deficient people, a situation that does not exist in the United Kingdom.

- ✔ **Anecdotes are not proof of the value of a treatment or test.** The favourable experience of one or even of a few people is not a substitute for a scientific study. If people did seem to respond to the drug, it may be for entirely different reasons than you think. For instance, many women going through the menopause swear by herbal remedies to improve their hot flushes. Several studies have been done to compare the effect of some of these herbal remedies with a placebo (a 'dummy pill' that doesn't contain any active ingredient, but the people taking it don't know that). All the trials show the same thing. Up to 30 per cent of women did report that their hot flushes got better with the herbal tablets, but exactly the same number swore that their hot flushes got better when they took a placebo. In other words, the women's symptoms improved because they *thought* they were taking an effective medicine. Mind over matter is a very powerful thing.

Getting information from the Internet

A lot of information on all sorts of subjects comes from the Internet, specifically the World Wide Web. In Appendix C, we provide the best resources currently available for diabetes from this amazing source.

The same rules apply when you consider the validity of claims made on the Web as those for any other claim, with a few new rules thrown in:

- ✔ **Don't rely on search engines.** Search engines do not check claims for validity.

- ✔ **Go to the site of the claim and check to see whether most of the information there makes sense.** A lot of silly information should alert you. If you still feel the treatment might work, ask the Webmaster for references. If none is forthcoming, forget about the idea.

- ✔ **Go to sites that you know are reliable to see whether you can find the same recommendations.** You can rely on the treatments listed on sites like Diabetes UK, the NSFs (National Service Frameworks), NICE (National Institute for Health and Clinical Excellence), and SIGN (Scottish Intercollegiate Guidelines Network). When you're not certain whether the advice or recommendation you're getting is a good one, these sites can usually help you figure out how trustworthy the information is.

- ✔ **Go to conferences put on by reputable experts.** The Diabetes UK Web site often has details of conferences.

Drugs That Don't Work

In the last decade, so many drugs have been touted as the cure for diabetes that you would think everyone would be cured by now. The fact is, as we have said again and again, you have the tools *right now* to control diabetes, but controlling your diabetes isn't as simple as taking a pill, contrary to what you may hear from other 'experts'. If a pill were all that you needed to control diabetes, this book wouldn't be necessary. In this section, we tell you about some drugs that have usually become well known because a few people claimed that they worked. The section above, on recognising a false claim or promise, can help you to understand why those people were convinced, even though the drug itself was not the reason for their improvement.

Chromium

In all kinds of magazines, newspapers, and on the Internet, you can find articles singing the praises of chromium for controlling the symptoms of diabetes. Should you take supplements of chromium?

The strongest case for chromium comes from a study of people with type 2 diabetes in China. These people were given high doses of chromium and then were found to have improved haemoglobin A1c, blood glucose, and cholesterol while reducing the amount of insulin they had to take. The 'evidence' sounds pretty impressive until you consider that these people were chromium deficient in the first place.

People in the United Kingdom and other countries where the diet is sufficient in chromium don't show chromium deficiency and don't show improvement in glucose tolerance when they take chromium. In addition, chromium is present in such small amounts normally that it is hard to measure even in people without chromium deficiency.

The amount of chromium a person needs in her diet is uncertain, but estimates put the level at 15–50 micrograms daily. People given much more than that tend to accumulate chromium in their liver, where it can be toxic. Some studies suggest that chromium can cause cancer in high doses.

For now, the evidence doesn't support the use of chromium in diabetes except where the person is known to be chromium deficient.

Aspirin

People who take the sulphonylurea drugs (see Chapter 10) sometimes have a greater drop in blood glucose when they take aspirin. This is because aspirin competes with the other drug for binding sites on the proteins that carry sulphonylureas in the blood. When they're bound to protein, the sulphonylureas aren't active, but when they're free, they are. Aspirin knocks the sulphonylureas off so that they're free. As a result, aspirin has been recommended as a drug to lower blood glucose.

By itself, aspirin has little effect on blood glucose. Its effect with sulphonylureas is so inconsistent that it can't be reliably depended on to lower the blood glucose.

Aspirin isn't useless in all respects; far from it. Aspirin is an amazingly effective tool for many high-risk people, both with and without diabetes, in the fight against heart disease and strokes. In fact, Diabetes UK recommends that most diabetics should take a small dose of 75 milligrams of aspirin every day. Just don't rely on aspirin for your glucose control.

Pancreas formula

Pancreas formula is sold on the Internet as a mixture of herbs, vitamins, and minerals that help diabetes. No clinical or experimental evidence shows that pancreas formula does anything of value in the human body. The claims that are made for this 'treatment' are not supported by factual evidence. Look for references in respected journals, and you won't find them. Save your money.

Fat Burner

You hear and read a lot of advertising for the Fat Burner product in reputable newspapers and on reputable radio stations. Advertising claims that you can 'burn fat without diet or exercise', and that the manufacturer even throws in, ABSOLUTELY FREE, a bottle of Spirulina to enhance your Fat Burner weight control programme. If you believe this is possible, I have a bridge that I would like to sell you, CHEAP – and I'll throw in a castle with every third bridge paid for, sight unseen. In order to burn fat, you must exercise and stop taking in large amounts of carbohydrates.

Gymnema silvestre

Gymnema silvestre is a plant found in India and Africa. It's promoted as a glucose-lowering agent as part of a type of alternative medical treatment called Ayurvedic medicine. Gymnema silvestre has never been tested in a controlled study in humans. One statement in its advertising is, 'For most people, blood sugar lowers to normal levels.' No evidence exists that this is the case.

Knowing the Dangers of Some Legal Drugs

Just because a drug is legal does not mean that it has no undesirable side effects. Several classes of drugs need to be used with caution.

In *Diabetes Care* (February 2004), four major medical associations warned that second-generation antipsychotic drugs, used to treat a variety of severe mental illnesses, can cause rapid weight gain, most of which is fat leading to pre-diabetes, diabetes, insulin resistance, and abnormal blood fats.

One drug that you don't need to worry about – Aspartame

You can find the statement that aspartame causes cancer in many news sources. Because aspartame is used so much in diabetes and by people who don't have diabetes, we want to emphasise the following:

Aspartame is an acceptable artificial sweetener with no known dangers to human beings. No evidence shows that aspartame causes cancer when used in normal amounts. The European Food Standards Agency (EFSA) has looked at all the research into aspartame, including a study in 2005 that found a possible link with cancer in rats. After examining all the evidence in great detail, the EFSA announced in May 2006 that there was no evidence of any link with cancer, even at the highest levels of aspartame that anyone uses.

The drugs differ in their risks, but clozapine (brand names Clozaril, Denzapine, and Zaponex), and olanzapine (brand name Zyprexa) appear to be the worst offenders. Other drugs named include risperidone (brand name Risperdal) and quetiapine (brand name Seroquel).

If you are taking one of these drugs, ask your doctor to screen and monitor you for evidence of weight gain and insulin resistance. The benefits of taking the drug may outweigh the risks. In the article, the panel suggests that baseline screening be done before using the drug. The following items should be part of your baseline screening:

- Personal and family history for obesity, diabetes, abnormal fats, high blood pressure, and cardiovascular disease
- Weight and height
- Waist circumference
- Blood pressure
- Fasting plasma glucose
- Fasting blood fat profile

If you are overweight or obese, you should receive nutritional and physical activity counselling if you take one of these drugs. If you are at risk for diabetes, your doctor should use the drug that is least associated with this problem.

Diets That Don't Work

If you walk into a reasonably large bookshop, you're overwhelmed by the number of diet books available. The books are way too numerous to list here, but they can be broken down into a few categories, as the following sections explain.

It's probably fair to say that the more books people write about a subject, the less we know for certain about that subject. Why would authors bother to come up with ten new books on dieting each year, if the solution rested in some older book? You can bet that word of mouth would have made that book the all-time bestseller in any category.

Diets that promote a lot of protein with little carbohydrate (including the Atkins)

The trouble with these diets is that they're not a healthy and balanced approach. Unless you use tofu as your source of protein, you're getting a lot of fat in your diet, much of it saturated fat, which isn't good for you. The diet is lacking in vitamins that a supplemental vitamin pill may or may not provide. Very few people stay on such a diet for long. How many people can eat chicken for breakfast, lunch, and supper? The diet is also lacking in potassium, an essential mineral.

People who do follow this kind of diet for a long time also find that they have problems with hair loss, cracking nails, and dry skin. Their breath and their urine smell of acetone because of all the fat breakdown. They become very dry and need to drink large quantities of beverages.

We see a place for this diet as a starter. Some people with type 2 diabetes who have high blood glucose levels show a rapid improvement when started on a diet like this. As the glucose comes under control, the diet can be changed to a more balanced one.

Diets that promote little or no fat

The people who can follow a diet that mandates less than 20 per cent fat deserve a new designation – *fatnatics* (fat fanatics). This kind of diet is extremely difficult to prepare and perhaps even more difficult to eat unless you're a squirrel. In order to make up the calories, people on this diet eat large amounts of carbohydrates. Chapter 8 makes clear why eating a lot of carbohydrates isn't a good idea for people with diabetes.

Like the protein diet, this diet may be lacking in essential vitamins and minerals, especially the fat-soluble vitamins. Rarely does someone stay on such a diet after she has left the confines of the spa or other sanctuary where the diet is promoted. However, this type of diet may be a good way to start a dietary programme for a person with type 2 diabetes, as long as the total calories are not greater than the daily needs of that individual.

Very low-calorie diets

These diets, in the form of little food or a liquid containing calories (which generally does not taste very good), are lacking in many essential nutrients. They must be supplemented by vitamins and minerals. They cannot form the basis of a permanent diet because the dieter would eventually become emaciated. Dieters who start this kind of programme do not last on it and regain every ounce they have lost and then some. (There are always exceptions, of course.)

We don't like this kind of diet even as a starter diet, because it is so unlike our usual eating habits that people rapidly find it intolerable. Eating is a basic part of human existence. You can eat alone, but it's more enjoyable in company. Eating is a source of great pleasure for human beings and other animals. A diet that takes away this fundamental activity cannot be tolerated for very long.

The transition from a very low-calorie diet to a balanced diet is a very difficult one and rarely succeeds.

A final word on diets

For the overweight person with type 2 diabetes, any diet that causes some weight loss helps for a time. But you have to ask yourself the following questions:

- ✔ Am I prepared to stay on this diet indefinitely?
- ✔ Is it a diet that is healthy if I stay on it?
- ✔ Does this diet combine all the features I need, namely weight loss, reduction of blood glucose, and reduction of blood fat levels, with palatability and reasonable cost?

If you can say yes to all those questions, then the diet will probably work for you.

Part V
The Part of Tens

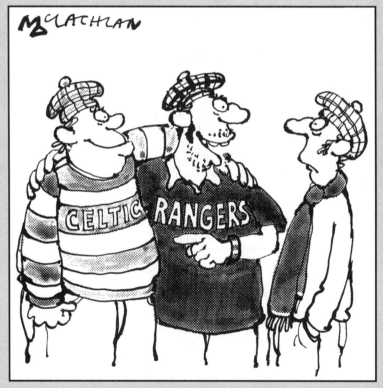

'But we're <u>both</u> diabetics!'

In this part . . .

In The Part of Tens, you discover the key techniques for managing diabetes. With just a little background from the other parts, you can use this section to really fine-tune your diabetes care. You find the ten commandments of excellent care, along with ten major myths about diabetes that you can discard. Finally, you find out how to utilise the skills and knowledge of the people around you, both the diabetes experts and your friends and family.

Chapter 18

Ten Ways to Prevent or Reverse the Effects of Diabetes

*I*f you read everything that came before this, congratulations. But we didn't really expect you to (this is a reference book, not a novel) and that's why we wrote this chapter. Follow the leaders' (that's us!) advice in this chapter, and you can be in great diabetic shape.

Monitoring Your Glucose Levels

If you use insulin, you should have a glucose meter. Now, what do you do with it? Most people don't like to stick needles into themselves and are reluctant to do so at first. But you can do this in so many ways, almost without pain, that you have no excuse for not using this great advance in diabetes care. How often you test is between you and your doctor, but the more you do it, the easier controlling your diabetes is. Monitoring gives you more insight into your body's response to food, exercise, and medications. (See Chapter 7 for more on monitoring.)

If you have type 1 diabetes or use insulin to control your type 2 diabetes, you should be using your blood glucose measurements to decide how much insulin you need. That means you should ideally be measuring your blood glucose before meals and at bedtime. If you don't take insulin, you and your doctor may have decided that you don't get much benefit from regular monitoring. Even if this is true most of the time, you should check your glucose when you're ill. That's because being ill for any reason can wreak havoc on your blood sugar control.

Paying Attention to Your Diet

If you are what you eat, then you have the choice of being controlled or uncontrolled depending on what you put into your mouth. If you gain weight, you gain insulin resistance, but you can reverse this situation by losing weight. The main point you should understand about a 'diabetic diet' is that it's a healthy diet for everyone, whether they have diabetes or not. You shouldn't feel like a social outcast because you're eating the right foods. You don't need special supplements – the diet is balanced and contains all the vitamins and minerals you require (although you want to be sure you're getting enough calcium).

You can follow a diabetic diet wherever you are, not just at home. Every menu has something on it that's appropriate for you. If you're invited to someone's home, let them know that you have diabetes and that the amount of carbohydrate and fat that you can eat is limited. If that fails, then limit the amount that you eat. And if that is somehow not possible, then accept the fact that your diet is not always perfect and go on from there. (See Chapter 8 for more on your diet.)

Doing Routine Health Tests

The people who make smoke detectors recommend that you change the battery without fail each time that you have a birthday. You can use the same simple trick to keep track of your diabetes testing. Every year around the same time, make sure that your doctor checks your urine for tiny amounts of protein and your feet for loss of sensation. Most general practices now have a diabetic register with a call and recall system. They should be inviting you regularly for check-ups, and for a more thorough check once a year.

The Cheat Sheet at the front of this book gives you the current testing recommendations. Check out these recommendations and make a copy for your doctor if he does not already have such a list. Demand that you get the tests when they are due. A doctor with a busy medical practice may forget whether you have had the tests you need, but you don't have an excuse for forgetting.

It takes five to ten years to develop the complications of diabetes. Sadly, about 50 per cent of people with type 2 diabetes have some complications by the time they're diagnosed. That's because many of them have lived with diabetes for years without knowing they have it, and without doing anything about it. But this certainly doesn't mean that you're ever too late to help yourself. Once you know that diabetes is present, you can do a lot to slow down its complications or even reverse them. Never has the saying been truer that 'an ounce of prevention is worth a pound of cure'. (For more on the complications you may develop, see Chapters 4 and 5.)

Making Time for Exercise

When you take insulin, controlling your diabetes is a little harder than taking pills, because you have to coordinate your food and the activity of the insulin. But we have patients who have had diabetes for decades and have little trouble balancing their food and insulin. They are the enthusiastic exercisers. They use exercise to burn up glucose in place of insulin. The result is a much more narrow range of blood glucose levels than is true of the insulin takers who do not exercise. They also have more leeway in their diet because the exercise makes up for slight excesses.

We're not talking about an hour of running or 50 miles on the bike. Moderate exercise like brisk walking can accomplish the same thing. The key is to exercise faithfully. (For more on exercise, see Chapter 9.)

Educating Yourself about Diabetes

When we see new patients who've had diabetes for some time, we're amazed how little they know about many fundamental areas of their disease. You may think that they want to know anything that can help them live more comfortably and avoid complications.

So much is going on in the field of diabetes that you need to be a lifelong learner if you want to be aware of the major advances made in diabetes care. Once you get past the shock of the diagnosis, you're ready to discover more.

This book contains a lot of basic stuff that you need to know. You can even take a good course in diabetes. Then you need to keep learning. Here are some suggestions:

- Become a member of Diabetes UK. Membership gives you access to Diabetes UK's excellent bi-monthly magazine, *Balance,* as well as all the other publications that the organisation produces.

- Go to meetings of one of the 400 local support groups set up by Diabetes UK.

- Go to the Web sites we list in Appendix C. Remember, however, that the Web contains a lot of misinformation, so be careful to check out a recommendation with your doctor before you start to follow any treatment. Even information on reliable sites may not be right for your particular problem.

Above all, never stop learning! The next thing you find out may be the thing that cures you.

Taking Your Medications Faithfully

Compliance means treating your disease in accordance with your doctor's instructions. The term has special relevance for the patient with a chronic disease like diabetes who must take medication day in and day out. Of course doing this is a pain (even if you could take insulin by mouth and not by injection). But the basic assumption in diabetes care is that you're taking your medication. Your doctor bases all his decisions on that assumption. Some very serious mistakes can be made if that assumption is false. Diabetes medication is pretty potent, and too much of a good thing can be bad for you. (For more on medication, see Chapter 10.)

Every time a study is done on why patients don't respond better to treatment, compliance is high up or leads the list of reasons. Do you make a conscious decision to skip your tablets, or do you forget? Whatever the reason, the best thing to do is to set up a system that forces you to remember. Make the system simple so that it works for you. Here are some ideas:

- Keep your pills in a dated container. Doing so lets you see at a glance whether you've taken your medication or not. You can even divide the pills by time of day.

- Get a dossette box from your pharmacist. These boxes let you organise your tablets for a week at a time. If you're housebound, your general practitioner can arrange for the district nurses to come in regularly to organise your tablets for you, if your pharmacist or carer can't do this.

✔ Ask your pharmacist about making up blister packs, which sort your tablets out for a month at a time.

Keep a Positive Attitude

Your approach to your disease can go a long way towards determining whether you live in diabetes heaven or diabetes hell. A positive attitude, treating diabetes as a challenge and an opportunity, not only makes managing your diabetes easier, but it also spurs your body to produce chemicals that make better management happen. A negative attitude, on the other hand, results in the kind of pessimism that leads to failure to diet, failure to exercise, and failure to take your medication. Plus, your body makes chemicals that are bad for you.

Diabetes is both a challenge (you have to think about certain things that other people never have to worry about) and an opportunity. It forces you to make healthy choices for your life, particularly regarding diet and exercise. As a result, you may well end up a lot healthier than your neighbour who doesn't have diabetes. A positive attitude spurs you on to make more and more healthy choices. As you do, you feel and test less and less like a person with diabetes.

Planning Ahead for the Unexpected

Life is full of surprises. That's why having a plan to deal with the unexpected is so important. Say you're invited to someone's home, and they serve something that you know raises your blood glucose significantly. What do you do? Or suppose that you go out to eat and the waiter gives you a menu of incredible choices, many of which are just not suitable for you. How do you handle that? You run into great stress at work or at home. Do you allow it to throw off your diet, your exercise, and taking your medication?

The key to these situations is being prepared with a plan. In the case of the friend who cooked the wrong thing for you, you can at least eat a small portion to limit the damage. When you go to restaurants, go prepared to order the food you know keeps you on your diet. Maybe you can carefully select the appropriate foods from the menu, or maybe you decide not to look at the menu at all and simply discuss with your waiter what the restaurant can offer you from your list of correct foods.

Taking Care of Your Feet

A recent headline read: 'Hospital sued by seven foot doctors.' We would certainly not like to treat any doctor with seven feet or even a doctor who is seven feet tall. Whether you have two feet or seven feet, you must take good care of them. The problem occurs when you can't feel with your feet because of neuropathy (see Chapter 5).

When you lose sensation in your feet, your eyes must replace the pain fibres that would otherwise tell you there is a problem. You need to examine your feet carefully every day, keep your toenails trimmed, and wear comfortable shoes. Your doctor should inspect your feet at every visit.

Although diabetes is the primary source of foot amputations, you can prevent such severe damage, but you must pay attention to your feet. Test bathwater by hand, shake your shoes out before you put them on, and wear new shoes for only a short while before checking for pressure spots. The future of your feet is in your hands.

The other aspect of fastidious foot care is making sure that the circulation in the blood vessels of your feet remains open. This is done by your doctor checking your feet out for signs and symptoms of peripheral arterial disease (see Chapter 5). This examination should be done once a year and quickly tells you and your doctor if there is a problem with your circulation.

Looking After Your Eyes

Caring for your eyes starts with a careful examination by a trained general practitioner, an ophthalmologist, or an optician. You need to have an exam at least once a year (or more often if necessary). If you've controlled your diabetes meticulously, the doctor finds two normal eyes. If not, signs of diabetic eye disease may show up (see Chapter 5). At that point, you need to control your diabetes, which means controlling your blood glucose. You also want to control your blood pressure, because high blood pressure contributes to worsening eye disease.

Although the final word is not in on the effects of smoking and excessive alcohol on eye disease in diabetes, if you smoke, consider quitting. Is it worth risking your sight for another puff of a cigarette? Even at this later stage, you can stop the progression of the eye disease or reverse some of the damage.

Chapter 19

Ten Myths about Diabetes That You Can Forget

....

In This Chapter

▶ Doing the exact right thing can yield a perfect glucose every time

▶ Eating a piece of cake can kill you

▶ More myths you shouldn't believe

....

*M*yths are a lot of fun. They're never completely true, but you can usu-ally find a tiny bit of truth in a myth – which is one reason (and the need for an explanation when 'science' fails to provide one) that we believe so many myths.

The trouble is that some myths can hurt you if you allow them to determine your medical care. This chapter is about those kinds of myths – the ones that lead you to fail to take your medication, fail to stay on your diet, or convince you to take things that may not be good for you. The ten myths in this chap-ter are only a small sample of all the myths that exist about diabetes, enough surely to fill up a whole book on their own. But the myths we describe in this chapter are some of the more important ones. Realising that these myths are false can help prevent you from making some serious mistakes about good diabetes care.

Perfect Treatment Yields Perfect Glucoses

Doctors are probably as responsible as their patients are for the myth that perfect treatment results in perfect glucoses. For decades, doctors measured the urine glucose and told their patients that if they just stayed on their diet, took their medication, and got their exercise, the urine would be negative for glucose. Doctors failed to account for the many variables that can result in a positive test for glucose in the urine, plus the fact that even if the urine was negative, the patient could still be suffering diabetic damage (because the urine becomes negative at a blood glucose of 10 mmol/l in most people, a level that still causes damage).

The same thing is true for the blood glucose. Although you can achieve normal blood glucose levels most of the time if you treat your diabetes properly, you can still have times when the glucose is not normal, sometimes for no apparent reason. So many factors – such as your diet, exercise, medication, and so on – determine the blood glucose level at any given time that this should hardly be a surprise.

The miracle is that the blood glucose is what you expect it to be as often as it is. Don't allow an occasional unexpected result to throw you. Keep on doing what you know to be right, and your overall control can be excellent.

Eating a Piece of Cake Can Kill You

Some people become fanatics when they develop diabetes. They think that they must be perfect in every aspect of their diabetes care. They often drive their family crazy with demands for exactly the right food at exactly the right time. Doctors, again, can be blamed for perpetuating this myth. They used to tell their patients that they must avoid sugar at all costs. Now, as Chapter 8 shows, doctors understand that a little sugar in the diet is not harmful, and that some foods, thought to be safe because they were 'complex' carbohydrates, can raise the blood glucose just as rapidly as table sugar.

This myth goes back again to the fact that science does not have all the answers. Knowledge is still evolving. It may never reach the point where the statement made to Woody Allen's character in the movie *Sleeper* is true. He wakes up after sleeping for 100 years and is told that scientists now realise that milkshakes and fatty meats are good for you. But who knows?

Unorthodox Methods Can Cure Diabetes

In Chapter 17, we talk about some treatments that don't work. The treatments included in that chapter are just the tip of the iceberg. Many more treatments exist that don't help you and may hurt you. Whenever a problem affects a huge number of people, others are eager to exploit this potential gold mine.

 How can you know whether what you read in your favourite magazine or see on the Internet is actually useful? Check the information out with your doctor, nurse, or another member of your team (see Chapter 11). These people know or can find out for you about any appropriate treatment. To date, diabetes has no simple cures. A book or organisation that promises an easy cure is not doing you any favours.

Diabetes Ends Spontaneity

You may think that your freedom to eat when you want and come and go as you please is gone once you have diabetes. This myth is far from the truth. If you have type 1 diabetes, you need to balance your insulin intake with your food intake, but the availability of newer insulins means that you can eat virtually when you want and take your short-acting insulin (see Chapter 10) just before or even during or right after you eat. If you're a heavy exerciser, you may not even need very much insulin. One of our type 1 patients takes only a few units of insulin because he is so physically active. The result is that he requires little insulin, and his blood glucose stays in a very normal range most of the time.

Newer oral agents for type 2 diabetes allow you to eat when you want and anticipate the blood glucose remaining normal. Exercise helps the type 2 patient as well.

Can you travel where you want with diabetes? Most certainly. You need to start a trip in good blood glucose control. You also need to make sure that you keep your medication with you so that if your luggage gets lost, your medicine doesn't go with it. Another reason for keeping your medication with you on plane journeys is that insulin is affected by the very low temperatures in the plane's hold. In addition, find out about doctors who speak your language where you're going. These three things are now simple to do and ensure that diabetes doesn't affect your trip.

Should you dance the night away even though you have diabetes? If you can dance, we see no practical reason not to. Cut back on your insulin because you're doing so much exercise and check your blood glucose once or twice during the night. Otherwise, go for it!

Hypoglycaemia Kills Brain Cells

Because hypoglycaemia often comes on so fast and leaves you with a headache or a general feeling of weakness and sometimes confusion, some people have thought that low blood glucose (see Chapter 4), especially if it occurs repeatedly, may destroy mental functioning. Tests of people who have had repeated episodes of hypoglycaemia have shown no loss of mental functioning. Children, on the other hand, may have different results because their brains are still developing, but adults have no loss of mental functioning.

Fortunately, your body is supplied with hormones to reverse hypoglycaemia. You need to check your blood glucose prior to heavy exercise and keep a supply of rapidly absorbable glucose nearby. Also let colleagues and loved ones know about your diabetes and how to recognise hypoglycaemia. If you're prone to frequent low blood glucose, wear an ID bracelet. But you do not have to fear for your grey matter. It can withstand some pretty low levels of blood glucose without complaint.

Needing Insulin Means That You're Doomed

Many people with type 2 diabetes believe that once they have to take insulin, they're on a rapid downhill course to death. This is not so. Once you're using insulin, it probably means that your pancreas has given up and cannot produce enough insulin to control your blood glucose, even when you stimulate it with oral drugs. But taking insulin is no more a death sentence for you than it is for the person with type 1 diabetes.

First of all, using insulin is often a temporary measure for when you're very sick with some other illness that makes your oral drugs ineffective. Once the illness is over, your insulin requirements end.

Secondly, we see more and more people with diabetes who have been on insulin for some time after 'failing' oral agents, who can now be taken off the insulin and given one of the newer oral agents, which actually controls their glucose better than the insulin. One typical patient came to us on 60 units of insulin and weighing 13 stone, with a haemoglobin A1c of 7.4. We gradually lowered his insulin as we added pioglitazone to his treatment. He lost 1½ stone, came off insulin entirely, and now has a haemoglobin A1c of 6.

Thirdly, elderly people with diabetes may need insulin to keep their blood glucose at a reasonable level, but don't need very tight control because their probable life span is shorter than the time it takes to develop complications. Their treatment can be kept very simple (you can find out more in Chapter 14). The insulin is being used to keep them 'out of trouble', not to prevent complications.

Finally, people with type 2 diabetes who truly need to be on insulin intensively need to check their blood glucose more often and live more like a person with type 1 diabetes. Hopefully, you realise that with today's methods, this level of intensive treatment means a much higher quality of life than it used to.

People with Diabetes Shouldn't Exercise

If any myth is really damaging to people with diabetes, it is this one: People with diabetes shouldn't exercise. The truth is exactly the opposite. Exercise is a major component of good diabetes management; one that, unfortunately, all too often gets the least time and effort on the part of the patient as well as her care providers.

Of course, if you have certain complications like haemorrhaging in your eye or severe neuropathy, you need to take precautions or not exercise at all for a time. Certainly, if you're older than 40 and have not exercised, you need to have an examination and start gradually. But except for these and a few other reasons (see Chapter 9), every person with diabetes should exercise regularly.

And we're not just talking about aerobic exercise where your heart is beating faster. Some form of muscle strengthening needs to be a part of your lifestyle. (See Chapter 9 to find out the benefits of muscle strengthening.)

If you have a muscle that you can move, move it!

You Can't Get Life and Private Medical Insurance

As the insurance industry recognises that people with diabetes take better care of themselves than those in the general population do, it is more and more willing to insure them. Some unenlightened insurance companies still exist, but most are seeing the light as the vital statistics of the diabetic population improves.

The old problem of a 'pre-existing condition' seems to be disappearing as well. Insurance companies are not being allowed to use this excuse to block you from getting new insurance when you change jobs.

Most Diabetes Is Inherited

Although type 2 diabetes runs in families, type 1 diabetes more often occurs as an isolated event in a family rather than being handed down from parent to child. (Chapter 3 explains why this is the case.) Even type 2 diabetes does not come out in every family member. It depends on such things as body weight, level of activity, and other factors.

If you're a parent of a small child who develops diabetes, you shouldn't feel guilty. Such feelings make it harder to perform the necessary functions that you must do until your child can do them herself. See Chapter 13 for information about children who have diabetes.

Diabetes Wrecks Your Sense of Humour

After the initial stages of accepting diabetes, your sense of humour should return. (See Chapter 1 for more on dealing with diabetes.) If your humour doesn't return, it's no laughing matter.

There is humour in every aspect of life. You just have to look for it. If you keep your eyes and ears open, you can see and hear much to laugh at.

The saying goes, 'Someday we'll laugh about this.' The question is, 'Why wait?'

Chapter 20

Ten Ways to Get Others to Help You

Diabetes is a social disease. No, we don't mean that you catch it like herpes. We mean that you can't continue very long with diabetes without calling on the help and expertise of others. Asking for help is not such a bad thing. People who regularly interact with others seem to live longer and have a higher quality of life.

In this chapter, you discover how to make use of the great resources that are available to you. So many knowledgeable people are out there. It is a shame not to take advantage of their information.

Teach Hypoglycaemia to Significant Others

If you take either insulin or one of the sulphonylurea medications (see Chapter 10), you may become hypoglycaemic. Occasionally, hypoglycaemia can be so severe that you're unaware of the problem. At that point, someone in your environment needs to know the symptoms of hypoglycaemia and how to treat it. Chapter 4 contains all that information.

You may want to make a list of the signs and symptoms of hypoglycaemia and pass it around to your family and friends. You should keep that list and an emergency kit to treat hypoglycaemia at home and at work. You may even want to wear a medical alert bracelet so that even a stranger can identify your problem when no one you know is around.

Follow the Standards of Care

Decades of following diabetes patients and advances in scientific knowledge have led to the establishment of 'standards of care' for the person with diabetes. These standards of care have now been produced in the form of national guidelines, which include the National Service Framework for Diabetes and the NICE (National Institute for Health and Clinical Excellence) guidelines. You can find details of how to access these guidelines on the Internet (you can look the address up in Appendix C). The standards of care include goals for treatment. If the standards are followed, the goals can be achieved. The goals of treatment give you a way of comparing your treatment with what is possible (though not necessarily certain).

By following the standards of care, you have a good chance of avoiding the short- and long-term complications of diabetes. If these complications have already occurred, you have a good chance of having them diagnosed while they are still treatable.

You're the one who needs to make sure that you get an annual eye examination, the necessary urine tests, the nerve tests, and all the other tests and studies that must be done regularly and routinely. (See Chapter 7 for more on these tests.) Don't expect your doctor to remember all these details. That job falls to you.

Make up a flow chart with a list of the important tests and studies in one column. The next columns are the dates on which these things have been done or will be done on a regular basis. Blank spaces on the flow chart should be obvious.

Find an Exercise Partner

Few people continue a regular exercise programme on their own. In contrast, when you know that someone is waiting for you, you tend to perform the exercise much more regularly. In our practices, we have many patients who are regular exercisers because we emphasise exercise so much. All of them exercise with a partner.

If you belong to a club, finding an exercise partner is easy. Just select the sport and then hang out in the place where the sport is played. Before long, you meet someone who can be your exercise partner.

If you're not a member of a club, finding an exercise partner is a little more difficult. Then you have to approach people with whom you work or your significant other. Most people are happy to walk with you, and some may run and cycle with you. Cyclists seem to like group activity, and you can usually find a cycling group to ride with. Check out listings at a local bike shop or look in your local newspaper in the activities section.

Use Your Chiropodist

Your chiropodist is your first line of defence against lesions of the foot. He knows what the foot should look like and notices problems very early when they're still reversible.

One of the most useful things the chiropodist can do is to cut your nails. It is too easy to cut your skin accidentally when you try to cut your own nails. If you have diabetes, the consequences can be serious. Should you notice an abnormality, you must get to the chiropodist as soon as possible. This is a situation where too much medical care is better than too little.

In the United Kingdom, there's a great deal of variation in the provision of National Health Service chiropody. You may want to check with your doctor or nurse about the availability of 'direct access' chiropody, which allows you to refer yourself urgently if you have a problem. Alternatively, your general practitioner may suggest that you contact him if you notice a foot problem, so that he can refer you on urgently.

Doctors recently did the first hand transplantation, which seems to be going well, but as far as we know no plans exist to do a foot transplantation. You'd better take good care of your feet because they have to last a lifetime. Your chiropodist can be your major ally in this endeavour.

Avoid Temptation

Ever since Adam and Eve, the problem of temptation has been on the front burner. And we're referring to exactly the same temptation: Eating food that's not good for you. In your case, of course, the food that's bad for you won't further your major diabetic goal, which is to control your blood glucose. The opportunities for messing up your diet are boundless. One way to stay on the right track is to enlist the help of a 'food partner'. Just like your exercise partner, your food partner can make staying on your diet a lot easier. This partner can help you in a number of ways. He can:

✔ **Prepare the right kinds of food.** To do this, your partner must know what to make and what to avoid (see Chapter 8). When you go to the dietician, take your food partner along.

Numerous books of recipes and meals are written specifically for the person with diabetes. The first cookbook you should look at is *Diabetes Cookbook For Dummies* (published by John Wiley & Sons, Ltd). You can also go on the Internet to find some good choices; see Appendix C for a list of great Web sites to visit. And check out Appendix A for some great recipes.

Knowing how much food to make is just as important as what to make for your meals. Again, that information is available in books, especially those published by Diabetes UK.

✔ **Steer you to restaurants where you can choose foods that work for you.** Once in the restaurant, he can point out the healthy choices.

✔ **Set an example for you.** Sticking to a diet is much easier if you see the same kinds of food across the table.

✔ **Inform your host of your special dietary restrictions** when you're asked to dinner in someone's home.

You're not the only one who'll benefit. By helping your food partner to discover more about the general principles of eating healthily, you'll enable them to get in better shape, too!

Don't turn your loved one into a nag. Don't ask him or her to remind you each time you stray from your diet, because this can lead to hostility.

Enjoy Your Favourite Foods

Years ago, when you got diabetes it meant that you had to make enormous changes in your diet. This was hard enough for people who ate the usual British diet, but much harder for people who came from another culture and had an entirely different diet. This has changed dramatically over the years. The new programme is to take your usual diet and fit it into a diabetic eating plan. Unless your diet consists of many bottles of sugary drinks or beer each day, you should be able to find a diet plan for you that you find palatable.

The dietician's job is to come up with a diabetic diet plan based on *your* food choices, not his own. If you have special dietary needs because of your culture, a dietician must be able to accommodate those needs if they are reasonable.

Don't be satisfied with a printed sheet of paper with the heading 'Diabetic Diet'. The keyword in diabetic diets is *individualisation*. You're not likely to stay on a diet that you don't enjoy.

Expand Your Education

The person who serves as your diabetes educator is the source of a huge amount of necessary and sometimes critical information. Every person with diabetes ought to go through a programme of education once the initial shock of the diagnosis is past (see Chapter 1). You need to know a lot of information, and the diabetes educator is most highly qualified to teach it to you. Never hesitate to ask a question, no matter how basic you think it may be. You may be surprised by how many other people want the same information.

Of course, every care giver should be a diabetes educator as well. Once you are past the formal diabetes education programme stage, ask your doctor, your dietician, or any of the other people in your team (see Chapter 11) when you have questions or concerns.

Knowledge in diabetes is expanding so fast that great advances are arriving almost daily. Some of these advances may be just what you need for your diabetes. Keep aware of them by checking with your diabetes educators on a regular basis.

Find Out about the Latest and Greatest

The specialist who knows the most about diabetes is the *diabetologist*, a physician with advanced training in diabetes care who maintains his edge by attending diabetes meetings regularly and keeping up with the literature by reading the most important clinical diabetes journals. In the modern world, an up-to-date specialist also has to be aware of what is on the Internet and how to differentiate reality from hype. This person can be a source of information about the latest advances in diabetes and should be the person you go to when things are not going the way you want them to.

If you get all your diabetic care from your general practice, the diabetic clinic should ideally be led by a general practitioner with a special interest in diabetes. Even if you see a different doctor in the practice for the rest of your medical care, you may want to contact the doctor who runs the diabetic clinic if you have questions about your diabetes.

The pace of advances in diabetes is amazing. A general physician, or a general practitioner without a special interest, cannot keep up with the changes. A general physician has to worry about heart disease, lung disease, liver disease, and so on. The diabetes specialist concentrates on diabetes, and that is to your benefit. If you're having problems with your diabetes and your general practitioner doesn't know the answers, you have a right to ask for a referral to a hospital diabetic clinic.

You have the right to insist on a thorough annual check once a year, just to make sure that you are benefiting from the 'latest and greatest' advances in knowledge. Be sure that you have your questions ready when you go. Write the questions down and check them off as you receive your answers.

Understand Your Medication

One of your most valuable and least utilised resources is your pharmacist. He is loaded with information about drug actions, interactions, side effects, proper dosage and administration, reasons to avoid certain medicines, and what to do in case of an overdose. Every time you get a new medication, you can have your pharmacist run it against the medication that you're already taking to see whether any problems may exist. Thanks to computers, this comparison takes only a few minutes. If you work with one pharmacy, you should be able to get a printout of your entire list of medication, which you can carry with you in case you ever need medical care.

Remember that the information in the pharmacist's computer tends to be all-inclusive. If a drug has ever had a side effect, no matter how rare, that information is probably in the computer. The drug manufacturer wants to be able to say that it warned you about every possibility. If a side effect or drug interaction is serious, you may want to discuss it with your physician before you start the new medication.

Your pharmacist also can tell you when a drug needs monitoring. For example, pioglitazone and rosiglitazone require liver function testing every two months for the first 12 months of use. If your doctor does not order the tests, the pharmacist often reminds you to remind the doctor.

Share This Book

If you really want your friends and loved ones to understand what you're going through, why not give them a copy of this book and ask them to read it? You can select the chapters that are most relevant to you. If they need to understand your diet, put a bookmark in Chapter 8. If they're unaware of the emotional adjustment you're going through, tell them to read Chapter 1. Your family and friends may well be delighted to have a resource they can understand, and you can expect a lot more help from them.

Part VI
Appendixes

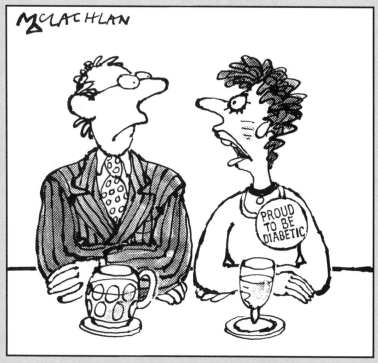

'And _don't_ call me "sugar"!'

In this part . . .

Appendix A is the *Diabetes For Dummies* Mini-Cookbook. Here, you can find some of the most delicious recipes that you can make. Appendix B shows you how to use diabetic exchanges to figure out a proper diabetic diet; this appendix is based on the information presented in Chapter 8. You know what and how much food you should eat to maintain normal weight and normal blood glucose levels, the key to preventing complications. And Appendix C presents an introduction to the magnificent World Wide Web and the almost limitless resources to be found there about diabetes. You may be amazed at how much is given away for free on the Web; some of it, however, is worth what you pay for it.

Appendix A

Mini-Cookbook

This appendix should make it clear to you that you can have great food from every corner of the world and still stay within the requirements of a diabetic diet. In a short appendix like this, we cannot include every possible type of food, so we have tried to select the foods that most people enjoy either at home or in a restaurant.

Sometimes we found it necessary to alter a recipe slightly to keep it appropriate for a diabetic diet, but we never did this without the approval of the chef who created the recipe. These chefs were a pleasure to work with and deserve great praise for their willingness to accommodate the needs of the diabetic patient. Some recipes may take a little longer to prepare than others, but all are worth the time and the effort.

Warm Asparagus and Morel Salad

This dish is perfect as the first or second course to any meal.

Preparation time: *1 hour*

Cooking time: *30 minutes*

Serves: *8*

48 asparagus spears	*Salt and pepper to taste*
250 ml balsamic vinegar	*2 heads of frisée*
225 g morel mushrooms	*1 to 2 tablespoons water*
1 tablespoon butter, plus 1 teaspoon to warm asparagus	*60 ml olive oil*

1 Peel each piece of asparagus 5 cm from the top to the base (you won't need to do this if you're using young, thin asparagus). Cut each spear, leaving a 7.5 to 10 cm tip. Use the remaining asparagus by slicing it into 5 cm rounds. Do not use the woody part of the asparagus. Keep tips and rounds separate.

2 Boil water, adding salt to taste. Add the asparagus tips to the boiling water. Once they are tender but still firm, about 2 minutes, place the asparagus in ice-cold water to cool. Proceed by blanching the asparagus rounds for another 2 to 3 minutes. Use the same process to cool them. Set the cooling tips and rounds aside, keeping them separate.

3 Over low heat, in a heavy-bottomed saucepan, cook the balsamic vinegar for 20 to 30 minutes, never allowing it to reach a boil. Once the balsamic vinegar reaches a syrupy consistency, remove it from the heat. This process requires attention – it is quite easy to burn the balsamic vinegar.

4 Slice the morel mushrooms into 5 cm rounds and place them in warm water to remove any excess dirt. Dry the mushrooms to get rid of the moisture. In a medium frying pan, heat the butter over a medium heat. When bubbly, add the mushrooms. Cook, occasionally stirring gently, until soft, about 4 to 5 minutes. Season with salt and pepper to taste. Set aside.

5 Remove all outside leaves from the frisée, leaving only the inner white leaves. Separate the leaves from the stem, rinse under cold water, and spin or pat dry. Set aside.

6 To serve: Drizzle the balsamic glaze decoratively on each plate. In a medium frying pan, warm the asparagus tips in the remaining butter mixed with 1 to 2 tablespoons water. Place the asparagus tips facing outwards towards the rim of the plate. In the same frying pan, heat the asparagus rounds with the morel slices. Then place the morels and asparagus rounds in a neat mound, slightly overlapping the ends of the asparagus tips. In a medium bowl, mix the frisée with the olive oil. Finally, top the mushrooms and asparagus with the frisée.

Nutrient analysis per serving: *133 calories; 3 grams protein, 13 grams carbohydrate, 9 grams fat, 2 grams saturated fat, 4 milligrams cholesterol, 3 grams fibre, 37 milligrams sodium.*

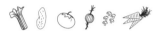

Cinnamon-Brandy Chicken

Looking for an alternative way to cook chicken? Here is a wonderful recipe brimming with flavour and easy to prepare. Serve with the rice pilaf and roasted vegetable dishes, later in this section.

Preparation time: *30 minutes*

Cooking time: *40 minutes*

Serves: *6*

125 ml brandy	4 garlic cloves, minced
1 tablespoon ground cinnamon	1 teaspoon salt
60 ml honey	½ teaspoon freshly ground black pepper
125 ml lemon juice	One 1.1 to 1.3 kg chicken, cut into pieces
125 ml orange juice	2 tablespoons vegetable oil

1 In a medium bowl, mix the brandy, cinnamon, honey, lemon and orange juices, garlic, salt, and pepper. Add the chicken and toss to coat evenly. Cover and marinate in the fridge 8 hours or overnight.

2 Preheat oven to 180°C/350°F/Gas mark 4. Remove the chicken, shaking off excess marinade. Pour the marinade into a small saucepan and bring to the boil. Boil for 5 to 10 minutes until it begins to thicken and about 250 ml remain.

3 Heat the oil in an ovenproof frying pan over a medium-high heat. Sear the chicken until golden on both sides. Pour the reduced marinade over the chicken and bake in the oven until just cooked through, for about 20 minutes, and then serve.

Nutrient analysis per serving: *506 calories; 42 grams protein, 16 grams carbohydrate, 25 grams fat, 7 grams saturated fat, 134 milligrams cholesterol, 0 grams fibre, 502 milligrams sodium.*

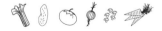

Grilled Swordfish with Worcestershire Vinaigrette and Roasted Vegetables

This dish is a delightful way to flavour both the fish and vegetables. It is a complete meal, but low enough in carbohydrate to include a couple of slices of French bread.

Preparation time: 40 minutes

Cooking time: 1 hour, 10 minutes

Serves: 8

8 swordfish steaks, approximately 170 g each

Vinaigrette

125 ml Worcestershire sauce

1 sprig rosemary, leaves only, chopped

2 tablespoons chopped chives

1 clove garlic, minced

1 tablespoon balsamic vinegar

Juice of ¼ lemon

250 ml extra-virgin olive oil

Roasted Vegetables

8 new potatoes, cut in half

16 baby beetroots, well rinsed and ends trimmed

24 baby carrots, peeled

16 shitake mushrooms, stems removed

16 shallots, unpeeled and cut in half

900 g red and yellow cherry tomatoes

3 tablespoons olive oil

Salt and pepper to taste

450 g rocket

1 *For vinaigrette:* Mix all ingredients together. This vinaigrette should be made 24 hours in advance. The nutritional analysis reflects only 2 tablespoons.

2 *For roasted vegetables:* Heat oven to 190°C/375°F/Gas mark 5. Keeping vegetables separate, in a large bowl, toss the potatoes, beetroots, carrots, mushrooms, shallots, tomatoes, 2 tablespoons olive oil, and salt and pepper, then transfer to a hot baking tray and roast in the oven until tender, for about 45 minutes. You can do this ahead of time and then reheat the vegetables when you're ready to cook the fish.

3 *For swordfish:* Reheat the vegetables in the oven if done ahead of time. Preheat the grill to a medium heat. Season the swordfish on both sides and cook under the grill until medium rare, about 3 minutes per side.

4 In a large frying pan, heat the remaining olive oil over a high heat. Add the rocket and cook, tossing or gently mixing with kitchen tongs, just until the greens start to wilt, about 1 minute. Mix the greens with the hot vegetables and place in the centre of each plate, dividing the vegetables evenly.

5 *To serve:* Place the swordfish on top of the vegetables. Drizzle 2 tablespoons of vinaigrette over each portion.

Nutrient analysis per serving: 519 calories; 48 grams protein, 36 grams carbohydrate, 22 grams fat, 3 grams saturated fat, 126 milligrams cholesterol, 3 grams fibre, 544 milligrams sodium.

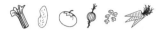

Marinated Grilled Duck Breast

Although duck is higher in fat than other types of poultry, it still can be served as a dish for special occasions. Round out this meal with a cup of wild rice and sautéed vegetables.

Preparation time: *30 minutes*

Cooking time: *1 hour*

Serves: *4*

250 ml balsamic vinegar	½ bunch flat-leaf parsley, chopped
225 ml Worcestershire sauce	½ bunch rosemary, chopped
60 ml honey	½ bunch chives, chopped
250 ml extra virgin olive oil	4 duck breasts
1 tablespoon chopped garlic	Salt and pepper to taste
½ tablespoon lemon juice	

1 *For marinade:* Place garlic, lemon juice, parsley, rosemary, and chives in a large bowl and mix well. Score the skin side of the duck breasts. Place the duck in the bowl, coat with marinade, and cover the bowl. Refrigerate and marinate for 24 hours.

2 Preheat grill to high. Remove the duck from the marinade and pat it dry with kitchen paper. Season with salt and pepper. Grill for 10 minutes on the skin side, turn, moving the breasts to a cooler part of the grill – usually a lower shelf – and cook for another 5 minutes, or until medium rare. Alternatively, to sauté the duck, place 2 nonstick pans over medium-high heat. When pans are hot, add the duck breasts, skin side down. Cook for 10 minutes. Reduce the heat, turn breasts over, and cook another 5 minutes or until medium rare. Slice just before serving.

Nutrient analysis per serving: 507 calories; 47 grams protein, 6 grams carbohydrate, 32 grams fat, 8 grams saturated fat, 177 milligrams cholesterol, 0 grams fibre, 300 milligrams sodium.

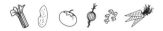

Miso Marinated Sea Bass

This unique marinade adds a tremendous amount of flavour without the use of fat. You can add a tossed green salad with your favourite vinaigrette. This dish is also low in carbohydrate, so complete the meal with a cup of rice.

Preparation time: *45 minutes*

Cooking time: *5 minutes*

Serves: *8*

115 g brown sugar

115 g sugar

225 g miso paste

60 ml soy sauce

250 ml sake

250 ml rice wine vinegar

8 x 170 g portions Chilean sea bass – normal sea bass can also be used

Vegetable oil

250 ml chicken stock

63 g mangetout

125 g thinly sliced carrots, boiled in salted water 3 to 4 minutes

225 g baby pak choi, boiled in salted water 1 to 2 minutes

5 radishes, thinly sliced

70 g shiitake mushrooms, sliced

1 x 225 g package enoki mushrooms

Salt and pepper

1 **For marinade:** In a large bowl, mix together the sugars, miso paste, soy sauce, sake, and rice wine vinegar. Place the fish in the bowl, coat it with marinade, and cover the bowl. Refrigerate and marinate for 24 hours.

2 Preheat the grill to high. Rub a shallow oven tray (large enough to fit the fish in a single layer) lightly with vegetable oil. Remove the sea bass fillets from the marinade, place them on the oven tray, and place under the grill. Cook until the fish begins to brown. Transfer the tray to the oven and cook the fish through for about 5 minutes, depending on the thickness of the fillets.

3 Combine the stock with the mangetout, carrots, pak choi, radishes, and shiitake and enoki mushrooms in a medium frying pan. Simmer, covered, until vegetables are warm. Season with the salt and pepper to taste. Place a mound of vegetables in the centre of each large plate or bowl, put a sea bass fillet on top, and spoon the stock around.

Nutrient analysis per serving: 295 calories; 37 grams protein, 26 grams carbohydrate, 4 grams fat, 0.5 grams saturated fat, 82 milligrams cholesterol, 2 grams fibre, 1,295 milligrams sodium.

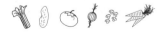

Lemon Braised Sea Bass with Star Anise and Baby Spinach

This meal is low in total carbohydrate and total fat, so you can complete the meal with a couple of servings of carbohydrate (such as a serving of French bread and rice) and a tossed green salad with vinaigrette dressing.

Preparation time: *30 minutes*

Cooking time: *15 minutes*

Serves: *4*

4 sea bass fillets (about 115 g each)

Salt and freshly ground pepper to taste

1 teaspoon olive oil

30 g celeriac, finely diced

40 g fennel bulb, finely diced

30 g carrot, finely diced

3 garlic cloves, peeled and chopped

4 star anise

60 ml freshly squeezed lemon juice

375 ml water

40 g cucumber, finely diced

65 g tomato, finely diced

15 g apple, finely diced

225 g baby spinach leaves

2 teaspoons extra virgin olive oil

Pinch mild cayenne powder

2 tablespoons chopped fresh chives

2 tablespoons chopped fresh parsley

1 Preheat oven to 240°C/475°F/Gas mark 9. Rub both sides of the sea bass fillets with salt and pepper and set aside.

2 Heat 1 teaspoon of olive oil in a large frying pan (preferably nonstick) over a high heat. Add the celeriac, fennel, carrot, garlic, and star anise and sauté until slightly caramelised, for 4 to 5 minutes. Soften the caramel with the lemon juice and cook for 1 minute.

3 Lay the sea bass fillets on top of the vegetables, add the water, and cover the pan. Bake just until the fish is cooked through (5 to 6 minutes). Remove the fillets of fish from the pan and set them aside, covered to keep warm.

4 Add the cucumber, tomato, and apple to the frying pan and place over high heat. Bring to the boil and cook for 1 to 2 minutes. Add the spinach, extra virgin olive oil, mild cayenne, and salt and pepper to taste. Cook just until the spinach wilts.

5 **To serve:** Into 4 shallow soup bowls, spoon an equal amount of the vegetables and juice from the pan. Lay a fish fillet on top of the vegetables and add a star anise to garnish. Sprinkle the chives and parsley over each portion and serve immediately.

Nutrient analysis per serving: 236 calories; 31 grams protein, 17 grams carbohydrate, 6 grams fat, 1 gram saturated fat, 77 milligrams cholesterol, 3 grams fibre, 240 milligrams sodium.

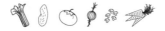

Red Roasted Root Vegetables

You can substitute any of your favourite root vegetables in this dish. It is a great side dish for chicken, fish, or meat.

Preparation time: 35 minutes

Cooking time: 40 minutes

Serves: 6

225 g turnips, peeled and cut into 2.5 cm chunks

225 g beetroot, peeled and cut into 2.5 cm chunks

225 g carrots, peeled and cut into 2.5 cm chunks

225 g butternut or other firm squash, peeled and cut into 2.5 cm chunks

1 onion, coarsely chopped

2 garlic cloves, minced

½ bunch fresh oregano leaves, coarsely chopped

75 ml olive oil

1 teaspoon salt

½ teaspoon freshly ground pepper

1 Preheat oven to 230°C/450°F/Gas mark 8. In a large bowl, toss together all the ingredients until well mixed.

2 Arrange the ingredients in a single layer in an enamelled casserole dish or baking tray. Cover and roast for 30 to 40 minutes, stirring every 10 minutes. The vegetables are done when golden, lightly caramelised on the edges, and easily pierced with the tip of a knife.

Nutrient analysis per serving: 171 calories; 2 grams protein, 15 grams carbohydrate, 11 grams fat, 2 grams saturated fat, 0 milligrams cholesterol, 4 grams fibre, 432 milligrams sodium.

Baked Apples

This dessert is a wonderful way to top off any meal. It is light, healthy, and low in calories.

Preparation time: 35 minutes

Cooking time: 1 hour

Serves: 6

250 ml plus 2 tablespoons apple juice

36 g raisins

60 ml apricot jam

30 g toasted chopped walnuts

2 tablespoons maple syrup

2 tablespoons brandy

6 medium apples, cored and the top third peeled

2 tablespoons unsalted butter

1 In a small saucepan, bring 2 tablespoons of apple juice and the raisins to a simmer and remove from heat. Let stand for 10 minutes.

2 Preheat the oven to 180°C/350°F/Gas mark 4. In a bowl, stir together the apricot jam, walnuts, maple syrup, brandy, and raisins with their juice and mix well.

3 Stuff the apples with the raisin mixture. Place the apples in a small oven tray and top each with a dab of butter. Pour the remaining 250 ml of apple juice into the pan and bake 50 to 60 minutes, or until tender but not split or mushy.

Nutrient analysis per serving: 218 calories; 2 grams protein, 38 grams carbohydrate, 8 grams fat, 3 grams saturated fat, 11 milligrams cholesterol, 4 grams fibre, 2 milligrams sodium.

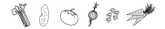

Maniche Al Pollo (Macaroni with Chicken)

This recipe is fairly concentrated in calories but is a delicious way to give chicken an Italian flavour. It makes a complete meal as written, but you can eat less pasta and replace it with a piece of bread if you prefer.

Preparation time: 10 minutes

Cooking time: 20 minutes

Serves: 4

2 tablespoons olive oil

340 g skinless chicken breasts, diced

Salt and pepper to taste

4 garlic cloves, sliced

125 ml white wine

280 g curved macaroni

4 sundried tomatoes

285 g fresh broccoli florets

4 tablespoons Parmesan cheese

1 Heat the oil in a large frying pan over a high heat. Add the diced chicken and salt and pepper. Sauté 2 to 3 minutes, or until cooked through. Add the garlic and brown lightly. Add the wine and cook until sauce is reduced to 1 to 2 tablespoons.

2 Boil the pasta according to the directions on the packet. Three minutes before the pasta is ready, add the sundried tomatoes and broccoli to the cooking water. When the pasta is cooked, drain and toss with the chicken, sauce, and Parmesan cheese.

Nutrient analysis per serving: 561 calories; 41 grams protein, 66 grams carbohydrate, 24 grams fat, 3 grams saturated fat, 70 milligrams cholesterol, 2.5 grams fibre, 283 milligrams sodium.

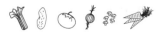

Baked Sea Bass

Here is a delightful way to season and bake fish. You can serve this with a rice pilaf and the roast vegetable dish given above for a complete meal.

Preparation time: *45 minutes*

Cooking time: *15 minutes*

Serves: *6*

6 115 g sea bass fillets

Salt and freshly ground pepper to taste

Salsa Verde

2 garlic cloves

2 jalapeño peppers, stemmed, seeded, and chopped

½ bunch coriander leaves, chopped

½ bunch flat-leaf parsley, chopped

6 spring onions, white and light green parts only, trimmed and chopped

6 green tomatoes, stalk removed, washed, and roasted

2 teaspoons dried oregano

75 ml chicken stock

2 tablespoons fruity olive oil

1 teaspoon salt

Lemon wedges for serving

1 Preheat the oven to 180°C/350°F/Gas mark 4. Season the fish all over with salt and pepper and place in an oiled ovenproof baking tray.

2 To make the salsa, combine all the ingredients in a blender or food processor and purée.

3 Pour the salsa over the fish in the pan and bake for 8 to 12 minutes, until the thickest part of the fish is cooked. Serve with lemon wedges and salsa spooned on top.

Nutrient analysis per serving: 158 calories; 22 grams protein, 2 grams carbohydrate, 9 grams fat, 1 gram saturated fat, 8 milligrams cholesterol, 0.2 grams fibre, 499 milligrams sodium.

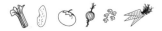

Roasted Tomatoes Stuffed with Couscous, Chicken, Chanterelles, and Pinenuts

You can serve this dish as a main course for lunch or as a side dish for dinner. If you serve this as a main course for lunch, you can round off the meal with a couple of slices of French bread and a tossed salad with 1 tablespoon of olive oil.

Preparation time: *1 hour, 15 minutes*

Cooking time: *15 minutes*

Serves: *4*

8 small tomatoes

2 tablesoons basil or olive oil

8 garlic cloves

8 thyme sprigs

8 bay leaves

8 large basil leaves

15g quartered chanterelle mushrooms

1 tablespoon olive oil

2 tablespoons sweetcorn kernels

360 g cooked couscous

2 tablespoons peeled, seeded, and diced tomatoes

2 tablespoons pinenuts

1 tablespoon peeled and finely diced cucumber

1 chicken breast, cooked and finely diced

2 teaspoons chopped chives

1 tablespoon chopped mixed fresh herbs (such as tarragon, mint, or basil)

Salt and pepper to taste

1 **For tomatoes:** Preheat oven to 130°C/250°F/Gas mark ½. Cut a small cross in the bottom of each tomato and drop into boiling water for 15 seconds. Remove the tomatoes from the water and peel off the skins. Cut a 2 cm slice off the bottom of each tomato, reserving the slices for lids. Scoop out the seeds and flesh from the tomatoes. Rub the insides with 1 tablespoon of the basil oil and place a clove of garlic, a sprig of thyme, a bay leaf, and a basil leaf in each tomato. Place the tomatoes in a small oven dish, put the lids on the tomatoes, and roast for 10 to 12 minutes, or until the tomatoes just begin to soften. Remove and discard the garlic and herbs.

2 **For filling:** In a medium frying pan, cook the mushrooms in 1 teaspoon of the olive oil over a medium heat for 3 minutes or until tender. Remove the mushrooms from the pan, add the sweetcorn kernels, and sauté for 2 minutes or until hot. Warm the couscous through and stir in the mushrooms, tomatoes, pinenuts, cucumber, chicken, and sweetcorn until thoroughly incorporated. Stir in the remaining 2 teaspoons of the olive oil, chives, and chopped mixed herbs, and season to taste with salt and pepper.

3 Rub the outsides of the tomatoes with the remaining 1 tablespoon of basil or olive oil and return to the oven for 3 minutes. Place 2 tomatoes in the centre of each plate. Spoon the filling loosely into the tomatoes, spooning the remaining filling around the base of the tomatoes, and serve.

Nutrient analysis per serving: *309 calories; 14 grams protein, 35 grams carbohydrate, 10 grams fat, 1 gram saturated fat, 18 milligrams cholesterol, 4 grams fibre, 504 milligrams sodium.*

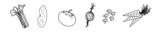

Scallops with Barley, Wild Mushroom Ragout, and Chicken Stock Reduction

This meal is low in carbohydrate, which allows you to have a couple of slices of bread too.

Preparation time: *1 hour*

Cooking time: *45 minutes*

Serves: *4*

3 tablespoons chopped fennel bulb	*125 ml Madeira*
3 tablespoons rapeseed oil	*Salt and pepper*
125 ml red wine	*1 teaspoon chopped parsley*
50 g peeled, seeded, and diced tomatoes	*1 teaspoon chopped tarragon*
750 ml chicken stock	*20 medium scallops*
565 g mixed wild mushrooms (shiitake, cepe, and so on)	*315 g cooked pearl barley, hot*

1 **For the reduction:** In a medium frying pan, cook the fennel in 1 tablespoon of the oil for 5 minutes or until thoroughly softened. Add the red wine and stir continuously until the wine is reduced to a glaze. Add the tomatoes and chicken stock and cook over a medium-low heat for 30 minutes or until reduced to 250 ml.

2 **For mushrooms:** Cut the mushrooms into large pieces (smaller ones can be used whole). In a medium nonstick frying pan, heat 1 tablespoon of the oil over a medium-low heat. Add the mushrooms and cook, tossing or stirring occasionally, for 10 minutes, or until mushrooms are tender and all the liquid has evaporated. Add the Madeira and cook until the liquid has completely evaporated. Season the mushrooms to taste with salt and pepper and add the parsley and tarragon. Set aside.

3 **For scallops:** Heat the remaining 1 tablespoon of the oil in a nonstick frying pan over a medium-high heat or until hot. Add the scallops and cook for 2 minutes, or until golden brown. Season the scallops with salt and pepper. Turn the scallops and cook for 1 minute.

4 **To serve:** Place the cooked pearl barley on each plate. Spoon some of the fennel sauce onto each plate, place a neat pile of mushrooms over the sauce, and surround with 5 scallops, leaning them against the mushrooms.

Nutrient analysis per serving: *398 calories; 27 grams protein, 36 grams carbohydrate, 20 grams fat, 5 grams saturated fat, 42 milligrams cholesterol, 2 grams fibre, 1,084 milligrams sodium.*

Onion Pie with Roquefort and Walnuts

This dish is a feast for the eyes as well as the tastebuds. Serve as a main course for lunch. A fresh fruit salad and a French bread roll are perfect complements to this meal.

Preparation time: *1 hour*

Cooking time: *15 minutes*

Serves: *8*

2 tablespoons olive oil

2 onions, very thinly sliced

60 ml water

85 g Roquefort cheese, crumbled into small pieces

Salt and freshly ground pepper to taste

80 g walnuts, coarsely chopped

1 tablespoon melted butter

Two puff pastry sheets (29 by 38 cm), fresh or thawed if frozen

1 egg, lightly beaten

8 slices prosciutto (about 15 g each)

Mixed greens to garnish

1 Place a baking tray with sides in the freezer.

2 In a frying pan over medium-high heat, warm the olive oil. Add the onions and sauté until golden brown (for about 10 minutes). Add the water and continue to sauté until all the moisture evaporates, for about 5 minutes longer. Reduce heat to medium-low. Add the Roquefort cheese and continue cooking, stirring occasionally, until melted, for about another 5 minutes. Season only lightly with salt, if needed, and add pepper to taste. Stir in the walnuts and then spread the mixture out onto the chilled tray. Replace in the freezer until the onions cool down completely (for about 10 minutes).

3 Preheat oven to 230°C/450°F/Gas mark 8 and evenly brush another baking tray with melted butter.

4 Place the puff pastry on a cutting board. Using the rim of a small plate about 12.5 cm in diameter as a guide, cut the pastry into 8 rounds and discard the scraps.

5 Place the rounds onto the buttered baking tray. Brush the outer rims and tops of the pastry with the beaten egg. Evenly distribute the cooled onion mixture in the middle of each of the 8 rounds, leaving 2.5 cm uncovered all around the edges. Place 1 prosciutto ham slice on top of each mound of the onion mixture. Fold over the pastry round to create a half-moon shape. Pinch down firmly around the edges to seal in the filling. Brush the top of each pie with more of the beaten egg. Using a sharp knife, pierce the top of each pie with a small slit.

6 Bake until the pastry is pale golden and fully puffed up, for 20 to 25 minutes.

Nutrient analysis per serving: 454 calories; 13 grams protein, 26 grams carbohydrate, 34 grams fat, 7 grams saturated fat, 47 milligrams cholesterol, 1 gram fibre, 562 milligrams sodium.

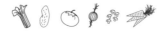

Green Rice Pilaf

This dish can accompany the chicken in the preceding recipe, or it can be served with meat or fish.

Preparation time: *40 minutes*

Cooking time: *25 minutes*

Serves: *6*

1½ tablespoons vegetable oil

1 small onion, finely diced

185 g long-grain white rice

500 ml hot vegetable or chicken stock, preferably homemade

½ teaspoon salt

3 medium chillis, roasted, peeled, seeded, and cut into strips

145 g fresh or frozen peas

75 g crumbled Mexican queso fresco or feta cheese

½ bunch flat-leaf parsley, finely chopped

½ bunch coriander, finely chopped

1 Heat the oil in a heavy saucepan over medium heat. Add the rice and onion and cook, stirring frequently, about 7 minutes, until the onion is softened but not browned.

2 Add the hot stock, salt, and chillis and bring to the boil. Reduce to a simmer and cook, covered, about 10 minutes.

3 Add the peas and simmer 5 minutes longer. Remove from heat and let stand, covered, about 10 minutes.

4 Add the cheese, parsley, and coriander, mix evenly, and fluff with a fork. Serve immediately.

Nutrient analysis per serving: 202 calories; 12 grams protein, 28 grams carbohydrate, 7 grams fat, 3 grams saturated fat, 1 milligram cholesterol, 2 grams fibre, 948 milligrams sodium.

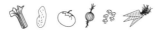

Lemon and Pernod Grilled Prawns with Couscous Salad

This meal is perfect for lunch or for dinner on warm summer evenings. Round out the meal with a bread roll, a chilled vegetable dish, and fresh fruit dessert.

Preparation time: *1 hour, 15 minutes*

Cooking time: *15 minutes*

Serves: *6*

Prawns

3 tablespoons Ricard or Pernod

3 tablespoons freshly squeezed lemon juice

4 garlic cloves, finely sliced

6 sprigs fresh thyme

½ teaspoon sea salt

¼ teaspoon freshly ground pepper

¼ teaspoon mild cayenne pepper

5 tablespoons extra virgin olive oil

450 g large raw prawns (about 24), peeled, and with the vein in the back of each removed

6-inch bamboo skewers

Couscous Salad

250 ml water

175 g couscous

120 g cucumber, peeled and finely diced

155 g pineapple, finely diced

1 large shallot, minced

4 tablespoons chopped fresh parsley

3 tablespoons chopped fresh mint

3 tablespoons fresh lemon juice

3 tablespoons extra virgin olive oil

Salt and pepper to taste

Pinch of mild cayenne pepper

1 **Marinade for prawns:** Combine Pernod, lemon juice, garlic, thyme, salt, pepper, cayenne, and olive oil in a mixing bowl; set aside. Insert 1 skewer, lengthwise, though the body of each prawn, starting with the tail end first, and working the skewer up though the head. In a shallow glass ovenproof dish, lay all the skewered prawns in a single layer. Pour the marinade over the prawns, making sure that they're thoroughly coated. Cover with clingfilm and set aside in the fridge for 2 to 3 hours, turning them over after 1 to 1 ½ hours.

2 **For the couscous:** Bring 250 ml of water to the boil. Add the couscous, stir, cover, and remove from heat. Allow to sit for 5 to 6 minutes and then fluff with a fork. Spread the couscous on a tray and place in the fridge to cool. In a large mixing bowl, combine the cucumber, pineapple, and shallots. Add the cooled couscous, parsley, mint, lemon juice, and olive oil and mix until well combined. Season with salt and pepper to taste.

3 Preheat an indoor grill or your barbecue to a hot temperature (but not smoking for barbecues). Place a small bed of couscous on the centre of each serving plate. Grill the prawns for 1 to 2 minutes on each side, depending on the size of the prawn. Remove from the grill and place on top of the couscous salad. Sprinkle with a pinch of cayenne and serve immediately.

Nutrient analysis per serving: *303 calories; 17 grams protein, 14 grams carbohydrate, 20 grams fat, 3 grams saturated fat, 115 milligrams cholesterol, 1 gram fibre, 311 milligrams sodium.*

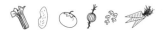

Drunken Pork Shoulder with Cabbage and Pears

This dish is a complete meal in itself. Luckily, it's low in carbohydrate, which leaves room for a couple of slices of French bread to dunk in the delicious sauce.

Preparation time: *3 hours*

Cooking time: *1 hour*

Serves: *6*

Bouquet garni (a seasoning), which comprises 4 parsley sprigs, 1 bay leaf, and 2 thyme sprigs tied together with kitchen string

2 onions, diced

2 carrots, peeled and diced

2 celery stalks, diced

3 garlic cloves

30 black peppercorns

1.2 litres dry red wine, such as Cabernet or Merlot

Salt to taste

900 g boneless pork shoulder, cut into 2.5 cm cubes

2 tablespoons olive oil

1 litre veal or chicken stock

1 head green cabbage, thinly sliced

1 tablespoon unsalted butter

¼ vanilla pod, split in half lengthwise

3 ripe but firm pears, such as Conference, cored, peeled, and cut into 2 cm cubes

3 tablespoons chopped fresh parsley

1 In a large nonmetallic dish, combine the bouquet garni, onions, carrots, celery, garlic, peppercorns, 1 litre of the red wine, and salt to taste. Stir to mix. Add pork and turn to coat evenly. Cover with clingfilm and marinate for at least 5 hours or as long as overnight.

2 Drain the meat and vegetables in a sieve, capturing the marinade in a small saucepan. Bring the marinade to a boil, remove from the heat, and set aside. Separate the meat from the vegetables and set both aside.

3 In a frying pan, over a high heat, warm the olive oil. Pat the meat dry with kitchen towels. Working in small batches, add the meat to the pan and brown on all sides, for about 2 minutes. Transfer the meat to a large saucepan.

4 To the same pan used for browning the meat, add the reserved vegetables and sauté over a medium-high heat until they begin to brown, for about 5 minutes.

5 Transfer the vegetables to the saucepan holding the meat. Add the reserved red wine marinade. Bring to the boil over a high heat and boil until reduced by half, for about 10 minutes. Add the veal stock and return to the boil. Reduce the heat to medium and simmer, uncovered, until the pork is tender, for 50 to 60 minutes.

6 Meanwhile, fill another large saucepan two-thirds full with water, add a pinch of salt, and bring to the boil. Add the cabbage, bring back to the boil, and cook until the cabbage is wilted, for about 2 minutes. Drain the cabbage, rinse with cold water, and drain again. In a frying pan over medium heat, melt the butter. Add the cabbage and sauté for 2 minutes. Remove from heat and set aside.

7 In another small saucepan, combine the remaining red wine (500 ml), the vanilla pod, and pears and bring to the boil. Reduce the heat to medium and simmer, turning the fruit every few minutes, for 5 to 10 minutes until tender.

8 Drain the meat and vegetables in a sieve, capturing the juices in a bowl. Cover the juices to keep them warm. Separate the pork from the vegetables; discard the vegetables.

9 *To serve:* Arrange a bed of the cabbage on a warmed platter. Place the pork on top of the cabbage and pour the juices over the top. Scatter the poached pear cubes around the meat. Garnish with the parsley and serve at once.

Nutrient analysis per serving: 610 calories; 32 grams protein, 25 grams carbohydrate, 30 grams fat, 10 grams saturated fat, 156 milligrams cholesterol, 5 grams fibre, 718 milligrams sodium.

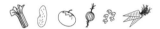

Saag (Spinach)

Here's a sure way of jazzing up a bland vegetable. This can provide one of the servings of vegetables to accompany the previous lamb, chicken, and fish dishes.

Preparation time: *15 minutes*

Cooking time: *15 minutes*

Serves: *6*

Two 300 g bags fresh spinach, trimmed and washed

2 teaspoons vegetable oil

½ teaspoon cumin seeds

10 garlic cloves, quartered

2 dried red chillis

Salt to taste

1 In a large saucepan of boiling salted water, blanch the spinach in batches for 30 seconds or until wilted. Drain and refresh in cold water. Squeeze the moisture from the leaves and chop finely.

2 Heat the vegetable oil over medium heat in a nonstick pan. Add the cumin seeds and stir for 5 seconds. Add the garlic and fry until soft, for 2 to 3 minutes. Add the chillis and cook for another minute. Add the spinach, toss well, and sauté until heated thoroughly and the liquid in the pan has evaporated. Season with salt, and serve hot.

Nutrient analysis per serving: 34.2 calories; 2.7 grams protein, 3.4 grams carbohydrate, 1.5 grams fat, 0.2 grams saturated fat, 0 milligrams cholesterol, 2 grams fibre, 63 milligrams sodium.

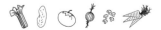

Seekh Kebab

Spices are a wonderful way of adding full flavour to a dish without using extra fats. This dish can be served as an entrée or as an appetiser. Combine this recipe with 185 g rice to provide the necessary carbohydrate. Two servings of vegetables, one of which could be the Saag, later in this section, complete the meal.

Preparation time: *30 minutes*

Cooking time: *10 minutes*

Serves: *6*

1 medium onion	*¼ teaspoon cayenne pepper*
2.5 cm fresh ginger	*½ teaspoon ground coriander*
2 garlic cloves	*½ teaspoon ground cumin*
2 teaspoons water	*¾ teaspoon garam masala*
1 teaspoon salt	*450 g lean minced lamb*

1 In a blender or mini-food processor, grind onion, ginger, and garlic with 2 teaspoons water. Transfer to a medium bowl and mix in salt, cayenne, coriander, cumin, and garam masala.

2 Add the minced lamb and mix until thoroughly combined. Let stand for 20 to 30 minutes in the fridge.

3 Preheat oven to 190°C/375°F/Gas mark 5. Divide the mixture into six equal portions. Lightly oil the skewers. Shape the lamb mixture into sausage shapes on the skewers, about 2.5 cm thick. Place skewers on a rack over a pan and bake for 15 to 20 minutes or until done. To grill, place skewers 7.5 to 10 cm from the heat and cook for approximately 7 minutes per side. Serve hot with a lemon garnish.

Tip: *If using wood or bamboo skewers, soak them overnight in water and oil them lightly. This step prevents the skewers burning while cooking.*

Nutrient analysis per serving: *144 calories; 12.6 grams protein, 2 grams carbohydrate, 9 grams fat, 42 milligrams cholesterol, 0.2 grams fibre, 419 milligrams sodium.*

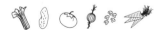

Chicken Tikka Kebab

Marinades can add great flavour to a meal without extra fat and/or sodium. Make this dish early in the day and grill right before serving. Combine this recipe with 185 g of rice to provide the necessary carbohydrate. Two servings of vegetables, one of which could be the Saag, later in this section, complete the meal.

Preparation time: *30 minutes*

Cooking time: *10 minutes*

Serves: *6*

2 tablespoons ginger, chopped

2 tablespoons garlic, chopped

60 ml low-fat yogurt

½ teaspoon ground white pepper

½ teaspoon ground cumin

¼ teaspoon ground nutmeg

¼ teaspoon ground cardamom

½ teaspoon cayenne pepper

½ teaspoon ground turmeric

¼ cup lemon juice

2 teaspoons vegetable oil

Salt to taste

3 whole chicken breasts, boned, skinned, and cut into 18 pieces

1 Combine the ginger, garlic, white pepper, yogurt, cumin, nutmeg, cardamom, cayenne pepper, turmeric, and lemon juice in a blender or food processor. With the motor running, drizzle in the oil.

2 Pour the marinade over the chicken in a bowl and mix thoroughly to coat. Cover and let marinade for 3 to 4 hours in the fridge.

3 Preheat oven to 190°C/375°F/Gas mark 5. Place chicken pieces on a skewer about 2.5 cm apart. Place skewers on a rack over a pan and bake for about 10 to 12 minutes or until cooked. Alternatively, to grill, place skewers 7.5 to 10 cm from the heat and grill for approximately 5 minutes per side. Serve hot with a lemon garnish.

Nutrient analysis per serving: 197 calories; 31.6 grams protein, 2.2 grams carbohydrate, 6 grams fat, 1.52 grams saturated fat, 14 milligrams cholesterol, 0.1 grams fibre, 8 milligrams sodium.

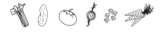

Summer Minestrone

This soup can be a complete meal. Serve with some crusty, fresh French bread, the salad in the preceding recipe, and a bowl of strawberries with a dash of cream.

Preparation time: *30 minutes*

Cooking time: *1 hour*

Serves: *6*

100 g dried red kidney beans, sorted and soaked overnight

1.5 litres cold water

2 bay leaves

2 fresh sage leaves

1 fresh oregano sprig

1 tablespoon extra virgin olive oil

1 medium red onion, diced, about 320 g

½ teaspoon salt

¼ teaspoon dried basil

Pepper to taste

6 garlic cloves, finely chopped

1 small carrot, diced, about 30 g

1 small red sweet pepper, diced, about 75 g

1 small courgette, diced, about 90 g

250 ml red wine

900 g fresh tomatoes, peeled, seeded, and coarsely chopped, or about 795 g canned tomatoes with juice, coarsely chopped

25 g small pasta, cooked al dente, drained, and rinsed

½ bunch fresh spinach or chard, cut into thin ribbons and washed, about 115 g

2 tablespoons chopped fresh basil

Grated Parmesan cheese

1 Drain and rinse beans. Place in a 2 litre saucepan with the water, 1 bay leaf, sage leaves, and oregano. Bring to the boil; reduce heat and simmer, uncovered, until the beans are tender, for about 45 minutes. Remove the herbs.

2 While the beans are cooking, heat the oil in a soup pot. Add the onion, ½ teaspoon salt, dried herbs, and a few pinches of pepper. Sauté the onion over medium heat until soft, for 5 to 7 minutes. Add the garlic, carrots, peppers, and courgette and sauté for 7 to 8 minutes, stirring often. Add the wine and cook for 1 to 2 minutes, until the pan is almost dry. Add the tomatoes and then add the pasta, spinach or chard, and beans with their stock. Season with salt and pepper to taste. Add the basil just before serving. Garnish each serving with a generous tablespoon of Parmesan cheese.

Nutrient analysis per serving: *98 calories; 4 grams protein, 17 grams carbohydrate, 2 grams fat, 0 grams saturated fat, 1 milligram cholesterol, 2 grams fibre, 652 milligrams sodium.*

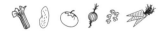

Sweet Pepper and Basil Frittata

You can serve this dish right out of the oven as a main course or let it cool and serve as a light lunch. You can also refrigerate the dish and cut it into small squares to serve as an hors d'oeuvre. Serve it with couscous and a tossed salad as a complete meal.

Preparation time: *30 minutes*

Cooking time: *25 minutes*

Serves: *10 servings*

2 tablespoons light olive oil	*1 bay leaf*
1 medium onion, thinly sliced, about 320 g	*6 eggs*
¾ teaspoon salt and ⅛ teaspoon pepper	*85 g Fontina cheese, grated*
4 medium sweet peppers, preferably a combination of red and yellow, thinly sliced, about 480 g	*55 g Parmesan cheese, grated*
	15 g fresh basil leaves, bundled and thinly sliced
4 garlic cloves, finely chopped	*3 tablespoons balsamic vinegar*

1 Preheat oven to 240°C/475°F/Gas mark 9. Heat 1 tablespoon of the olive oil in a large frying pan, add the onion, ½ teaspoon of the salt, and a few pinches of pepper. Sauté the onion over medium heat until it begins to soften, for 4 to 5 minutes. Add the sweet peppers, garlic, and bay leaf; stew the onion and peppers together for about 15 minutes, until the peppers are tender. Set the vegetables aside to cool. Remove the bay leaf.

2 Beat the eggs in a bowl and add the onion–pepper mixture, cheeses, and basil. Season with the remaining salt and the ⅛ teaspoon pepper.

3 In a 9-inch/23-cm nonstick frying pan with an ovenproof handle, heat the remaining tablespoon of olive oil until almost smoking. Swirl the oil around the side of the pan to coat. Turn the heat down to low and then immediately pour the frittata mixture into the pan. The pan should be hot enough so that the eggs sizzle when they touch the oil. Cook the frittata over a low heat for 2 to 3 minutes, until the sides begin to set; transfer to the oven and bake, uncovered, for 6 to 8 minutes, until firm and the eggs are completely cooked.

4 Loosen the fritatta gently with a rubber-ended spatula; the bottom will tend to stick to the pan. Place a plate over the pan, flip it over, and put it on a plate. Brush the bottom and sides of the frittata with the vinegar and cut into wedges. Serve warm or at room temperature.

Nutrient analysis per serving: *149 calories; 9.6 grams protein, 45 grams carbohydrate, 10 grams fat, 4 grams saturated fat, 159 milligrams cholesterol, 1 gram fibre, 349 milligrams sodium.*

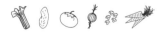

Rhubarb-Strawberry Cobbler

This wonderful dessert is easy to make. You can make it with less sugar if you use strawberries alone. In that case, you need about 750 grams of strawberries, washed, hulled, and cut into halves or left whole if small. You can serve the cobbler warm topped with a touch of whipped cream.

Preparation time: *40 minutes*

Cooking time: *40 minutes*

Serves: *6*

Cobbler filling

565 g rhubarb	2½ tablespoons plain flour
225 g strawberries	Rind of 1 small orange
granulated sugar	

Cobbler topping

185 g unbleached flour	2 tablespoons sugar
¼ teaspoon salt	4 tablespoons unsalted butter
1 tablespoon baking powder	250 ml double cream

1 Preheat oven to 190°C/375°F/Gas mark 5. Wash the rhubarb well, cutting off any brown spots or leaves still on the stalks. If the stalks are especially thick, cut them in half lengthwise before slicing them 1.5 cm thick so that all the pieces are approximately the same size.

2 Wash the strawberries, pat dry, and hull. Cut them into halves or leave whole if small.

3 Toss the fruit with the sugar, flour, and orange rind; place in an 8-inch/20-cm square baking dish, a 9-inch/23-cm round cake pan, or 6 to 8 individual ovenproof dishes.

4 Make the cobbler topping by combining the dry ingredients. Cut in the butter with a food processor, electric mixer, or two knives until the mixture has a coarse consistency. Add the cream and mix lightly, just until the dry ingredients are moistened.

5 Cover the fruit with tablespoon-size dollops of cobbler topping, using all the topping. Bake for 25 to 30 minutes, until the topping is browned and cooked through and the fruit is bubbling. Individual cobblers take about 20 minutes.

Nutrient analysis per serving: 328 calories; 5 grams protein, 60 grams carbohydrate, 8 grams fat, 5 grams saturated fat, 21 milligrams cholesterol, 2 grams fibre, 425 milligrams sodium.

Shiitake Mushrooms with Baby Pak Choi

This recipe makes a great vegetable side dish.

Preparation time: *30 minutes*

Cooking time: *15 minutes*

Serves: *4*

1.5 cm piece ginger root, peeled and crushed

Pinch of sugar

Pinch of salt

1 tablespoon plus 1 teaspoon vegetable oil

1 litre water

2 bunches baby pak choi

Salt to season

250 ml chicken stock

1 tablespoon oyster sauce

1 tablespoon dark mushroom soy sauce

1 tablespoon sherry

1 teaspoon sugar

225 g shiitake mushrooms, cleaned, stemmed, and poached until tender

1 tablespoon cornflour mixed with 125 ml cold water

1 Place the crushed ginger root, a pinch of sugar and salt, 1 teaspoon vegetable oil, and water in a large pan and bring to the boil. After 1 minute, remove the ginger. Set aside to cool slightly and then grate.

2 Add the baby pak choi to the simmering water and cook for 1 minute. Drain. Set aside.

3 Heat the remaining vegetable oil in a wok and add the baby pak choi and grated ginger. Season with salt and stir-fry for 1 minute. Arrange the baby pak choi on a platter.

4 Pour the chicken stock, oyster sauce, soy sauce, sherry, and 1 teaspoon sugar into a hot wok and bring to the boil. Add the shiitake mushrooms and cook until they are heated through. Stir the cornflour–water mixture into the mushrooms in the wok, simmering 2 to 3 minutes, until thickened.

5 Pour the sauce over the baby pak choi on the platter and serve immediately.

Nutrient analysis per serving: 98 calories; 7.3 grams protein, 22 grams carbohydrate, 4.7 grams fat, 2.5 grams saturated fat, 0 milligrams cholesterol, 4 grams fibre, 1,294 milligrams sodium.

Scallopine Al Funghi (Veal with Mushrooms)

This recipe makes delicious use of veal, but you can substitute chicken breasts for the veal. Just marinate the chicken with chopped sage and rosemary. Try using different types of mushrooms, which gives the recipe a different taste: button mushrooms, shiitake, chanterelle, or porcini. The necessary carbohydrate can come from 70 g of any cooked pasta (or, if you prefer, a slice of bread and 35 g of pasta).

Preparation time: *25 minutes*

Cooking time: *15 minutes*

Serves: *4*

8 x 55–85 g veal escalopes	*1 garlic clove, chopped*
Salt and pepper to taste	*70 g mixed mushrooms, sliced*
1 tablespoon plain flour	*125 ml white wine*
2 tablespoons butter	*10 leaves flat-leaf parsley*
2 tablespoons olive oil	*60 ml vegetable stock*

1 Place the veal escalopes two at a time between sheets of cling film and pound them with a meat mallet until 5 cm thick. Season them with salt and pepper. Cover the veal escalopes with flour, shaking off the excess. Heat the butter in a frying pan. Add the veal and cook for 2 minutes on each side. Transfer veal to a plate.

2 To the same pan add the oil, garlic, mushrooms, white wine, and parsley. Cook for a few minutes and add the veal and stock. Simmer for about 5 minutes.

3 Set the veal on a plate and top with the mushroom sauce.

Nutrient analysis per serving: *442 calories; 49 grams protein, 2 grams carbohydrate, 22 grams fat, 7 grams saturated fat, 179 milligrams cholesterol, 0.5 grams fibre, 175 milligrams sodium.*

Potato Gnocchi with Spring Peas and Prosciutto

This recipe makes a wonderful side dish, or you can serve it as a main course. If you choose to serve the gnocchi as an entrée, serve it with a tossed green salad, a fresh dinner roll, and fresh fruit for dessert.

Preparation time: *1 hour, 30 minutes*

Cooking time: *15 minutes*

Serves: *6*

450 g potatoes, unpeeled

2 litres water

1 egg

2 egg whites

1 cup plain flour, or more if needed

1 teaspoon salt

1 teaspoon ground black pepper

125 ml chicken or vegetable stock, prepared without added salt and all fat removed

60 ml double cream

225 g fresh peas, shelled and blanched in boiling water for 2 minutes

1 tablespoon butter

115 g prosciutto or Parma ham, sliced into strips

1 Put the potatoes in a pan with water. Bring the water to the boil and simmer the potatoes for 20 minutes or until tender. Drain the water from the pan and let the potatoes cool for only a few minutes before you begin to pull the skins from the potatoes. Discard the potato skins and, while still hot, pass the potatoes through a dicer or mash into a bowl.

2 *For gnocchi:* To the diced potatoes, add the egg and egg whites, season with salt and pepper, and using a rubber spatula or wooden spoon, mix until just combined. Add the flour in two stages so that only the amount that is necessary is used to bind the potato (use additional flour if necessary) and mix well to form a dough. Divide the dough in half and, on a floured work surface, roll the first half of the dough into a log 2.5 cm thick. Cut the log into 1.5 cm thick pieces. Lay the pieces out and, with your thumb, make an indentation on one side. Set aside and refrigerate until needed.

3 *For sauce:* Heat the chicken or vegetable stock and cream together in a saucepan, add the peas, and allow to simmer several minutes. Remove from heat and add the butter to the cream, whisking to incorporate well. Stir in the prosciutto. Set aside, keeping the sauce warm.

4 *For gnocchi:* Cook the gnocchi as you do pasta in several litres of boiling, salted water. They cook very quickly and are cooked when they float to the surface, after about 2 to 3 minutes.

5 *To serve:* Pour the sauce over the drained gnocchi, stir gently in a large serving bowl and serve immediately.

Nutrient analysis per serving: 241 calories; 10 grams protein, 32 grams carbohydrate, 8 grams fat, 4 grams saturated fat, 64 milligrams cholesterol, 2 grams fibre, 614 milligrams sodium.

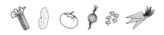

Clam Chowder

This soup is a wonderful start to any meal. Make sure that you have some crusty French bread on the table, so that you and your friends can clean out the soup bowl.

Preparation time: *45 minutes*

Cooking time: *1 hour, 30 minutes*

Serves: *6*

1 tablespoon olive oil

2 tablespoons rindless unsmoked streaky bacon, diced

4 carrots, peeled and diced, about 250 g

1 large onion, peeled and diced, about 160 g

4 celery stalks, diced, 120 g

3 tablespoons chopped fresh oregano

3 tablespoons fresh thyme leaves

2 bay leaves

2 tablespoons garlic, chopped

¼ teaspoon cayenne pepper

200 g canned plum tomatoes, drained and crushed

2 litres water

2 potatoes (about 340 g), cleaned, peeled, and diced

2 dozen large clams, steamed open, cleaned, chopped, and juices reserved

Salt and freshly ground black pepper to taste

1 In a heavy-bottomed pan, heat the olive oil, add the bacon, and cook until its fat begins to flow, about 5 minutes.

2 Add the carrots, onions, and celery to the pan and cook, stirring often, over low heat until tender, about 15 minutes.

3 Add the oregano, thyme, bay leaves, garlic, and cayenne and stir to combine.

4 Add the crushed tomatoes and water and bring to the boil. Reduce the heat and simmer for 1 hour.

5 Add the potatoes and continue to simmer for another half hour. Stir in the chopped clams with their juice and continue to cook for 2 minutes.

6 Season with salt and freshly ground pepper. Serve hot, with plain crackers and freshly grated horseradish as a garnish.

Nutrient analysis per serving: *77 calories; 4 grams protein, 10 grams carbohydrate, 3 grams fat, 0.7 grams saturated fat, 92 milligrams cholesterol, 2 grams fibre, 604 milligrams sodium.*

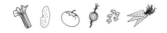

Chicken Thighs Braised in Apple Cider

This meal is low in carbohydrate as well as calories. You can even enjoy a couple of servings of starch. Why not serve with the potato gnocchi (recipe follows) and a fresh bread roll. Top off the meal with a serving of strawberries and a dollop of cream.

Preparation time: *30 minutes*

Cooking time: *1 hour*

Serves: *6*

6 chicken leg-thigh sections, skin and excess fat removed

Salt and pepper to taste

2 tablespoons olive oil

1 large onion, diced, about 160 g

3 carrots, diced

2 Granny Smith or other tart apples, peeled, cored, and cut into eighths

1 tablespoon curry powder

1 tablespoon plain flour

60 ml Calvados or cider

125 ml apple juice

125 ml hot chicken stock

1 Preheat oven to 180°C/350°F/Gas mark 4. Season chicken thighs with salt and pepper. Heat a large ovenproof frying pan or flameproof casserole over medium heat with the olive oil. Add the chicken thighs and cook 4 to 5 minutes, until well browned. Then turn and brown on the other side. When chicken is browned, remove and set aside.

2 Add the onion to the pan and cook over medium heat to a golden brown before adding the carrot. Cook the carrot for 2 to 3 minutes, add the apple slices, and begin to caramelise them.

3 Sprinkle the curry powder over the vegetables and apple and then sprinkle on the flour. Stir to combine well and begin to toast the curry–flour combination for 1 minute.

4 Return the chicken to the pan, remove the pan from the heat, and carefully pour in the Calvados. Let the brandy bubble and begin to evaporate in the hot casserole before returning it to the heat.

5 Add the apple juice and chicken stock, bring quickly to the boil, reduce the heat to a slow simmer, cover the pan with a tight-fitting lid, and place in the oven for 35 minutes. When chicken is fully cooked, remove from the oven, carefully ladle off any fat, and serve.

Nutrient analysis per serving: 236 calories; 14 grams protein, 16 grams carbohydrate, 10 grams fat, 2 grams saturated fat, 48 milligrams cholesterol, 3 grams fibre, 618 milligrams sodium.

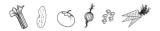

Spaghetti Gamberi e Zucchine
(Spaghetti with Prawns
and Courgettes)

The delicious taste of prawns is combined with a favourite Italian vegetable. This recipe is a complete meal. If you prefer to have a slice of bread, reduce the amount of pasta in the dish.

Preparation time: *20 minutes*

Cooking time: *20 minutes*

Serves: *4*

4 tablespoons extra virgin olive oil

450 g shelled raw prawns

Salt and pepper to taste

4 garlic cloves, sliced

4 small courgettes, diced

4 ripe plum tomatoes, peeled and diced

20 leaves flat-leaf parsley

1 pinch chilli flakes

4 tablespoons brandy

125 ml white wine

340 g spaghetti or other pasta

1 In a large frying pan, heat the oil over a high heat. Add the prawns and season with salt and pepper to taste. Sauté about 1 minute per side and then add the garlic and courgettes. Cook, tossing or gently stirring, for another minute. Add the tomatoes, parsley, chilli flakes, brandy, and wine. Simmer 4 to 5 minutes, until the sauce thickens and the courgette is tender.

2 Boil the spaghetti in salted water until cooked tender but firm. Drain and toss with prawn sauce.

Nutrient analysis per serving: 562 calories; 31 grams protein, 60 grams carbohydrate, 15 grams fat, 2 grams saturated fat, 229 milligrams cholesterol, 3 grams fibre, 297 milligrams sodium.

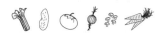

Risotto ai Vegetali (Italian Rice with Vegetables)

A serving of this recipe provides all the carbohydrates for a full meal. It contains the vegetables you need as well. It lacks protein, which you can make up with a small serving of chicken or fish. Use whatever vegetables are in season, including courgette, artichokes, asparagus, and mushrooms. Be aware of the number of servings you have when you make this dish. Overeating is easy if you're not careful!

Preparation time: *10 minutes*

Cooking time: *1 hour*

Serves: *10*

3 tablespoons butter	*125 ml white wine*
1 large shallot, diced	*2 litres vegetable stock*
370 g seasonal vegetables, diced	*½ tablespoon grated Parmesan cheese*
370 g Italian Arborio rice	*Salt and pepper to taste*

1 In a 4 to 6 litre heavy-bottomed saucepan, heat 1 tablespoon of the butter over a low-medium heat. Stir in the shallots and cook slowly for 4 minutes or until the onions are soft and transparent, but not brown. Increase the heat to medium, add the vegetables, and cook, stirring, for 1 to 2 minutes. Stir in the rice and cook, gently stirring, for 1 to 2 minutes. Pour in the white wine and cook until it is almost completely reduced. Add the stock, 250 ml at a time, and cook at a low boil, stirring often, until absorbed. Each 250 ml of stock must be absorbed before the next is added. After 15 minutes, taste a grain of rice – it should have a slight resistance to the bite. If it seems too hard, add a little more stock and continue cooking for a couple more minutes.

2 When rice is ready, remove from heat. Add remaining butter and Parmesan cheese. Season with salt and pepper to taste and mix with a wooden spoon until creamy in texture.

Nutrient analysis per serving: *204 calories; 4.6 grams protein, 34 grams carbohydrate, 5 grams fat, 2.3 grams saturated fat, 9 milligrams cholesterol, 1.6 grams fibre, 625 milligrams sodium.*

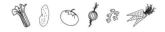

Appendix B

Exchange Lists

. . . .

. . . .

*I*n this appendix, you discover the method that dieticians have been using for many years to help their clients eat the right number of calories from the correct energy sources while permitting them to vary their foods.

Listing the Foods

Thousands of different foods are available, but each one can be broken down on the basis of the energy source (carbohydrate, protein, or fat) that is most prevalent in the food. Fortunately, the food content of one type of fish is just about the same as another type of fish (just don't tell a fish that – they're very sensitive creatures!). Therefore, a diet that calls for one fish exchange (such as salmon) can use any one of a number of choices or exchanges (such as halibut). You can exchange one for the other, so your diet is never boring.

The starches list

The starch exchanges are listed in Tables B-1 and B-2. Each exchange contains 15 grams of carbohydrate plus 3 grams of protein and 0 to 1 gram of fat, which amounts to 80 kilocalories per exchange. If the produce contains whole grains, it has about 2 grams of fibre.

Table B-1	Starch Exchanges	
Cereals, Grains, Pasta	*Bread*	*Dried Beans, Peas, Lentils (Higher in Fibre)*
Bran cereals, 10 g	Bagel, ½	Beans and peas, 55 g (cooked)
Cooked cereals, 115 g	Breadsticks, 2	Lentils, 65 g (cooked)
Grape Nuts, 3 tablespoons	Muffin, ½	Baked beans, 65 g
Pasta (cooked), 70 g	Beef burger roll, ½	Broad beans, 90 g
Puffed rice cereal, 20 g	Pitta, 15 cm across, ½	Peas, green, 70 g
Rice (cooked), 65 g	Currant bread, 1 slice	
Shredded wheat, 20 g	Tortilla, 15 cm across, 1 piece	
	White bread, 1 slice	
	Wholemeal bread, 1 slice	

Table B-2	More Starch Exchanges	
Crackers/Snacks	*Starchy Vegetables*	*Starchy Foods with Fats*
Matzoh, 20 g	Potato, baked, 1	Chips, 10 (85 g)
Melba toast, 5 slices	Potato, mashed, 100 g (add a fat exchange)	Sweet muffin, 1
Popcorn (unsweetened, no fat), 35 g	Squash, 110 g	
Wholemeal cracker, 4		

Meat and meat substitutes list

One exchange contains no carbohydrate, 7 grams of protein, and 1 to 8 grams of fat. Thus the kilocalories vary from 35 to 100 per exchange.

Lean meat and substitutes:

- Beef: Lean, such as rump steak, sirloin, and flank steak, fillet steak, 30 g
- Pork: Lean, such as fresh, canned, cured, or boiled ham, 30 g
- Veal: All cuts but veal escalopes, 30 g
- Poultry: Chicken, turkey, and poussins (no skin), 30 g

Fish:

- ✔ All fresh and frozen fish, 30 g
- ✔ Oysters, 6 medium
- ✔ Tuna (canned in water) 150 g
- ✔ Sardines (canned), 2 medium

Wild game:

- ✔ Venison, and rabbit 30 g
- ✔ Pheasant, duck, and goose 30 g

Cheese:

- ✔ Any cottage cheese, 55 g
- ✔ Grated Parmesan, 2 tablespoons
- ✔ Diet cheeses, 30 g

Other:

- ✔ Egg whites, 3

Medium-fat meat and substitutes:

- ✔ Beef: Minced, roast, and steak 30 g
- ✔ Pork: Chops, loin, and escalopes, 30 g
- ✔ Lamb: Chops, leg, and roast, 30 g
- ✔ Veal: Escalopes, 30 g
- ✔ Poultry: Chicken with skin, minced turkey, 30 g
- ✔ Fish: Tuna in oil, 30 g, salmon (canned) 60 g
- ✔ Cheese: Skimmed or semi-skimmed milk cheese like ricotta, 60 g, and mozzarella and diet cheeses, 30 g

High-fat meat and substitutes:

- ✔ Beef: Prime cuts like ribs, 30 g
- ✔ Pork: Spare ribs, minced pork, and fresh pork sausage, 30 g
- ✔ Lamb: Minced, 30 g
- ✔ Fish: Any fried fish, 30 g
- ✔ Cheese: All regular cheeses like Emmenthal and Cheddar, 30 g
- ✔ Other: Cured meat like salami, 30 g; sausage, 30 g; frankfurter, 1; and peanut butter, 1 tablespoon

Fruit list

Each exchange in Table B-3 contains carbohydrate (60 kilocalories) but no protein or fat. The list includes fresh, frozen, canned, and dried fruit and juice.

Table B-3	Fruit Exchanges	
Fruit	*Dried Fruit*	*Fruit Juice*
Apple, 115 g	Apple, 4 rings	Apple, 125 ml
Apple sauce, 130 g	Apricots, 7 halves	Cranberry, 75 ml
Apricots, 4	Dates, 2 ½	Grapefruit, 125 ml
Apricots, 130 g	Figs, 1 ½	Grape, 75 ml
Banana (23 cm), ½	Prunes, 3	Orange, 75 ml
Blackberries, 110 g	Raisins, 2 tablespoons	Pineapple, 125 ml
Blueberries, 110 g		Prune, 75 ml
Cantaloupe, ⅓ melon (12.5 cm diameter)		
Cherries, 12		
Cherries (canned), 125 g		
Figs, 2		
Fruit cocktail, 125 g		
Grapefruit, ½		
Grapes, 15		
Honeydew, ⅛ melon		
Kiwi, 1		
Mango, ½		
Nectarine, 1		
Orange, 1		
Papaya, 210 g		
Peach, 1		
Peaches (canned), 130 g		

Fruit	Dried Fruit	Fruit Juice
Pear, 1 small		
Pears (canned), 130 g		
Persimmon, 2		
Pineapple, 150 g		
Pineapple (canned), 80 g		
Plums, 2		
Raspberries, 125 g		
Strawberries, 185 g		
Tangerines, 2		
Watermelon, 385 g		

Vegetable list

Each exchange has 5 grams of carbohydrate and 2 grams of protein, which equals 25 kilocalories. Vegetables have 2 to 3 grams of fibre. Remember that the starchy vegetables like lentils, corn, and potatoes are on the starches list, earlier in this chapter. The serving size for all is 90 grams of cooked vegetables or 100 grams of raw vegetables.

- Artichoke (½ medium)
- Asparagus
- Fresh beans
- Bean sprouts
- Cabbage
- Carrots
- Cauliflower
- Aubergine
- Greens (chard, chicory)
- Kohlrabi
- Okra
- Onions
- Pea pods

- ✔ Peppers (green)
- ✔ Swede
- ✔ Sauerkraut
- ✔ Turnips
- ✔ Water chestnuts
- ✔ Courgettes

Fats list

These foods have 5 grams of fat and little or no protein or carbohydrate per portion. The calorie count is, therefore, 45 kilocalories. The important thing in this category is to notice the foods that are high in cholesterol and saturated fats and avoid them. See Table B-4.

Table B-4	Fat Exchanges
Unsaturated Fats	*Saturated Fats*
Avocado, ⅛ medium	Butter, 1 teaspoon
Salad dressing, 1 tablespoon	Bacon, 1 slice
Margarine, 1 teaspoon	Coconut, 2 tablespoons
Salad dressing, low fat, 2 tablespoons	Cream, 2 tablespoons
Margarine, low fat, 1 tablespoon	Cream, sour, 2 tablespoons
Mayonnaise, 1 teaspoon	Cream, double, 1 tablespoon
Almonds, 6	Cream cheese, 1 tablespoon
Cashews, 1 tablespoon	
Pecans, 2 whole	
Peanuts, 10 large	
Walnuts, 2 whole	
Seeds (pinenuts, sunflower) 1 tablespoon	
Seeds (pumpkin) 2 teaspoons	
Oil (corn, olive, sunflower, peanut), 1 teaspoon	
Olives, 10 small	

Other carbohydrates

This new list (as of 1997) contains cakes, pies, puddings, and other foods with lots of carbohydrate (and often fat). They're considered to have 15 grams of carbohydrate and a variable amount of fat and given the kilocalorie value of 60 per exchange. Examples are too numerous to list but include, for example:

- ✔ Ice cream, 65 g

Free foods

These foods contain less than 20 calories per serving, so you can eat as much of them as you want without worrying about overeating and without worrying about serving size.

- ✔ **Drinks:** Sugar-free drinks, sparkling water, coffee, and tea
- ✔ **Salad greens:** Endive, any type of lettuce, and spinach
- ✔ **Sweet substitutes:** Sugar-free sweets, sugar-free chewing gum, sugar-free jam, and sugar substitutes such as saccharin and aspartame
- ✔ **Fruit:** Cranberries, unsweetened, and rhubarb
- ✔ **Vegetables:** Cabbage, celery, cucumber, spring onions, capsicums, mushrooms, and radishes
- ✔ **Condiments:** Tomato ketchup (1 tablespoon), horseradish, mustard, pickles (unsweetened), low-calorie salad dressing, salsa, and vinegar
- ✔ **Seasonings:** Basil, lemon juice, lime, cinnamon, mint, chilli powder, chives, oregano, curry, paprika, dill, pepper, flavouring extracts (vanilla, for example), pimiento, garlic, spices, garlic salt, soy sauce, herbs, wine (used in cooking), lemon, and Worcestershire sauce

Using Exchanges to Create a Diet

Having all foods in exchange lists makes it easy to create a diet with great variation. The following menus have been adjusted to reflect the lower carbohydrate and higher protein that we recommend. Here are the amounts for diets of 1,500 and 1,800 kilocalories. See Table B-5.

Table B-5	1,500 kilocalories
Breakfast	*Lunch*
1 fruit exchange	3 lean meat exchanges
1 starch exchange	1 vegetable exchange
1 medium-fat meat exchange	2 fat exchanges
1 fat exchange	1 starch exchange
	2 fruit exchanges
Dinner	*Snack*
4 lean meat exchanges	1 bread exchange
2 vegetable exchanges	1 lean meat exchange
1 fruit exchange	
2 fat exchanges	

This diet provides 150 grams of carbohydrate, 125 grams of protein, and 45 grams of fat, keeping it in line with the 40 per cent carbohydrate, 30 per cent protein, and 30 per cent fat programme.

Translating this into food, you can have the menu in Table B-6 on one day:

Table B-6	A Sample Menu
Breakfast	*Lunch*
125 ml apple juice	85 g skinless chicken
1 piece toast	90 g cooked green beans
1 teaspoon margarine	4 walnuts
1 egg	1 slice bread
1 cup skimmed milk	
Dinner	*Snack*
115 g lean beef	55 g cottage cheese
1 piece bread	½ muffin
90 g peas	125 ml skimmed milk

Dinner	Snack
90 g broccoli	
⅓ cantaloupe	
2 tablespoons salad dressing	
salad of free foods	
115 g low-fat yogurt	

For an 1,800 kilocalorie diet, you have the menu in Table B-7:

Table B-7	1,800 kilocalories
Breakfast	**Lunch**
1 fruit exchange	3 lean meat exchanges
1 starch exchange	1 vegetable exchange
1 medium-fat meat exchange	2 fat exchanges
2 fat exchanges	2 starch exchanges
	2 fruit exchanges
Dinner	**Snack**
4 lean meat exchanges	2 bread exchanges
2 starch exchanges	2 lean meat exchanges
2 vegetable exchanges	
1 fruit exchange	
3 fat exchanges	

This diet provides 180 grams of carbohydrate, 135 grams of protein, and 60 grams of fat, again maintaining the 40:30:30 division of calories.

Using the example of the 1,500 kilocalorie diet, you should be able to make up an 1,800 kilocalorie diet at this point.

Appendix C

Dr WW Web

*I*n just a few years the World Wide Web has gone from providing little or no information to offering more than anyone can digest. This appendix presents the best places for you to check. You should be able to get answers to just about any question that you have, but you must be cautious about the source of the advice. Do not make any major changes in your diabetes care without checking with your doctor. In Chapter 19, you can find advice about how to differentiate between useful and useless information on the Web. Sometimes free advice is worth no more than you pay for it. Remember that the Web is constantly changing and growing, but these addresses are valid at least on the day that we list them.

General Sites

These sites tell you about diabetes from A to Z. They run the gamut from well-known organisations to individual doctors who specialise in diabetes. Sometimes the sites get a little technical, so keep this book handy for reference.

Diabetes UK

Diabetes UK is the largest organisation in the United Kingdom working for people with diabetes, funding research, campaigning, and helping people live with the condition. This site covers just about everything you need to know about living with diabetes in Britain.

```
www.diabetes.org.uk
```

Juvenile Diabetes Research Foundation (JDRF)

The JDRF is the leading charity and advocate regarding juvenile (type 1) diabetes research worldwide. You can find what you want to know about the latest programmes that emphasise finding a cure for diabetes.

```
www.jdrf.org
```

NHS Direct Online

NHS Direct Online provides online healthcare information and advice. Its health encyclopaedia covers many conditions and has lots of information on diabetes. The service is also available in Welsh.

```
www.nhsdirect.nhs.uk
```

National Electronic Library for Health

This electronic library aims to provide healthcare professionals and the public with knowledge and know-how to support healthcare-related decisions. The site has a great diabetes section containing lots of information.

```
www.nelh.nhs.uk
```

Diabetes Insight

This site aims to give people living with diabetes and their families a better understanding of diabetes. You can find an e-mail support forum where people can share information and discuss all of the personal and medical aspects of diabetes and how it affects their lives.

```
www.diabetes-insight.info
```

NetDoctor.co.uk

Netdoctor.co.uk is the United Kingdom's leading independent health Web site written by doctors and health professionals. The section on diabetes includes fact sheets, health information, and a drug information database.

```
www.netdoctor.co.uk/diabetes/index.shtml
```

BBC Health Diabetes Guide

This BBC guide explains what diabetes is, outlines what its main causes and symptoms are, and gives information on the treatments currently available.

```
www.bbc.co.uk/health/diabetes
```

Diabetes Travel Information

This Web site is for people who love to travel and have diabetes treated with insulin, or who may be travelling with someone who has. It provides tips and information to make your journey enjoyable and trouble free.

```
www.diabetes-travel.co.uk
```

MedicAlert

MedicAlert is a registered charity providing identification jewellery for people with hidden medical conditions and allergies. It provides a 24-hour emergency telephone number that can access the jewellery wearer's details from anywhere in the world in over 100 languages.

```
www.medicalert.co.uk
```

Dr Rubin

Here you can find general information and advice about diabetes, daily tips, new developments, and answers to questions.

```
www.drrubin.com
```

Diabetes and Driving

The Driver and Vehicle Licensing Agency (DVLA) has a variety of 'at-a-glance' pages designed to take you through all the regulations relating to driving when you have diabetes. Be warned, however – the information is only 'at a glance' if you have a photographic memory! The regulations are extremely complicated, but you can narrow down your search by looking within the site for your kind of diabetes and the type of vehicle you want to drive.

```
http://www.dvla.gov.uk/at_a_glance/ch3_diabetes.htm
```

Government Web Sites

These sites provide lots of authoritative information about diabetes while telling you all about the latest government programmes.

The National Institute for Health and Clinical Excellence (NICE)

NICE is part of the National Health Service (NHS) and its role is to provide patients and health professionals with authoritative and reliable guidance on current best practice in diabetes care. The information on this site is also available in Welsh, and there is a text version for the visually impaired.

```
www.NICE.org.uk
```

National Service Framework for Diabetes

This Department of Health site features the National Service Framework for Diabetes, which recognises the importance of raising the standards of diabetes care and support in the United Kingdom.

```
www.doh.gov.uk/nsf/diabetes/index.htm
```

Diabetes Exercise and Sports Association

The Diabetes Exercise and Sports Association is a place where you can find out about many different kinds of exercise, how much exercise you can and should do, and whether you face any limitations on exercise because of your diabetes. You can also find other people who share your interests.

```
www.diabetes-exercise.org
```

Regional Sites

The Diabetes Federation of Ireland

The Diabetes Federation of Ireland is dedicated to helping people with diabetes and their families living in Ireland.

```
www.diabetesireland.ie
```

Health of Wales Information Service (HOWIS)

HOWIS is the official Web site of NHS Wales and brings together information sources about the health and lifestyle of the population of Wales.

```
www.wales.nhs.uk
```

Diabetes in Scotland

This NHS Scotland Web site gives lots of information on diabetes and its treatment.

```
www.diabetesinscotland.org
```

The Tayside Diabetes Network

This is an excellent Web site covering many aspects of diabetes, with lots of great downloadable patient leaflets.

```
www.diabetes-healthnet.ac.uk
```

Diabetes Information in Other Languages

Not everyone speaks and reads English. Diabetes educational sites exist in many languages. The following ones account for only the most common languages, but you can find many others.

- **French:** www.diabetenet.com
- **German:** www.diabetes-deutschland.de
- **Italian:** www.publinet.it/diabete
- **Korean:** www.diabetes.or.kr
- **Russian:** www.diabet.ru
- **Spanish:** www.feaed.org
- **Bengali, Cantonese, Gujarati, Hindi, Punjabi, Urdu, and Welsh –** the Diabetes UK Web site provides information in all of these languages: www.diabetes.org.uk/risk/index.html

Sites for the Visually Impaired

If diabetes is not controlled it can have a major impact on vision. You can find lots of information on every issue related to visual impairment at these sites.

Royal National Institute for the Blind (RNIB)

The RNIB offers practical support and advice to anyone with a sight problem. You can find resources, information, research, talking books, and imaginative and practical solutions to the everyday challenges of living with a visual impairment.

```
www.rnib.org.uk
```

Diabetic Retinopathy

This Web site is a partnership between the Good Hope Hospital and the University of Birmingham. You can find out all you need to know about diabetic retinopathy and get information on prevention, treatment, and research.

```
www.diabeticretinopathy.org.uk
```

Eye Library

This site gives you information on every aspect of sight problems. It gives useful coverage on how diabetes affects the eyes and how eye screening works.

www.cgeye.org

Diabetic Foot Care

Feet for Life – Society of Chiropodists and Podiatrists

The Society of Chiropodists and Podiatrists' site is packed with foot health information and has a section dedicated to foot health and diabetes. The site also features a searchable database to help you find a chiropodist.

www.feetforlife.org

Dr Foot

Dr Foot gives comprehensive and detailed information on all major foot conditions. The site is compiled by a group of state-registered chiropodists and includes an 'Ask Dr Foot a Question' section for e-mail advice.

www.drfoot.co.uk

Diabetic Foot

This site is designed to assist healthcare professionals who look after the foot problems of diabetic patients, but is also of interest to diabetics themselves. You can download foot-care advice leaflets in 29 languages from here.

www.diabeticfoot.org.uk

Diabetes Care in Pregnancy

Pregnancy and diabetes

A section on the Diabetes UK Web site highlights the healthcare issues that need to be considered before and during pregnancy if you have diabetes. It also provides answers to some of the frequently asked questions on gestational diabetes.

    www.diabetes.org.uk/pregnancy

Animals with Diabetes

Yes, your dog and cat (and many other pets) can get diabetes, too. Here are sites for Fido and Tiddles (but you might need to help them to read the longer words!).

Dogs

This site tells you how to manage your canine with diabetes.

    www.petdiabetes.org

Cats

This site has helpful information for anyone who has a diabetic cat.

    www.felinediabetes.com

Recipe Web Sites for People with Diabetes

You can find a number of excellent recipe sites on the Internet. You can generally count on the recipes in books to contain the nutrients they list, but on the Web, you need to evaluate the site before accepting the recipes. These are the best of the currently available Web sites that provide recipes appropriate for a person with diabetes. Things change so frequently on the Internet that keeping up to date is difficult, so check back on your favourite site often.

✔ Leicester has a large ethnic population, and the city's NHS Trust has created an excellent Web site that includes South Asian, Caribbean, and British recipes in a variety of languages, including English, Hindi, Punjabi, and Urdu.

www.leicestershirediabetes.org.uk

✔ The nutrition section of Diabetes UK contains information about nutrition as well as lots of great recipes.

www.diabetes.org.uk/eatwell/index.html

✔ The Vegetarian Society maintains a large site filled with information for vegetarians. Its 'Beating Diabetes' section has information on vegetarian diets for diabetics and features some recipes at

www.vegsoc.org/cordonvert/recipes/diabetic.html

✔ Children with Diabetes is an American site that includes a large amount of information on meal planning, sugar substitutes, and the food guide pyramid, as well as lots of recipe ideas at

www.childrenwithdiabetes.com

Index

• F •

• S •

• *T* •

• *U* •

• *V* •

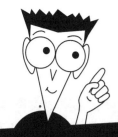

FOR DUMMIES®

Do Anything. Just Add Dummies

PROPERTY

UK editions

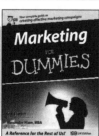

Buying and Selling a Home

0-7645-7027-7

Renting Out Your Property

0-470-02921-8

Buying a Property in Eastern Europe

0-7645-7047-1

PERSONAL FINANCE

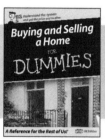

Investing

0-7645-7023-4

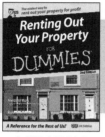

Paying Less Tax 2006/2007

0-470-02860-2

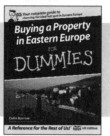

Sorting Out Your Finances

0-7645-7039-0

BUSINESS

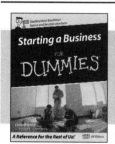

Starting a Business

0-7645-7018-8

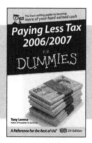

Marketing

0-7645-7056-0

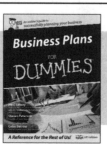

Business Plans

0-7645-7026-9

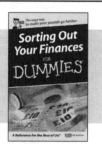
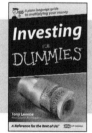

Answering Tough Interview Questions For Dummies
(0-470-01903-4)

Arthritis For Dummies
(0-470-02582-4)

Being the Best Man For Dummies
(0-470-02657-X)

British History For Dummies
(0-470-03536-6)

Building Confidence For Dummies
(0-470-01669-8)

Buying a Home on a Budget For Dummies
(0-7645-7035-8)

Children's Health For Dummies
(0-470-02735-5)

Cognitive Behavioural Therapy For Dummies
(0-470-01838-0)

Cricket For Dummies
(0-470-03454-8)

CVs For Dummies
(0-7645-7017-X)

Detox For Dummies
(0-470-01908-5)

Diabetes For Dummies
(0-7645-7019-6)

Divorce For Dummies
(0-7645-7030-7)

DJing For Dummies
(0-470-03275-8)

eBay.co.uk For Dummies
(0-7645-7059-5)

European History For Dummies
(0-7645-7060-9)

Gardening For Dummies
(0-470-01843-7)

Genealogy Online For Dummies
(0-7645-7061-7)

Golf For Dummies
(0-470-01811-9)

Hypnotherapy For Dummies
(0-470-01930-1)

Irish History For Dummies
(0-7645-7040-4)

Neuro-linguistic Programming For Dummies
(0-7645-7028-5)

Nutrition For Dummies
(0-7645-7058-7)

Parenting For Dummies
(0-470-02714-2)

Pregnancy For Dummies
(0-7645-7042-0)

Retiring Wealthy For Dummies
(0-470-02632-4)

Rugby Union For Dummies
(0-470-03537-4)

Small Business Employment Law For Dummies
(0-7645-7052-8)

Starting a Business on eBay.co.uk For Dummies
(0-470-02666-9)

Su Doku For Dummies
(0-470-01892-5)

The GL Diet For Dummies
(0-470-02753-3)

The Romans For Dummies
(0-470-03077-1)

Thyroid For Dummies
(0-470-03172-7)

UK Law and Your Rights For Dummies
(0-470-02796-7)

Winning on Betfair For Dummies
(0-470-02856-4)

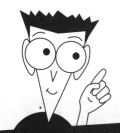

FOR DUMMIES®

Do Anything. Just Add Dummies

HOBBIES

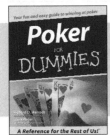

Poker
0-7645-5232-5

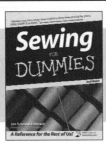

Sewing
0-7645-6847-7

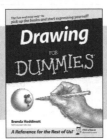

Drawing
0-7645-5476-X

Also available:

Art For Dummies
(0-7645-5104-3)
Aromatherapy For Dummies
(0-7645-5171-X)
Bridge For Dummies
(0-471-92426-1)
Card Games For Dummies
(0-7645-9910-0)
Chess For Dummies
(0-7645-8404-9)

Improving Your Memory
For Dummies
(0-7645-5435-2)
Massage For Dummies
(0-7645-5172-8)
Meditation For Dummies
(0-471-77774-9)
Photography For Dummies
(0-7645-4116-1)
Quilting For Dummies
(0-7645-9799-X)

EDUCATION

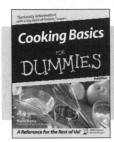

Cooking Basics
0-7645-7206-7

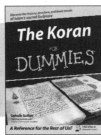

The Koran
0-7645-5581-2

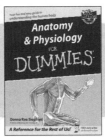

Anatomy & Physiology
0-7645-5422-0

Also available:

Algebra For Dummies
(0-7645-5325-9)
Algebra II For Dummies
(0-471-77581-9)
Astronomy For Dummies
(0-7645-8465-0)
Buddhism For Dummies
(0-7645-5359-3)
Calculus For Dummies
(0-7645-2498-4)

Forensics For Dummies
(0-7645-5580-4)
Islam For Dummies
(0-7645-5503-0)
Philosophy For Dummies
(0-7645-5153-1)
Religion For Dummies
(0-7645-5264-3)
Trigonometry For Dummies
(0-7645-6903-1)

PETS

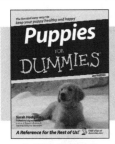

Puppies
0-470-03717-2

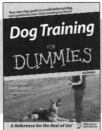

Dog Training
0-7645-8418-9

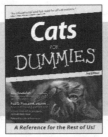

Cats
0-7645-5275-9

Also available:

Labrador Retrievers
For Dummies
(0-7645-5281-3)
Aquariums For Dummies
(0-7645-5156-6)
Birds For Dummies
(0-7645-5139-6)
Dogs For Dummies
(0-7645-5274-0)
Ferrets For Dummies
(0-7645-5259-7)

Golden Retrievers
For Dummies
(0-7645-5267-8)
Horses For Dummies
(0-7645-9797-3)
Jack Russell Terriers
For Dummies
(0-7645-5268-6)
Puppies Raising & Training
Diary For Dummies
(0-7645-0876-8)
